THE ULTIMATE HUMANITAS UNIVERSITY MEDICINE ADMISSIONS TEST GUIDE

UniAdmissions

ISBN 978-1-915091-29-1

Published by *RAR Medical Services Limited*
www.uniadmissions.co.uk
info@uniadmissions.co.uk
Tel: +44 (0) 208 068 0438

THE ULTIMATE HUMANITAS UNIVERSITY MEDICAL ADMISSIONS TEST GUIDE

DR ROHAN AGARWAL

DR MATTHEW WILLIAMS

DR WIRAAJ AGNIHOTRI

UniAdmissions

ABOUT THE AUTHORS

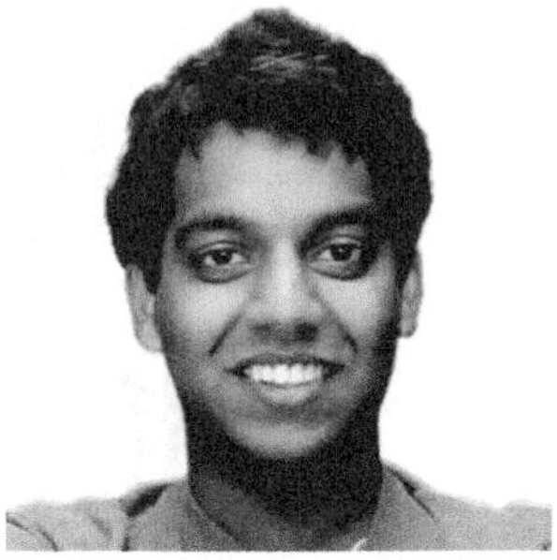

Rohan is the **Director of Operations** at *UniAdmissions* and is responsible for its technical and commercial arms. He graduated from Gonville and Caius College, Cambridge and is a fully qualified doctor. Over the last five years, he has tutored hundreds of successful Oxbridge and Medical applicants. He has also authored ten books on admissions tests and interviews.

Rohan has taught physiology to undergraduates and interviewed medical school applicants for Cambridge. He has published research on bone physiology and writes education articles for the Independent and Huffington Post. In his spare time, Rohan enjoys playing the piano and table tennis.

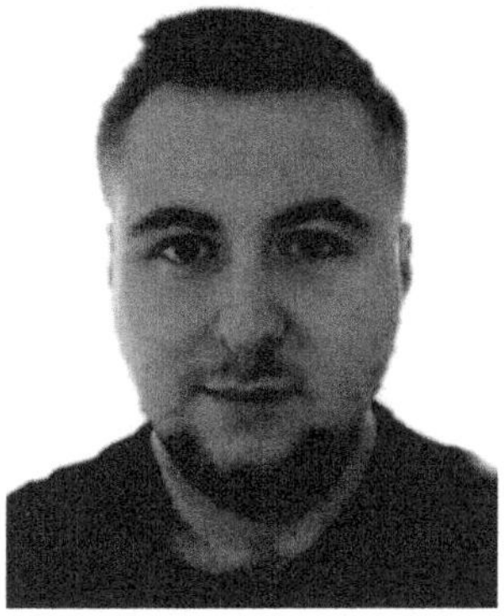

Matthew is **Resources Editor** at *UniAdmissions* and a 5th year medical student at St Catherine's College, Oxford. As the first student from Barry Comprehensive School in South Wales to receive a place on the Oxford medicine course he embraced all aspects of university life, both social and academic. Matt Scored in the **top 5% for his UCAT and BMAT** to secure his offer at the University of Oxford.

Matt has worked with UniAdmissions since 2014 – tutoring several applicants successfully into Oxbridge and Russell group universities. His work has been published in international scientific journals and he has presented his research at conferences across the globe. In his spare time, Matt enjoys playing rugby and golf.

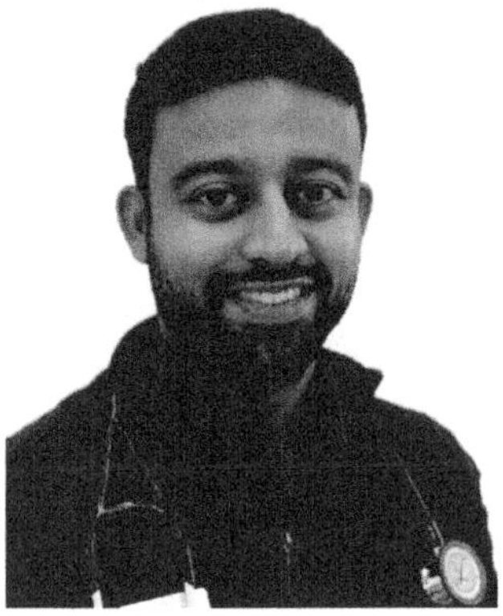

Wiraaj graduated in 2012 with an honours degree in Natural Sciences from Pembroke College, Cambridge where he was selected to receive annual scholarship funding from the Cambridge Trusts. In his final year at Cambridge, he specialised in the rigorous Mechanisms of Disease option during which he wrote an independent research dissertation on autoimmune thyroid disease.

Wiraaj subsequently completed graduate medical studies (MBBS) at the University of Sydney in 2016. He is currently a resident medical officer in Sydney where he plans to pursue further clinical specialisation as an internal medicine physician.

With a longstanding passion for teaching, Wiraaj has been heavily involved in tutoring students at various stages of their education. Over the years Wiraaj has successfully coached a great number of students into Medical Schools globally. Outside of medicine and education, Wiraaj enjoys playing jazz, guitar and football.

TABLE OF CONTENTS

PREFACE

First of all, I'd like to thank you for trusting UniAdmissions to help you with your university application.

It's a tough and confusing process to approach in many ways. As time has passed, the application has become more competitive and convoluted with the introduction of Admissions Tests and an extremely high calibre of students applying, making differentiating yourself increasingly challenging.

When I was applying to Cambridge, there weren't any good resources that I felt I could trust my future with. Unsurprisingly, many of my peers felt the same way and UniAdmissions was born! We started in 2013 and have had an amazing response from the thousands of students we support with their applications each year.

Since UniAdmissions' inception in 2013, we have made it our mission to improve our students' Oxbridge acceptance rate year on year. We've been quite successful in doing that; while the average Oxbridge acceptance rate stands at around 18%, UniAdmissions' success rate is consistently at 61% - triple the national average. Everyone here at UniAdmissions is always looking at how we can push this success rate even higher.

Overwhelmingly, our focus is on applications to highly competitive universities and courses. These are world-renowned and draw the brightest and best pupils from around to globe to their gates. To set yourself apart from this exceptional group of applicants, you must show yourself to be truly remarkable. Over the years, we have made great headway to cracking this formula – as evidenced with our success rates, which we're extremely proud of.

The purpose of this book is to help you prepare for your upcoming admissions test and, ultimately, help you gain your place to study at great universities like Oxford or Cambridge, or on your dream course. I sincerely believe this book will help you prepare, but words on a page can only take you so far.

In the past we have offered our students books, physical courses, tuition, mock interviews, online resources and much more. All of these forms of support make their mark on your application, although what we have discovered is that a holistic approach works much better. Which is why, nowadays, we have shifted our focus at UniAdmissions completely towards our Oxbridge and Medical Programmes. The Programmes each represent a structured syllabus that covers everything you need to know and practice in order to get your dream offer.

The support we provide splits broadly into four key categories: one-to-one teaching, intensive courses, materials, and enrichment seminars. Each represents a different style of learning which has its own positives and negatives.

We believe in offering the very best support we can provide to each student who entrusts a portion of their application to us, as you have with this book. One of the key tenets of our support comes in the form of intensive courses. In order to help you get your dream offer, we're offering you the opportunity to **attend one of our intensive courses – completely free of charge.**

The course is a half-day affair that is led by an expert instructor for your test. You'll be taken through the ins-and-outs of the exam, learn valuable time-saving tips and vital strategies to score marks that most students won't.

The idea behind UniAdmissions was always to help each student get their dream offer. Now that we have the resources available to widen our support, we're delighted to offer you this opportunity at no cost.

All that's left is for you to read on, I hope you enjoy this book and I wish you the very best of luck! **– Dr Rohan Agarwal**

THE ULTIMATE HUMANITAS UNIVERSITY MEDICAL ADMISSIONS TEST GUIDE

THE BASICS

What is the HUMAT?

The Humanitas University Medical Admissions Test (HUMAT) is a 2-hour written exam for medical students who are applying for the Humanitas University in Italy.

What does the HUMAT consist of?

Section	SKILLS TESTED	Questions	Timing
ONE: Scientific Thinking	Problem-solving skills, procedural thinking and analysing patterns. Visual Thinking – examining shapes and structures in three dimensions. Mathematical thinking – using algebra, graphs, and GCSE level mathematics.	30 MCQs	60 minutes
TWO: Academic Literacy	Ability to recall, understand and apply GCSE level principles of biology, chemistry, physics and maths. Usually the section that students find the hardest.	30 MCQs	60 minutes

Why is the HUMAT used?

Medical applicants to Humanitas tend to be very aspirational. For a number of years, the IMAT test was used to filter out the best candidates from a pool of applicants all with great grades. In time, the IMAT was phased out and replaced with a brand new test devised just for Humanitas, in order to allow applicants to show the skills which Humanitas particularly value.

When can I sit HUMAT?

The HUMAT is sat once a year, in February. In 2022, it's the 17th and 18th. You register online, through Humantias's MyPORTAL site – you can usually choose either available date to sit the test, which is currently taken online. Be sure to contact Humanitas directly if you have any disabilities or learning disabilities as far in advance as possible, to allow for any reasonable accommodations to be made.

Who has to sit the HUMAT?

Anyone applying to Humanitas University Medical School.

How is the HUMAT Scored?

Section 1 and Section 2 both have maximums of 90 marks, giving a total of 180 marks for the entire exam. In section one, there are three sections, Procedural Thinking, Visual Thinking, and Mathematical thinking. Each one has ten questions, and each correct answer gives you three marks, giving a total of 30 possible marks for each subsection of section 1.

Each wrong answer is worth -1 mark. This means that you are penalised for entering an incorrect answer and should try, whenever possible, to avoid *guessing* answers to questions. Not submitting an answer will provide zero marks, and is the safest bet if you have no idea what the correct answer is to a question. The marks in section 1 and section 2 are weighted equally – and they each have the same *minimum* mark threshold. That is: If you score below a certain mark in section 1 OR section 2, you will fail the whole test, regardless of your mark in the other section. In the HUMAT, the minimum mark is currently 20. That means that you could score a perfect 90 in the Scientific Thinking section, and 19 in the Academic Literacy section, and fail the test, while someone who got 21 in both sections would not.

If you and another candidate get the same score – the 'winner' will be the candidate who has the smallest difference between both sections. Meaning that it is very important to try and perform equally well in both sections where you can, rather than focusing your efforts on one, over the other, during your preparation in this guide.

Can I resit the HUMAT if I'm unhappy with my score?

No, you can only sit the HUMAT once per admissions cycle. You can resit the HUMAT if you apply for medicine again in the future.

Do I have to resit the HUMAT if I reapply?

You must resit the HUMAT with each admissions cycle, if you applying to a university that requires it. You cannot use your score from any previous attempts.

Where do I sit the HUMAT?

Currently, the HUMAT is taken online. You take it on your own computer, invigilated by Proctor software.

When do I get my results?

Results are usually published at the end of February, that is, usually a week or two after you took the test, with a public ranking from top to bottom.

GENERAL ADVICE

Start Early

It is much easier to prepare and do well if you practice little and often. Start your preparation well in advance; ideally by mid November but at the latest by early December. This way you will have plenty of time to complete as much practice as you wish in order to feel comfortable with the exam content and style and won't have to panic and cram just before the test, which is a much less effective and more stressful way to learn. In general, an early start will give you the opportunity to identify the complex issues and work at your own pace to better your understanding of the material.

Prioritise

Some questions can be long and complex – and given the intense time pressure in the HUMAT you need to know your limits. It is essential that you don't get stuck and waste valuable time on very difficult questions. If a question looks particularly long or complex, mark it for review and move on. You don't want to be caught 5 questions short at the end just because you took more than 3 minutes in answering a maths question worth the same marks as a visual thinking question that you could have done in 30 seconds. If a question is taking too long, mark for review if you have time later, and move on. Remember that each question carries equal weighting and therefore, you should adjust your timing accordingly. With some disciplined practice under timed conditions, you can get very good at this and learn to maximise your efficiency. In short, exam technique is a crucial part of the HUMAT, and matters almost as much as learning the content, so it is wise to spend your preparation time developing a consistent approach to the exam.

Marking

There are penalties for incorrect answers in the HUMAT; you will gain three marks for each right answer, and lose one mark for a wrong answer. Unanswered questions will net you zero. While this means that you are not punished as severely for a mistake as you are rewarded for a success – it does mean that you need to be careful with choosing answers which you aren't completely sure of. Too many incorrect answers will massively drain your final score. Since each question provides you with 5 possible answers, you have a 20% chance of guessing correctly. What that means, is that you also have an 80% chance of losing a mark, on every question you guess, with a 20% chance of gaining 3 marks – guessing with no idea about the correct answer is, as a result, never the right thing to do. You should only venture an educated guess on a question if you are *reasonably* certain of the answer, based on clear logic, your understanding of the topic, and common sense. Even then, we strongly advise caution, because the odds are against you unless you can clearly work out the answer. Therefore, preparation, revision, and practice is all the more important.

It is important also to try to avoid losing easy marks on other questions because of poor exam technique. The HUMAT is very time pressured, so you must attempt to get through as many questions as you can by doing plenty of practice under timed conditions well in advance of the exam. If you have failed to finish the exam on the day, don't panic and guess the remaining questions – leave them blank, and remember that each correct answer nets you three marks.

Practice

This is the best way to familiarise yourself with the style of questions and the timing for HUMAT. Although the HUMAT thinking skills, rather than specific knowledge, you must make sure you revise the question types and various skills required to excel in the exam. The best way to do this, is by practicing using this book – but revising your GCSE science and mathematics syllabi is also a good idea. Due to the nature of the HUMAT, you will be required to apply principles rather than knowledge acquired from rote-learning, so it is important to ensure you fully understand the material on the test specification.

Practising questions will put you at ease and make you more comfortable with the exam. The more comfortable you are, the less you will panic on the test day when confronted with tricky questions, and the more likely you are to score highly. Initially, work through the questions at your own pace, and spend time carefully reading the questions and looking at any additional data provided on the test paper. As you get closer to the test, **make sure you practice the questions under exam conditions**.

Past Papers

There are no HUMAT past papers to work from, however – there are two specimen papers available on the Humanitas website – these should be used as your final practice before the exam, as they are the closest thing you will get to the paper you are about to sit. Worked solutions for these papers are not available from Humanitas, but are coming soon from UniAdmissions.

Repeat Questions

When checking through your answers to practice questions, pay particular attention to questions you have got wrong. Look through the worked solution carefully until you feel confident that you understand the reasoning, and then repeat the question without help to check that you can do it. If only the answer is given, have another look at the question and try to work out why that answer is correct. You can refer to worked solutions for similar types of questions for some pointers if the answer doesn't seem obvious. This is the best way to learn from your mistakes, and means you are less likely to make similar mistakes when it comes to the real HUMAT. The same applies for questions which you were unsure of and made an educated guess which was correct, even if you got it right. When working through this book, **make sure you highlight any questions you are unsure of**, to ensure you know to spend more time looking over them once marked.

No Calculators

You aren't permitted to use a calculator in the HUMAT – thus, it is essential that you have strong numerical skills and feel confident manipulating figures with pen and paper. For instance, you should be able to rapidly convert between percentages, decimals and fractions. You will seldom get questions that you might reasonably expect to need a calculator but you would be expected to be able to arrive at a sensible estimate. Consider for example:

Estimate 3.962 x 2.322;

3.962 is approximately 4 and 2.323 is approximately 2.33 = 7/3.

Thus, $3.962 \text{ x } 2.322 \approx 4\, x \frac{7}{3} = \frac{28}{3} = 9.33$

It is important part of exam technique to know that in the HUMAT you will rarely be asked to perform difficult calculations. In fact, you can use this as a marker of whether you are tackling a question correctly.

For example, when solving a physics question, if you end up having to divide values such as 8,079 by 357- this should raise alarm bells as calculations in the HUMAT are rarely this difficult.

A word on timing...
"If you had all day to do your HUMAT, you would get 100%. But you don't."
Whilst this isn't completely true, it illustrates a very important point. Once you've practiced and know how to answer the questions, the clock is your biggest enemy. This seemingly obvious statement has one very important consequence. The way to improve your HUMAT score is to improve your speed. There is no magic bullet. But there are a great number of techniques that, with practice, will give you significant time gains, allowing you to answer more questions and score more marks.

> ***Top tip!*** In general, students tend to improve the fastest in Section 1 and slowest in Section 2; Remember that you must score above 20 points in BOTH sections to pass the test, so make sure to plan your preparation accordingly if you are finding one section harder than the other.

Timing is tight throughout the HUMAT – mastering the timing of each section is the first key to success. Some candidates choose to work as quickly as possible through every question to save up time at the end to check their answers, but this is generally not the best approach.

HUMAT questions can have a lot of information in them – each time you start answering a question it takes time to get familiar with the instructions and information given. By splitting the question into two sessions (the first run-through and the return-to-check) you double the amount of time you spend familiarising yourself with the data, as you have to do it twice instead of only once. This costs valuable time. In addition, candidates who do check back may spend 2–3 minutes doing so and yet not make any actual changes.

While this can feel reassuring in a high stakes exam, it is actually false reassurance as this approach is unlikely to have a significant impact on your actual score. Therefore it is usually best to pace yourself very steadily, aiming to spend the same amount of time on each question and finish the final question in a section just as time runs out. This reduces the time spent on re-familiarising yourself with the content of the questions and maximises the time spent arriving at the answer. This approach is the most efficient way to gain the maximum marks you are capable of.

It is essential that you don't get stuck with the hardest questions – no doubt there will be some tough ones scattered through both sections of the HUMAT. In the time you might spend attempting to answer only one of these questions you could miss out on answering three easier questions, worth three times as many marks! If a question is taking too long, and you don't have a good idea of what the answer is, leave it blank and move on. Never see this as giving up or in any way failing – rather, it is the smart way to approach a high stakes test with a tight time limit. With practice and discipline, you can get very good at this and learn to maximise your efficiency. It is not about being a hero and aiming for full marks – this is almost impossible and very much unnecessary for an offer. It is about maximising your efficiency and gaining the maximum possible number of marks within the time you have. In summary, perfecting your exam timing and technique is an important way for you to give yourself the best chance of achieving a score that will secure you an interview at medical school.

Top tip! Ensure that you take a watch that can show you the time in seconds into the exam. This will allow you have a much more accurate idea of the time you're spending on a question. In general, if you've spent >150 seconds on a section 1 question or >90 seconds on a section 2 questions – move on regardless of how close you think you are to solving it, to ensure you have enough time to answer all the other questions too.

Use the Options:
Some questions may try to overload you with information. You could see this as a distraction technique designed to intimidate candidates, so knowing what to do in this situation is critical.
When presented with large tables and data, it's essential that you look at the answer options so you can focus your mind. This can allow you to reach the correct answer a lot more quickly. Consider the example below:

The table below shows the results of a study investigating antibiotic resistance in staphylococcus population. A single staphylococcus bacterium is chosen at random from a similar population. Resistance to any one antibiotic is independent of resistance to others.

Calculate the probability that the bacterium selected will be resistant to all four drugs.

Antibiotic	Number of Bacteria tested	Number of Resistant Bacteria
Benzyl-penicillin	10^{11}	98
Chloramphenicol	10^{9}	1200
Metronidazole	10^{8}	256
Erythromycin	10^{5}	2

A. 1 in 10^{6}
B. 1 in 10^{12}
C. 1 in 10^{20}
D. 1 in 10^{25}
E. 1 in 10^{30}
F. 1 in 10^{35}

Looking at the answer options first makes it obvious that there is **no need to calculate exact values-** only in powers of 10. This makes your life a lot easier. If you hadn't noticed this, you might have spent well over 90 seconds trying to calculate the exact value when it wasn't even being asked for.

In other cases, you may actually be able to use the answer options to arrive at the solution quicker than if you had tried to solve the question from scratch as you normally would. Consider the example below:

A region is defined by the two inequalities: $x - y^2 > 1$ *and* $xy > 1$. Which of the following points is in the defined region?

A. (10,3)
B. (10,2)
C. (-10,3)
D. (-10,2)
E. (-10,-3)

Whilst it's possible to solve this question both algebraically or graphically by manipulating the identities, by far **the quickest way is to simply use the options given to you in the question**.

Note that options C, D and E violate the second inequality, narrowing down to answer to either A or B. For A: $10 - 3^2 = 1$ and thus this point is on the boundary of the defined region and not actually in the region. Thus the answer is B (as 10 - 4 = 6 > 1)

In general, it pays dividends to look at the answer options briefly to see if they can be help you arrive at the solution more quickly. Get into this habit early on in your HUMAT preparation – it may feel unnatural at first but it's guaranteed to save you time in the long run.

Key Words

If you're stuck on a question; pay particular attention to the options that contain key modifiers like "**always**", "**only**", "**all**" as examiners like using them to test if there are any gaps in your knowledge. For example, the statement "arteries carry oxygenated blood" would normally be true. However the statement "<u>**all**</u> arteries carry oxygenated blood" would be false because there is an exception: the pulmonary artery carries deoxygenated blood.

SECTION 1: SCIENTIFIC THINKING

This is the first section of the HUMAT and as you begin, it is inevitable that you will feel nervous. Make sure that you have been to the toilet prior to the exam because once it starts you cannot simply pause and go due to the time pressure. Take a few deep breaths and calm yourself down. Remember that panicking will not help and may negatively affect your marks - so try and avoid this as much as possible.

You have one hour to answer 30 questions in section 1. The questions fall into three categories:

- Procedural Thinking
- Visual Thinking
- Mathematical Thinking

Whilst this section of the HUMAT is renowned for being difficult to prepare for, there are a number of powerful shortcuts and techniques that you can use. Learning specific exam techniques and practising plenty of example questions will train you to work efficiently and make the best of the time available for Section 1.

You have approximately 120 seconds per question. Although this may initially sound like plenty of time the questions in Section 1 often require you to read and analyse passages or graphs to find the correct answer, meaning it is important to work as quickly and efficiently as possible. Some questions in Section 1 are very tricky and can be a big drain on your limited time. **The people who fail to complete section 1 are those who get bogged down on a particular question**.

Therefore, it is vital that you start to get a feel for which questions are going to be easy and quick to do and which ones should be left until the end. The best way to do this is through practice and the questions in this book will offer extensive opportunities for you to do so.

SECTION 1: PROCEDURAL THINKING

HUMAT procedural thinking questions require you to demonstrate your ability to intelligently analyse, absorb, conceptualise, and manipulate data. They can be broken down into six main skill areas, requiring you to:

- understand the components of a complex text, or treatise
- combine data from multiple streams in order to answer a question
- correctly process and understand algorithms
- compare evidence to a theory and see if they support each other
- predict the outcome of an alteration to a described system
- to select relevant data from a complex table or graph.

Having a good grasp of language and being able to filter unnecessary information quickly and efficiently is a vital skill in medical school – you simply do not have the time to sit and read vast numbers of textbooks cover to cover. Instead, you will need to be able to filter the information to quickly identify the key points. Ultimately this skill will contribute to your success in your studies, which is why it forms part of the HUMAT.

Selecting the most relevant pieces of information from a larger passage is also a key skill for qualified doctors, who simply do not have the time to read pages and pages of notes on the wards to make important healthcare decisions. As such, it is important not to underestimate the importance of getting to grips with verbal reasoning skills at this stage and throughout university.

Key Tips & Tricks for Section 1

1. Only use the data.
Your answer must only be based on the information available in the data provided by the question, whether it is a passage, a graph, or an equation. Do not try and guess the answer based on your general knowledge as this can be a trap. For example, if the passage says that spring is followed by winter, then take this as true even though you know that spring is followed by summer.

2. Take your time
Because you are negatively marked for wrong answers, it is important that you try not to rush. Practice means that you will be able to work accurately and quickly, but you must ensure that you are giving yourself the time needed to analyse the flow chart, or text, or table etc correctly.

PROCEDURAL THINKING QUESTION TYPES

UNDERSTANDING THE COMPONENTS OF A TEXT

Here, you have to study a short text of around 300 words – and then demonstrate that you have understood the relationships described within it. Usually, in the HUMAT this is done by either asking you to identify a particular element (i.e. "Which of these people is the most widely respected by the other individuals in the passage") or by asking you to select one of five concept maps which most accurately summarises the text.

You are presented with a passage, upon which you answer questions. The total number of texts you will have to examine will vary from exam to exam, though there are typically two. Remember that you are answering based *ONLY* on the passage and not on any of your own knowledge. A clear thought process and careful reading is key to doing well in these questions – as it is better to read a passage carefully once, than rush through it multiple times because you're unsure of the answer. You will have the opportunity to build your accuracy and speed that up through practice questions until you're answering like a pro!

How to Approach This Section

You should look carefully to see what the question is asking. Often it's best to read the question before reading the passage. Then when reading the passage you're likely to find the information you need much more quickly.

Sometimes the question will simply need you to find a phrase in the text. In other instances, your critical thinking skills will be needed and you'll have to carefully analyse the information presented to you.

Be a Lawyer

Put on your most critical and analytical hat for these questions! Carefully analyse the statements like you're in a court room. Then look for the evidence! **Examine the passage closely, looking for evidence** that directly addresses the question, or which matches elements in the concept map.

Read the Question First

Follow our top tip and read the question before the passage. By reading the statement or question first, you can understand what it is that is required of you and can then pick out the appropriate area in the passage.

Find the Keywords

The keyword is the most important word to help you relate the question to the passage; sometimes there might be two keywords in a question – concept maps will often give you a great idea of what words or names to be looking out for. When you read the passage, focus in on the keywords straight away. This gives you something to look for in the passage to identify the right place to work from. It is usually easy to find the keyword/s, and you'll become even better with practice. When you find it, go back a line and read from the line before through the keyword to the end of the line after. Usually, this contains enough relevant information to give you the answer.

Use only the Passage

Your answer ***must*** only be based on the information available in the passage. Do not try and guess the answer based on your general knowledge as this can be a trap. For example, if the question asks who the first person was to walk on the moon, then states "the three crew members of the first lunar mission were Edwin Aldrin, Neil Armstrong and Michael Collins". The correct answer is "can't tell" – even though you know it was Neil Armstrong and see his name, the passage itself does not tell you who left the landing craft first. Likewise, if there is a quotation or an extract from a book which is factually inaccurate, you should answer based on the information available to you rather than what you know to be true.

Concept maps

Some of these questions will require you to choose one of five concept maps, these are, in effect, flow charts which describe a process or a set of relationships – and you will need to choose the map which most closely reflects the relationships or processes described in the passage. This requires close reading of the text.

> ***Top tip!*** Though it might initially sound counter-intuitive, it is often best to read the question ***before*** reading the passage. Then you'll have a much better idea of what you're looking for in the text and are therefore likely to pick out the relevant information quickly.

A concept map for a passage describing relationships in the British royal family might look like this:

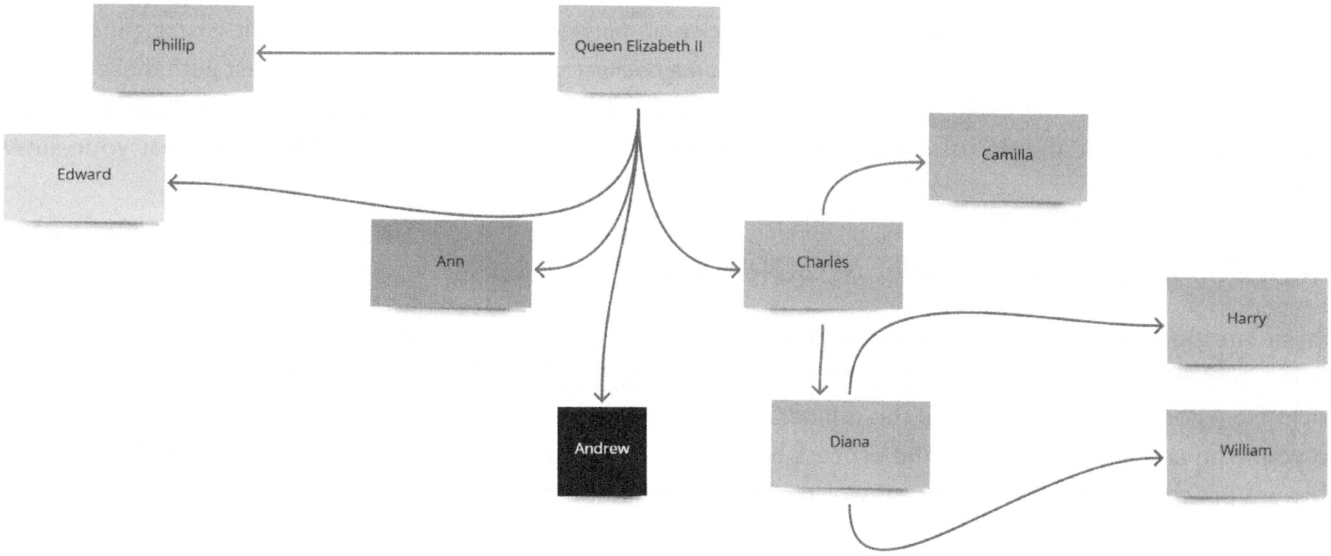

You will be presented with a detailed passage and a number of different concept maps, many of them may look similar but only one will reflect what is described in the passage. Remember to use only the passage, and identify the one which matches it for the full three marks. A useful trick here is to examine the available options and look for errors, often – there will be clear contradictions between a couple of the maps and what the passage says, and this lets you narrow down the correct option quickly. Another trick is to compare the options to each other – you'll often find that three or four of the options have a lot in common between them – identify any outliers and examine them. If one of the maps is vastly different to the others, you can either quickly disregard it, or all of the other options!

COMBINING DATA FROM MULTIPLE STREAMS

These are fairly straightforward data handling questions in the Procedural Thinking section, which require you to examine a set of information, and then draw conclusions based on consideration of that whole set. For example:

Paul has four hamster cages, each containing four hamsters. He has numbered each one, for the sake of keeping track of them. He needs to take one hamster from each cage for entry into a hamster pageant.

Cage 1: Hamster 7, Hamster 14, Hamster 12, Hamster 3
Cage 2: Hamster 9, Hamster 11, Hamster 10, Hamster 1
Cage 3: Hamster 2, Hamster 4, Hamster 13, Hamster 16
Cage 4: Hamster 15, Hamster 6, Hamster 8, Hamster 5

Which combination of hamsters could **never** be entered into the pageant?

A) 10, 15, 13, 14
B) 7, 5, 11, 13
C) 9, 13, 14, 15
D) 12, 1, 3, 6
E) 3, 8, 4, 10

As with understanding the text – the key is to carefully examine the information. Often, with questions like this, you can very quickly filter out irrelevant data. With practice, in particular, you should find that it is straightforward to glance through the data streams provided and decide on a correct answer. You can get very fast with these questions by the time you get to the exam, but it is easy to make simple mistakes. The questions are not designed to catch you out, but they can and do use tricks like re-arranging the order of the streams. Make sure that your answer makes sense!

PROCESS AND UNDERSTAND ALGORITHMS

These questions, put simply, are all about flow charts. You must study a diagram of a process, or an algorithmic chain – and answer a question about either the input or output of the process. You can use some of the tips and tricks from concept maps here – but this is fundamentally about your ability to quickly process information presented to you in an unconventional way. The process being described could be from medicine, but is more likely to be an abstract process not rooted in the real world – their expectation is that you will study the chart and answer it in a vacuum.

With a flow chart – it is tempting to rush to the final levels – the output, and try to work out what answer to pick from there. Usually though, candidates trip up here, because the final level of a flow chart is always dependent on a large number of other steps in the HUMAT – and they end up working backwards. This wastes time, and you'll get to your answer much more quickly if you start from the top of the process, and work down.

The first thing, as with most HUMAT questions, is to read the question. Once you understand what the question wants, you can analyse the process/data provided, and as you work through it in your head, you already know what to look for. This can save valuable time. Particularly with flow charts, this is a valuable tactic because if you know what the desired output is, you can limit how much time you spend on streams of the chart, or algorithm, which don't relate to the output or input which the question is asking for.

COMPARE EVIDENCE TO A THEORY

These questions are very similar to the understanding components of a text questions – you'll be presented with a short text of around 300 words, and asked a question about it. The difference is that how, rather than being asked to identify a particular element, or the most accurate concept map – you will be asked which conclusion is the most valid, on the basis of the evidence provided in the passage.

Just like before, take the time to carefully examine the passage, and determine which of the options provided is the most relevant or most likely to be true, based on what you have been told. The passage will contain a lot of detail, much of which may well be superfluous to the question so again, as always, read the question first, and then examine the passage. Disregard data which is not relevant to you. Doctors have to be good at pulling out important information from a lot of data very quickly, and if you can do this here, you'll do well. Be aware that these kinds of questions will often have an answer option which is "Can't tell" "None of the above" or similar – these are not a red herring, sometimes there is not enough data provided to be able to answer, or none of the other answers match up with the data, don't be afraid to use this one if you find this to be the case, and don't worry about re-reading the passage in great detail if the evidence doesn't match any of the theories on offer.

PREDICT THE OUTCOME OF AN ALTERATION

These questions look just like the process/flow chart questions, and you can go about them in a similar way. You'll be provided with data about a process – like a cycle, algorithm, workflow, or programme – and you will be told in the question that one element of that process has been changed – one step in the workflow is inverted, for example. You'll then be asked to select from one of five options the output of the process which would result from this change.

Note that they aren't asking for the output of the original process – lots of candidates are presented with a process, study it, determine what the output would be, and look for that in the answers. You have an extra step with these questions – once you have studied the process, you must then *change* one of the components, and work out in your head how all the subsequent steps would be altered as a result. When presented with a question like this – remember that you can disregard all steps of the process BEFORE your alteration. Sometimes, the alteration will be in the initial input, so you can't ignore anything, but usually you'll have a change inside the process. Save time, and maximise your marks by only focusing on the parts of the process after the change – hold only those parts in your mind when visualising the change.

If you are struggling to visualise the change, you can always make a note on pen and paper – sketching it out. Be aware that while the exam is being invigilated online, you may have limitations on what you can do using a pen and paper, and you should always check with Humanitas directly if you have concerns.

SELECTING RELEVANT DATA

Relevant Data questions show a great variation in type and difficulty. The best way to improve with these questions is to do lots of practice questions in order to familiarise yourself with the style of questions.

Options First

Despite the fact that you may have lots of data to contend with, the rule about looking at the question and options first still stands. This will allow you to register what type of calculation you are required to make and what data you might need to look at for this. Remember, here you want Options → Question → Data/Passage.

Working with Numbers

Percentages frequently make an appearance in this section and it's vital that you're able to work comfortably with them. For example, you should be comfortable increasing and decreasing by percentages, and working out inverse percentages too. When dealing with complex percentages, break them down into their components. For example, 17.5% = 10% + 5% + 2.5%.

Graphs and Tables

When you're working with graphs and tables, it's important that you take a few seconds to check the following before actually extracting data from it.

Table	Graph
Read any rubric or instructions	Read any rubric or instructions
Look at the Headings	Look at the Axes
Look at the Units	Look at the Units
Look at the Data - are there any obvious patterns?	Look at the Plot - are there any obvious trends?

Get into the habit of doing this whenever you are faced with data and you'll find it much easier to approach these questions under time pressure.

SECTION 1: VISUAL THINKING

The visual thinking questions in section 1 of the HUMAT is focused on assessing your spatial awareness and ability to imagine complex shapes and re-orient them in your head.

The questions are very similar in nature to UCAT Abstract Reasoning questions, if you're preparing for that exam as well – and will generally be trying to assess your ability to perform the following skills:

- Think in three dimensions
- Find complementary shapes
- Identify visual patterns
- Localise objects in relation to other objects.
- Identify an image from a written description

The Basics

The idea behind this section of the paper is to test how well the candidate is able to respond to questions that may go beyond the scope of their knowledge or require them to apply their existing knowledge in an unusual way. This is thought to be helpful in determining how well a student will be able to interpret information such as scans, X-rays or other test results as a clinician.

This section of the test examines pattern recognition and the logical approach to a series of symbols in order to match symbols to one group or another. There are a number of different question types, but all require one key skill – the ability to recognise patterns in a set of shapes.

Think of it in terms of the image sets. There can be one question per image set, or several. By far the hardest task is deducing the rules – once you have them, matching the options to the correct set is straightforward.

Timings

As with the rest of the test, you have to keep an eye on the time to keep track of how you're doing. Make sure that you stay within your time limit of 120 seconds per question. Your **practice will increase both your speed and overall likelihood of finding the rule**, but despite thorough preparation, you still may fail to spot the pattern. If you can't see it, don't despair – simply move swiftly on.

Top tip! Give yourself plenty of time to systematically work out the rules. Once you have found them, answering the questions will be quick.

Pattern Recognition

By far the most important ability in this section is to correctly identify patterns, as regardless of question style the matching process is straightforward once you have identified the rules. Some people are naturally better at this than others. You might be the sort of person who sees these patterns easily and can quickly put a name to the rule, or you might be the sort of person who finds it takes them more time and effort to work out what's going on. In reality, everyone lies at a different position on this scale, but one thing is certain. **You can improve your speed and accuracy on this section by having a methodical system** that can be repeated and applied to all shape-sets. One such system is the **NSPCC** system. This provides a logical structure for working through each set of images and looking for different components of a possible pattern.

In this system, the letters stand for:

N̲umber ➔ S̲ize ➔ P̲osition ➔ C̲olour ➔ C̲onformation

Using this system, you consider each of the following aspects of the images in sequence, looking each time for commonly used patterns. We recommend this because it begins by looking for the simplest and most common potential patterns – if they are present, you are sure to get the pattern quickly and easily. If the first few patterns you look for are not present, then you look further on in the sequence to check for harder and less commonly tested patterns until you arrive at the answer.

Practice

It's very important to practice for this section as the style of questions are unlikely to be familiar. **Practicing well gives you three key advantages**. Firstly, you get used to the types of patterns which are likely to be asked in the real exam. This makes it more likely you will spot the patterns quickly as you will have seen them before, and it also trains up your implicit recognition system, meaning that if you take an 'educated guess' you are more likely to be right. Secondly, it gives you practice implementing a pattern recognition system, like **NSPCC**. With practice you will become better at using the system, and therefore quicker and more accurate overall. Thirdly, you will gain a feeling for the time it takes to answer different types of questions. This will allow you to better plan your time on the day, making the most out of every second you have.

Guessing

In the HUMAT, guessing should be kept to an absolute minimum, however… Whilst the best way to answer these questions correctly is to formally deduce the rule and apply it (using a pattern recognition system like **NSPCC** helps), humans *do* have an innate instinct for pattern recognition. This innate instinct is not necessarily right and can lead you astray, but in a situation where you cannot be certain of the answer, but *think* you may be right – the Visual Thinking questions are the most likely to reward you in this case.

That is to say, in some questions the overall look of the image will feel as though it should be placed in a particular set – you wouldn't be able to say exactly why, but to you it would look much more like one group than the other. Learning to harness this power can help give you a much better guessing accuracy. This is a simple example to demonstrate:

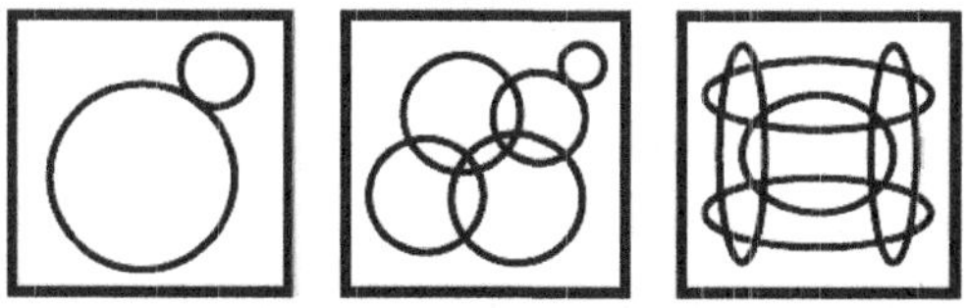

By quickly looking at the images provided for Set A and B, you get a general feel for what the contents are like. If asked which set the question image belongs to, you might be tempted to say Set B – it kind of looks more complicated and cluttered then Set A. It just looks more like the image. Now whilst this reasoning does not provide a comprehensive rule, in instances like this it can lead you to the correct answer quickly – even if you don't properly identify the underlying pattern.

Using the NSPCC system

The **NSPCC** system is a good way of working through possible patterns in a structured way. Whilst no structured response can be perfect, this system will solve over 90% of patterns quicker and more reliably than by trusting intuition alone.

Using the system, it is important that you are thorough. Sometimes the pattern can be subtle, and you could easily miss out on it if not taking care. You have to examine the details closely: count corners, sides of shapes, check where they are, etc. **You shouldn't be looking AT the shapes; you should be looking FOR patterns**. You should be working quickly, checking one thing, and if it's not that checking the next item in your list until you find the rule. Now to look at the system step-by-step.....

Number

Looking at 'number' is about counting as many things as possible. How many dots? How many squares? How many sides? How many corners? How many right angles? Also have a look at how many different types of shapes you can find in the frames. Sometimes you might find one type of shape only in Set A and not in Set B for example. A good rule of thumb: block arrows have 7 sides, so don't count all the sides individually every time you see one!

Size

It is quite common to find patterns in the size of the shapes. Is one shape always bigger than the others? Is there always a big shape in the centre, or in the corner? Are there smaller shapes inside larger ones?

Position

Look for patterns in where shapes are positioned. You might, for instance, always find a square in the top right corner in one set and a circle in the top right corner of the other set. Look also for touching and overlap of shapes – when you see this, make careful note of the type of contact. Is it tangential? Does it cut the shape in equal pieces, or is it off centre? Is there a certain shape that always makes this contact?

Colour

The shading of different shapes can constitute a pattern. Whilst this is often the easiest pattern to spot, it takes its place lower down in the system as it can often be a distracter. Most diagrams contain some amount of shading, but only occasionally is the primary pattern centred upon this. Look for shapes that are always shaded. Are all triangles black in one set and all circles black in the other, for example? On the other hand, are some shapes never shaded?

Conformation

These are the hardest patterns to spot, as they are the more complex patterns that can't be found by looking at the more geometric aspects. Conformation describes the pattern by which the shapes are arranged within the box – so you have to take a step back and look at the box as a whole in order to spot them. Look for patterns to the arrangement, like shapes arranged in a horizontal, vertical or diagonal line. Look also for the influence of one shape on another. For example, the presence of a white circle might signal a 90 degrees clockwise rotation of one shape and the presence of a black circle might signal a 90 degrees anticlockwise rotation, for example. When there are arrows, look at where they are pointing: are they all pointing in the same direction or at the same thing? You're looking for second order patterns, how things change with other aspects of the image.

VISUAL THINKING QUESTION TYPES

THINKING IN THREE DIMENSIONS

For questions which require you to **think in three dimensions** – you'll be presented with a written description of a three dimensional shape – this may have unique properties, like different colours or images on each surface. You'll then be presented with five options, each one an image of this shape, and you'll be asked to identify which image corresponds to the description, requiring you to convert the written description into an image. To answer this question well – examine the description and create rules. If you know that the surface of a pyramid has no green faces, for example – quickly establish that the correct answer cannot contain green. If the red face must be opposite the blue face, then establish a rule that you cannot see both colours at once, etc. Then work through the answers, with your rules, and quickly eliminate every answer which breaks them.

FINDING COMPLEMENTARY SHAPES

For questions requiring you to **find complementary shapes** you will be given an image right away, rather than a description of a shape. This shape will usually be quite complicated – and may remind you of active bonding sites on enzymes and other kinds of biological receptors. You will be presented with five different shapes as options, and asked to choose the shape which would fit into the shape provided in the question. For questions like this, it is best to start by focusing on one area and expanding as needed. Many candidates find it easiest to start at one end of the shape. Identify three or four unique traits at one end of the provided shape, and then examine each option for the mirror image of that. Being able to recognise mirror images and inversions is extremely useful, and can come up in a range of questions – this skill hinges on being able to hold the image in your head and imagine it inverted – if you struggle with this, the best bet is to practice visual thinking questions, and carry out activities which improve your spatial awareness and handling of geometry, like 'brain training' games.

IDENTIFYING PATTERNS AND LOCALISING OBJECTS IN RELATION TO OTHERS

For questions which require you to **identify patterns or localise objects in relation to others**, you will be presented with a sequence of shapes. You may then be asked to choose the next shape in the sequence out of five options, or to identify from a list of five possible rules a rule which fits the sequence. This style of question is normally quicker to answer, as it is more intuitive. In addition, you have transition points that you can compare to each other to help deduce whether you have correctly identified the rule.

To answer this style of question well, start by scanning quickly across the provided shapes – this gives you a general understanding of what is happening in the sequence. Then, focus on the element that is changing and apply your system to find out exactly *how* it is changing. You may also be asked to examine the shapes which you have been presented with – and answer a question about the arrangement of the shapes *from a different perspective*. Like the rotation and complementary shapes questions, these require you to rotate or invert the shapes in your mind, and determine which answer best reflects the altered shapes. It is particularly useful here to pay attention to how the provided shapes are grouped together, and use this grouping when considering your answer. If all the shapes along the top are circles, that would still be true if it was flipped on the horizontal axis, for example.

IDENTIFYING IMAGES FROM DESCRIPTIONS

For questions which require you to **identify an image from a description** you will be presented with a text description of a shape – with or without an accompanying visual aid. This description will lay out the rules for the shape which govern its layout and orientation. You'll be provided with five options which will all depict images of that shape – and you'll be asked which image is the shape described or, if you have been provided with a visual aid in the question, which image is the shape mirrored, rotated, or inverted. You can also be asked to do the inverse of this, on rare occasions. You will be presented with an image of a complex shape, and be asked to pick from one of five descriptions, which fits it best. Occasionally, the question may require you to rotate or invert the shape first, so as always, be sure to read the question and study the options closely before examining the data.

Example 1

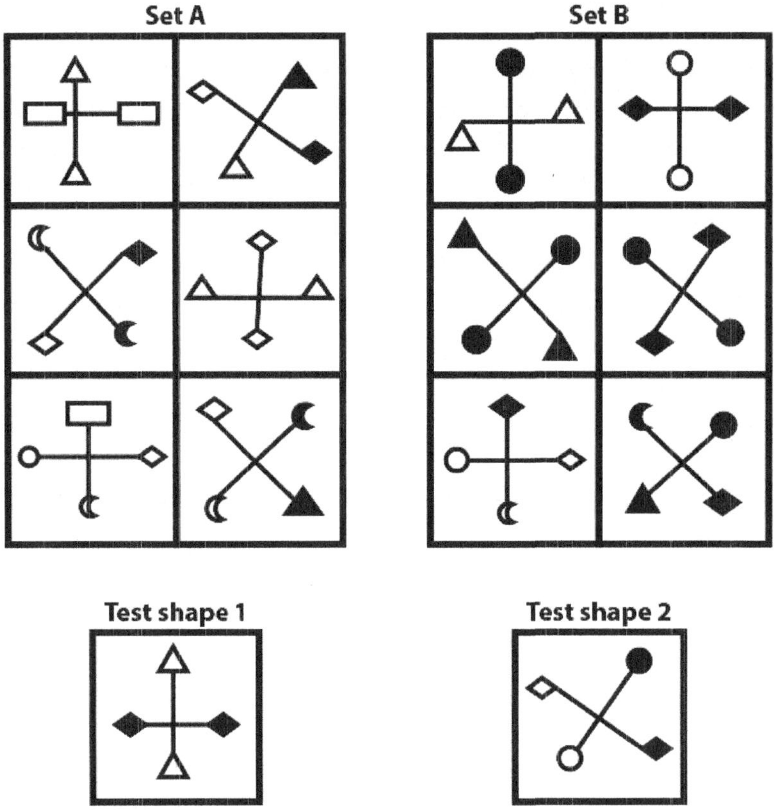

Start by applying the NSPCC system.
Number: count the number of shapes, sides, angles and so on looking for a pattern (can't see one in this example).
Size: are all shapes the same size (yes they are).
Position: is there a pattern to where certain shapes are (not obviously).
Colour: is there a pattern to the shading (yes, the shading is dependent upon the shape of the cross). If you didn't get that, look back now to identify what the pattern is before reading on.
We can use our observations to devise the following rules:
Set A: (+)-shaped crosses have four white shapes, and (X)-shaped crosses have two white and two black shapes.

Set B: (+)-shaped crosses have two white and two black shapes, and (X)-shaped crosses have four black shapes.

Applying these rules tells us Test Shape 1 belongs to Set B and Test Shape 2 belongs to Set A.

A Final Word

This section is all about pattern recognition. The more you see the better you will become. Once you're familiar with the main types of patterns which come up, you'll be able to solve the majority of questions without difficulty. Remember that **you're looking to identify a rule** for each set of boxes, something which links them all together. Then, you can decide which set each question item fits into (or indeed neither). Start using the **NSPCC** system, then practice makes perfect!

SECTION 1: MATHEMATICAL THINKING

Section 1 Maths questions are overwhelmingly focused on your mental arithmetic skills, and ability to work flexibly with equations and interpreting data. Revising GCSE maths will be valuable to you here, particularly the areas of maths which can be applied to real-world scenarios. Focus should be especially applied to indices, surds, rearranging equations to give a specific subject, proportionality and ratio, percentages and fractions, probability, and forming equations. Forming equations is of special significance and many HUMAT questions in the mathematical thinking section rely on your ability to use, interpret, and manipulate equations. Algebra I and Algebra II from American syllabi are a great place to start preparation. It is vital for your success in this section that you are very comfortable with carrying out quick, accurate calculations, and that you're comfortable with converting units and interpreting graphs.

We know that we don't need to go into pages of detail explaining how ratios, percentages, fractions, and equations work – you've known that for years, but some of the more advanced concepts here could be valuable for you to revise specifically, so we've included an overview below.

MATHEMATICS BASICS

1. Surd rules – including rationalising the denominator.

$\sqrt{a} \times \sqrt{a} = a$
$\sqrt{a} \times \sqrt{b} = \sqrt{ab}$
$a\sqrt{b} \times c\sqrt{d} = ac\sqrt{bd}$
$\frac{\sqrt{a}}{\sqrt{b}} = \sqrt{\frac{a}{b}}$

$\frac{\sqrt{a}}{\sqrt{b}} = \frac{\sqrt{a}}{\sqrt{b}} \times \left(\frac{\sqrt{b}}{\sqrt{b}}\right) = \frac{\sqrt{ab}}{b}$
$\frac{\sqrt{a}}{b+\sqrt{c}} = \frac{\sqrt{a}}{b+\sqrt{c}} \times \frac{b-\sqrt{c}}{b-\sqrt{c}} = \frac{\sqrt{a}(b-\sqrt{c})}{b^2-c}$

2.. Index laws.

$a^m \times a^n = a^{m+n}$
$\frac{a^m}{a^n} = a^{m-n}$
$(a^m)^n = a^{mn}$

$a^0 = 1$
$a^1 = a$
$a^{-m} = \frac{1}{a^m}$

$a^{\frac{1}{m}} = \sqrt[m]{a}$
$a^{\frac{m}{n}} = \sqrt[n]{a^m} = (\sqrt[n]{a})^m$

$a^n \times b^n = (ab)^n$
$\frac{a^n}{b^n} = \left(\frac{a}{b}\right)^n$

3. Common 'probability' definitions.

Mutually exclusive – events which can't both happen (e.g. both raining and not raining at all on one day)
Mutually inclusive – events which must both happen (e.g if I marry my husband, he must marry me)

Independent – the probability of one event happening is unaffected by the outcome of another event (e.g. the chance of rolling a 6 on a die is unaffected by the chance of getting a heads or tails on a coin flip)

Dependent – the probability of one event happening is affected by the outcome of another event (e.g. the chance of me doing well on a test at school is affected by the chance of me missing the bus and being late)
Conditional probabilities are the probability of a certain event occurring based on prior knowledge about some other event (e.g. the probability of it raining today *given* it rained yesterday is likely to be higher than the probability of it raining today if it was sunny yesterday)

4. AND & OR Rules

The probability of event A AND event B happening, $P(A \cap B)$, is given by $P(A) \times P(B)$, provided that A and B are independent.
The probability of event A OR event B happening, $P(A \cup B)$, is given by $P(A) + P(B)$, provided that A and B are mutually exclusive.
If they aren't mutually exclusive $P(A \cup B) = P(A) + P(B) - P(A \cap B)$. *(Which is just a more generalised version of the rule above if you think about it!)*
The probability of NOT A happening (also called the complement of A) is $P(A^C) = 1 - P(A)$

5. How to create and use Probability Trees

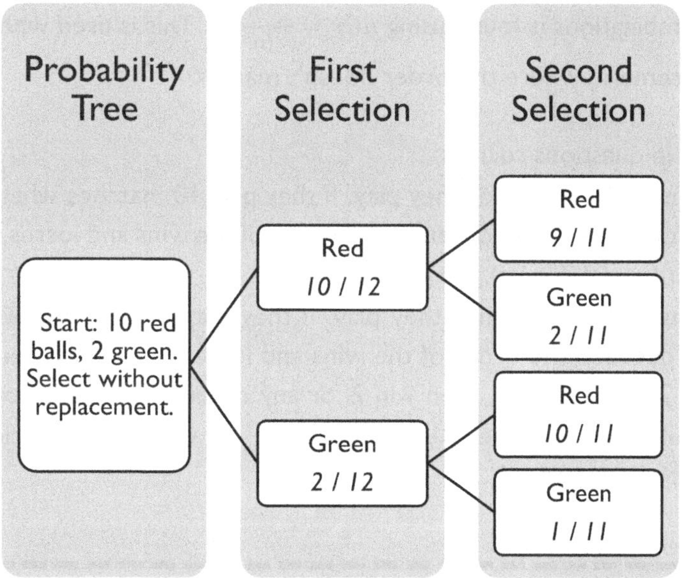

To find the probability of red followed by red multiply along the branches (to give $\frac{90}{132}$).
The sum of the probabilities calculated for each branch must total 1 (e.g. 'red & red + red & green + green & red + green & green = 1').

6, How to create and use Probability Tables.

	Revised	Didn't Revise	Total
Passed Test	15	5	20
Didn't Pass Test	2	8	10
Total	17	13	30

The probability that someone picked at random revised for the test is $\frac{N(revised)}{N(total)} = \frac{17}{30}$

The probability that someone picked at random revised & passed the test is $\frac{N(revised\ \&\ passed)}{N(total)} = \frac{15}{30} = \frac{1}{2}$

The *conditional* probability that someone passed *given that* they revised is $\frac{N(passed)}{N(revised)} = \frac{15}{17}$

7. Permutations & Combinations (including Factorial Notation).

The number of possible permutations is found using $nPr = \frac{n!}{(n-r)!}$. This is used when choosing 'r' things from a set of 'n' things (without replacement) where the order matters.

The number of possible combinations is found using $nCr = \frac{n!}{r!(n-r)!}$. This is used when choosing 'r' things from a set of 'n' things (without replacement) where the order doesn't matter.

You can see the difference in questions such as:

- A tennis player wins 75% of matches they play. If they play 10 matches what is the probability they win the first 5 and lose the next 5? For this question the order of the wins and losses matters, so the equation would be $WWWWWLLLLL = (0.75^5)(0.25^5)$
- A tennis player wins 75% of matches they play. If they play 10 matches what is the probability they win exactly 5? For this question the order of the wins and losses doesn't matter, they could win 5 then lose 5, or they could lose 2, win 3, lose 3, then win 2, or any other combination of wins and losses which works. The equation would therefore be $10C5(0.75^5)(0.25^5)$ which is 252 times larger than the previous probability where order mattered.

Check Your Knowledge:

A bag contains y yellow balls, and g green balls. A ball is taken from the bag (and removed), followed by two more balls (all with removal). What is the probability that all three balls are the same colour? *Assume that there are more than 3 balls of each colour available in the bag.* [3]

Answer: $P = \frac{g(g-1)(g-2)+y(y-1)(y-2)}{(g+y)(g+y-1)(g+y-2)}$

8. How to Estimate

If a question in the PAT resulted in a calculation such as 3.962×2.322 you should consider this to be approximately $4\left(\frac{7}{3}\right) = \frac{28}{3} \approx 9$.
This is incredibly important to make sure that you don't lose marks for silly calculator typing errors when your method is otherwise sound. Make sure you know what a sensible answer would be before you type it in!

9. How to Round (including Significant Figures).

You need to be able to accurately round to both a given number of decimal places, or significant figures.
You should also follow the convention that you should *never* give an answer to more significant figures than you were given in the question (e.g. if the values in the question have 2, 3, and 4 s.f. then your answer should be to the minimum number, 2s.f).

Our earlier section on interpreting data is relevant here as well, as Mathematical Thinking questions can be identical to selecting relevant data questions from procedural thinking.

10. Constructing Equations

Some of the problems in Section 1 are quite complex and you'll need to be comfortable with turning prose into equations and manipulating them. For example, when you read "Mark is twice as old as Jon" – this should immediately register as $M = 2J$. Once you get comfortable forming equations, you can start to approach some of the harder questions in this book (and past papers) which may require you to form and solve simultaneous equations. Consider the example:

Nick has a sleigh that contains toy horses and clowns and counts 44 heads and 132 legs in his sleigh. Given that horses have one head and four legs, and clowns have one head and two legs, calculate the difference between the number of horses and clowns.

A. 0 B. 5 C. 22 D. 28 E. 132 F. More information is needed.

To start with, let C = Clowns and H = Horses.
For Heads: $C + \mathrm{H} = 44$
For Legs: $2\mathrm{C} + 4\mathrm{H} = 132$
This now sets up your two equations that you can solve simultaneously.
$\mathrm{C} = 44 - \mathrm{H}$
So $2(44 - \mathrm{H}) + 4\mathrm{H} = 132$
Thus, $88 - 2\mathrm{H} + 4\mathrm{H} = 132$;
Therefore, $2\mathrm{H} = 44$; $\mathrm{H} = 22$
Substitute back in to give $\mathrm{C} = 44 - \mathrm{H} = 44 - 22 = 22$
Thus, the difference between horses and clowns $= \mathrm{C} - \mathrm{H} = 22 - 22 = 0$

It's important you are able to do these types of questions quickly and **without resorting to trial & error** as they are commonplace in section 1.

SECTION 2: ACADEMIC LITERACY

The Academic Literacy section of the HUMAT is markedly different from section 1 in a number of key ways. The focus is on longer extracts from text as your data, and each text has a number of different questions asked about it. Unlike section 1 then, this means that you will have the opportunity to spend some time analysing the data, and then answering multiple questions about the data in quick succession. Another difference is that the academic literacy section is not broken down into multiple subsections.

However, there are similarities – the questions will require you to critically engage with and interpret the texts provided, just as the procedural thinking questions did – and there will be a range of different types of questions being asked.

These can be boiled down into two categories, critical thinking, and logical reasoning. Critical Thinking questions will all revolve around being able to identify conclusions of the passage. Logical reasoning questions require you to examine the passage and choose the answer option which best finished a sentence begun in the question, for example "In the first paragraph, Shakespeare describes the two houses as…"

Some Logical reasoning questions will include a particular quotation from the passage, and will ask you to explain what those particular words mean, or refer to. Overwhelmingly, answering this will hinge on a point made in another part of the text.

In order to get the best outcomes here – you need to make sure that you are familiar with the entirety of the text. Texts in the HUMAT are long, around 700 words, and you need to take time to work through them. There are five texts to work through in an hour – each with six questions. That means that you have twelve minutes per text – but this doesn't equal two minutes per question. The bulk of this time should be spent carefully reading the text at the start of your time for the question. Once you have taken time to comprehend it, answering the questions should be very quick. Similarly, because many of the questions use language from the text, it is impractical to read them and the options closely before studying the text – as you'll often struggle to hold that information in your head meaningfully before you have a context to apply it to. We'd suggest, then, that for each text you spend about six minutes carefully reading it, and then the remaining six minutes for each text working through the six answers.

Remember, mark distribution is 3 for a correct answer, 0 for no answer, and -1 for an incorrect answer – so don't just guess if you don't know.

A top tip to remember is that every question can be answered with *only information from the text.* Every single question can, then, be answered if you have read the text and understood it sufficiently, and that's why giving yourself plenty of time to study the text is important.

PRACTICE QUESTIONS:

SECTION 1 PROCEDURAL THINKING QUESTIONS

SET I

The country of Ecunemia has a somewhat complicated tax code. There are four states that make up Ecunemia: Asteria, Bolovia, Casova and Derivia. Each state has its own tax code, including different tax rates on different items. The table below represents the tax a **customer** has to pay when they purchase an item from a store.
E.g. a £100 coat in Asteria would cost £110.

	Asteria	Bolovia	Casova	Derivia
Clothes	10%	15%	10%	10%
Food	5%	0%	10%	0%
Imports from other states	20%	5%	10%	15%

The customer must add the tax onto the advertised purchase price. In the case of an item falling into multiple categories (for example, in the case of Imported Food), the higher tax rate is paid and the lower rate is ignored.

Question 1:
A shopper visits a certain supermarket. Without tax, the shopper spends $50 on food, $30 on clothes and nothing on imported items. She spends $88 in total. Which state is this supermarket in?

A. Asteria B. Bolovia C. Casova D. Derivia

Question 2:
Someone runs a supplier in Bolovia, supplying supermarkets in each state in Ecumenia. Each year they supply each state with 250 items of clothing, which the supermarket sells for $40 (including tax), and the supplier gets all of this revenue, minus the tax paid. A competitor in Asteria goes out of business, and this supplier has the opportunity to buy the manufacturing plant for $20,000, and transfer to this state.

If the supplier purchases the site, and moves to Asteria, how many years will it take to make back the cost of purchasing the site?

A. 5 years B. 12 years C. 23 years D. 26 years

Question 3:
John goes into a store and spends $100. Of this, $12 is tax. Which of the following is possible?

A. He shopped in Asteria and bought no imported goods.
B. He shopped in Casova.
C. He shopped in Derivia and bought at least $50 of food (excluding tax).
D. He shopped in Bolovia and spent $10 on imported goods (excluding tax).

Question 4:

Sibella is on a road trip through Ecunemia, driving through different states. On the journey she buys $100 of the finest Asterian ham, $30 of the finest Bolovian caviar, a $10 case of Casovan orange juice and spends $100 on a Derivian dress (all of these prices without tax). Which of the following cannot have been the total amount Sibella spent, including tax?

A. $256 B. $264 C. $273 D. $288

SET 2

As a probe drops through the ocean, the pressure it experiences increases. For every 10 metres the probe drops down, the pressure it experiences increases by 10,000 Pascals (Pa).

Question 5:

A particular probe can survive 200 pounds per square inch without incurring damage. Given that the conversion factor between these units is 7000 Pa = 1 pound per square inch and assuming that pressure at sea level is 0 Pascals, how deep can the probe drop into the ocean without incurring damage?

A. 14 m B. 140 m C. 1.4 km D. 14 km

Question 6:

A different probe is dropped into the ocean and falls downward. This probe can withstand 300,000 Pa of pressure without breaking. A model of the effect of the fluid states that the object's depth in the fluid is $d = \frac{1}{2}\sqrt{(t^3)}$, where d is depth in metres and t is time in seconds. How long will it take for this probe to break?

A. 65 seconds B. 71 seconds C. 75 seconds D. 78 seconds

SET 3

The fictional drug Cordrazine is used to treat four separate conditions. The following table gives the amount of drug used in each case to treat each condition, written in the form *x* mg/kg: i.e. for every kilogram you weigh, you take *x* mg of the drug. The recommended course for the drug is also listed, in the form of number of times a day and how many weeks you need to take the drug.

Condition	Dosage	Course
Black Trump Virus	4 mg/kg	3 times daily for 4 weeks
Swamp Fever	3 mg/kg	Once daily, 1 week
Yellow Tick	1 mg/kg	2 times daily for 12 weeks
Red Rage	5 mg/kg	2 times daily, 3 weeks

Question 7:

Over the course of treatment, John, an 80 kg male, takes 26.88 grams of the drug. Which disease was he prescribed the drug for?

A. Black Trump Virus B. Swamp Fever C. Yellow Tick D. Red Rage

Question 8:

Carol is a 60 kg female who is prescribed the drug (precisely and at different times) three times in one year. Two of the cases are for Yellow Tick. In total she takes 40.32 grams of the drug. Which was the third disease she was prescribed the drug for?

A. Black Trump Virus B. Swamp Fever C. Yellow Tick D. Red Rage

Question 9:

Clarence takes the drug twice in his life. Once he takes it for Swamp Fever at age 18, when he weighs 80 kg, and he takes it later in life at age 40 for Black Trump Virus, when he weighs 110 kg. What is the ratio of the amount he takes each time?

A. 1:23 B. 1:22 C. 1:21 D. 1:20

Question 10:

Danny has liver disease. His system cannot cope with more than 15.5 grams of Cordrazine every 4 weeks. Danny has a medical condition usually treated with Cordrazine, but doctors have advised him to not complete a course of the treatment, as he would exceed the dose that his system is able to cope with. Which of the following statements is possible?

A. Danny suffers from Red Rage and weighs 75 kg.
B. Danny suffers from Swamp Fever and weighs 100 kg.
C. Danny suffers from Black Trump and weighs 45 kg.
D. Danny suffers from Yellow Tick and weighs 75 kg.

Question 11:

Eileen has kidney failure. Her system cannot cope with more than 10 grams of Cordrazine every 4 weeks. She suffers from Red Rage, but doctors have recommended she does not use Cordrazine to treat it, as this would exceed the 10 g dosage her system can cope with. Which of the following weights is the minimum that would support this recommendation?

A. 40.34 kg B. 42.53 kg C. 45.81 kg D. 47.62 kg

SET 4

A bakery sells four varieties of cakes. The cakes contain the following ingredients:

	Sponge (520g)	Madeira (825g)	Pound (710g)	Chocolate (885g)
Flour (g)	125	250	150	200
Butter (g)	125	175	185	175
Egg (g)	120	180	180	120
Milk (g)	25	45	45	150
Sugar (g)	125	175	150	200
Cocoa (g)	-	-	-	40

Question 12:

Which cake contains the highest proportion of flour?

A. Sponge B. Madeira C. Pound D. Chocolate.

Question 13:

The cake recipes are scaled up for a large order. One cake weighs 2.6 kg and contains 625 g of flour. What variety of cake is it?

A. Sponge B. Madeira C. Pound D. Chocolate

Question 14:

Eliza is having a wedding and wants to produce a 4-tiered wedding cake. She wishes each tier to be of different size, and scaled such that that the bottom cake is 50% heavier than normal (e.g. the cake contains 50% more ingredients), the second cake is 25% heavier than normal, the third cake is 10% heavier than normal and the top cake is normal-sized, where each cake is of the same type. Which of the following is a possible weight of sugar for the cake (rounded to 2 s.f.)?

A. 940 g B. 970 g C. 1,000 g D. 1,030 g

Question 15:

It is known that flour costs £0.55 per 1.5 kg and sugar costs £0.70 per 1 kg. Which of the following is the closest to the cost ratio of flour to sugar in a Madeira cake?

A. 1:2 B. 3:4 C. 4:5 D. 5:6

Question 16:

Milk costs £0.44 per kilogram and flour costs £0.55 per 1.5 kg. What is the cost ratio of flour to milk in a chocolate cake?

A. 1:1 B. 2:3 C. 8:7 D. 10:9

SET 5

The Kryptos Virus is particularly virulent. The infection rate is dependent upon the gender of the recipient. A random sample of 100 men and 100 women are taken from a population and tested for the Kryptos virus using Test A. The results of Test A are displayed below:

	Men	Women
Have virus	45	63
Do not have virus	55	37

Question 17:

What percentage of people tested have the virus?

A. 45% B. 54% C. 55% D. 63%

Question 18:
A population of 231,768 is divided: 53% women, 47% men. Use the data in the table to estimate the number of people in the population that have the Kryptos virus. Assume that the infection rates in each gender will be the same as for the sample population in Test A. Which of the following is the number of people expected to be infected with Kryptos virus in this population?

A. 123,587 B. 123,589 C. 125,541 D. 126,406

Question: 19
3/9 of the men and 5/7 of the women testing positive for Kryptos in Test A have visited the city of Atlantis. Which of the following is the correct percentage of people in the test group testing positive for Kryptos who have NOT visited Atlantis?

A. 40% B. 44% C. 50% D. 55%

Question 20:
It is known that Test A is not always correct. Test B is a more accurate test. The 45 men who tested positive for the Kryptos virus using Test A were then re-tested with Test B – only 20 tested positive. Assuming the same proportion of men and women experienced false positive results with Test A, how many women in the test group do we expect to actually have the Kryptos virus?

A. 20 B. 28 C. 35 D. 42

Question 21:
It is decided the women who tested positive under test A should be retested using test B. This time 29 women test positive for the Kryptos Virus. Considering both the men and women tested, what percentage of people who tested positive in Test A also tested positive in Test B (to the nearest whole number)?

A. 40% B. 45% C. 50% D. 55%

SET 6
A business has 3 manufacturing plants and 3 stores. Each plant can ship to each store, and the following table shows the flat rate cost, in pounds sterling (£), of the business sending a truck from the plant to the store.

	Store 1	Store 2	Store 3
Plant A	100	190	530
Plant B	120	180	600
Plant C	140	200	450

Question 22:
Currently the businesses strategy is to send material from Plant A to store 2, from Plant B to store 3 and from Plant C to store 1. One truck is sufficient for a day's delivery. What is the daily cost of this plan?

A. £850 B. £930 C. £970 D. £1,030

Question 23:

The store wishes to optimise their shipping costs by sending material from Plant C to store 3, noticing that the delivery cost is lower. They then choose the two other options that save the most money. What percentage saving is achieved by this strategy relative to the strategy in the previous question (to the nearest whole number)?

A. 18% B. 20% C. 22% D. 24%

SET 7

The table below shows the number of books sold by a bookshop in one day:

	Below 18	Above 18
Non-Fiction	12	30
Horror	50	45
Sci-Fi/Fantasy	23	90
Other Fiction	103	159

Question 24:

The shop also ran an author's visit event in the evening in which 106 people purchased the author's book. These books are **NOT** counted in the above table. What proportion of the books sold on this particular day were sold at the author's visit event (to the nearest whole number)?

A. 13% B. 17% C. 21% D. 25%

Question 25:

Non-fiction books cost, on average, £10, and fiction books cost, on average, £6. What percentage of the shop's revenue (excluding the author's visit event) came from non-fiction books?

A. 10% B. 13% C. 19% D. 23%

Question 26:

Assume that the shop makes this number of sales of each type of book every day. One week, the shop adopts a new marketing strategy and markets non-fiction books more heavily. The result is that the number of non-fiction sales double during this week, but all of the other book sales stay in line with previous sales. How much does the shop earn this week?

A. £24,250 B. £25,620 C. £26,950 D. £27,890

Question 27:

The following week, the shop decides to market the horror books more heavily, resulting in the sales of horror books doubling, and the sales of non-fiction books returning to the normal level. How much does the shop's income increase this week compared to the non-fiction marketing week? Sales of all other books assumed to be the same as un-marketed weeks.

A. 1% B. 2% C. 3% D. 4%

SET 8

The following table shows the taxing structure for Italian city hotels. Unless specifically mentioned, assume that all of the people below are aged 18 or over.

City	Tax
Venice	1 euro per star per room per night. Rooms with children under 16 are tax exempt.
Rome	Per person, per night: 5 euros for 3-star, 6 euros for 4-star, 7 euros for 5-star, up to a maximum of ten nights worth, after which no tax is charged. Children under age 10 are tax exempt.
Padua	Per person, per night: 2 euros for 3-star or below, 3 euros for 4-star or above. Rooms with children under 16 are tax exempt.
Siena	2 euros per person per night in high season, 1 euro per person per night in low season. Children under 12 are tax exempt.

Question 28:

A family goes on a tour of Italy in the high season. They are 2 adults and 2 children, aged 9 and 13. They spend two nights in each of Venice, Rome, Padua and Siena. They stay in 3-star hotels for the entire trip and have two rooms (an adult room and a child room). How much tax do they pay for their trip?

A. 35 euros B. 56 euros C. 60 euros D. 65 euros

Question 29:

Claude is comparing cities. He can either spend 7 nights in Rome in a 4-star hotel, or 8 nights in Padua in a 5-star hotel. Which of the following is the ratio between the tax he pays in Rome and the tax he pays in Padua?

A. 8:3 B. 7:4 C. 6:2 D. 1:4

Question 30:

Alice goes on a trip for 2 days to Venice in a 3-star hotel and for 3 days to Padua in a 4-star hotel. What is the percentage more tax she pays in Padua relative to Venice?

A. 25% B. 50% C. 75% D. 100%

Question: 31

How long does Reuben have to stay in a 4-star hotel in Rome so that the tax would be less than or equal to the tax he incurs if staying the same length of time in a 4-star hotel in Padua?

A. 10 days B. 15 days C. 20 days D. 25 days

SET 9

Peter is building a house that contains rooms of different sizes. The sitting room is 10m x 20m, the hallway is 3m x 10m, and the master bedroom is 15m x 15m. In addition, the house has another square-shaped bedroom, a kitchen and a bathroom.

Question 32:
Assuming that the second bedroom walls are 60% of the length of the master bedroom, what is the area of the second bedroom?

A. 64 m^2 B. 81 m^2 C. 100 m^2 D. 121 m^2

Question 33:
Suppose the kitchen has a floor area of 100 m^2 and the bathroom has a floor area of 4 m^2, and the second bedroom has the floor area calculated in the previous question. What percentage of the area of the house is taken up by the master bedroom?

A. 30% B. 35% C. 40% D. 45%

Question 34:
After building the house, Peter decides to add an extension to the sitting room, turning it into a combined lounge and dining room. He extends the room by increasing the length of the longer wall by 5 metres. The lounge is 3 metres high. How much extra wall (in m^2) does Peter have to build, assuming that he is extending directly outwards and cannot move or re-use any wall?

A. 15m^2 B. 30m^2 C. 45m^2 D. 60m^2

Question 35:
A larger extension is considered, and two builders offer Peter separate quotes. The first builder offers to build wall at a cost of £15 per m^2, but there is also a flat fee of £200 just for starting the job. The second builder offers to build wall at a cost of £16 per m^2 but with no flat fee at the start. If Peter builds 300 m^2 of wall, what is the ratio of builder 1 cost to builder 2 cost (to 3 s.f.)?

A. 1.00:1.00 B. 1.00:1.02 C. 1.02:1.00 D. 2.00:3.00

SET 10
The table below shows the service prices for competing mobile phone plans A-D. Any SMSs or call minutes beyond those free with the plan are charged individually at listed price.

	A	B	C	D
Monthly fee	£0	£5	£10	£15
# Free SMSs	0	200	1000	Unlimited
# Free call minutes	0	0	100	Unlimited
Price/SMS	10p	20p	20p	-
Price/call minute	10p	20p	20p	-

Question 36:
John buys Plan B for one month. He calls for 15 minutes and sends 207 SMSs. How much does he pay this month?

A. £5.00 B. £6.60 C. £7.80 D. £9.40 E. £11.20

Question 37:
Robin buys Plan A and makes no calls. How many SMSs can Robin send before Plan B would have been cheaper?
A. 6 B. 21 C. 51 D. 101 E. 121

Question 38:
Mary wants to call for 5 minutes and send 5 SMSs every day in September. Which plan should she choose for the lowest cost?
A. Plan A
B. Plan B
C. Plan C
D. Plan D
E. Plan A and Plan B are both the lowest

Question 39:
Evan buys Plan B but Chris buys Plan C. Which of these options is cheaper for Evan than Chris per month?
A. They each call for 29 minutes and send no SMSs.
B. They each call for 26 minutes and send 174 SMSs.
C. They each send 351 SMSs and call for 8 minutes.
D. They each call for 4 minutes every day of the month.
E. They each send 223 SMSs and make no calls.

Question 40:
Rachel doesn't send any SMSs and buys Plan C. What is the maximum percentage by which she can exceed her free call minutes allowance without Plan D being cheaper?
A. 5% B. 10% C. 25% D. 50% E. 75%

SET 11
A muffin recipe calls for ingredients in the amounts listed in the table below:

Ingredient	Density	Amount
Flour	600 gram/dm^3	2 cups
Sugar	850 gram/dm^3	1 cup
Milk	1050 gram/dm^3	½ cup
Butter	950 gram/dm^3	4 tablespoons

1 cup = 2.5 decilitres (dl); 1 tablespoon = 15 millilitres (ml); 1 cubic decimetre (dm^3) = 1 litre

Question 41:
How many cups of ingredients are called for overall by the recipe (to 2 decimal places)?
A. 3.54 B. 3.66 C. 3.74 D. 3.82 E. 3.86

Question 42:
What weight ratio of milk to butter does the recipe call for (to 1 decimal place)?
A. 2.3:1 B. 2.7:1 C. 3.1:1 D. 3.4:1 E. 3.9:1

Question 43:
Jane wants to use only a ½ cup measure for baking. What is the smallest number of cups of flour she would need for it to be possible to measure all required ingredients in ½ cups?
A. 2 B. 10 C. 25 D. 30 E. 50

Question 44:
To make pancakes, the amount of flour and milk are reversed. What is the average density of pancake batter, assuming that there are no interactions that change the densities of the individual ingredients when they are mixed?
A. 930 grams/dm^3
B. 970 grams/dm^3
C. 1,050 grams/dm^3
D. 1,070 grams/dm^3
E. 1,100 grams/dm^3

Question 45:
If Peter wanted to make 10 muffins weighing 100 grams each, how much butter would he need to 1 decimal place? Assume that the finished product weighs the same as the initial dough.
A. 55.1 grams B. 62.3 grams C. 70.7 grams D. 76.4 grams E. 81.3 grams

Question 46:
When Peter's ten 100-gram muffins are done, assuming no losses to cooking, what percentage of the weight will be made up by flour, to the nearest whole number?
A. 35% B. 39% C. 43% D. 46% E. 52%

SET 12
New ocean crust is formed at spreading ridges. The area of the crust formed is dependent on temperature. The volume of crust formed in a given time interval depends on the **crust cross sectional area** and on the spreading rate (the rate at which newly formed crust moves away from the spreading ridge, an independent variable).

The relationship between **crust volume** formed in a time interval, **cross sectional area** and **spreading rate** is:
Crust volume per time = cross sectional area x spreading rate

The table below gives the crustal cross sectional area, spreading rate and temperature at Locations A-D:

	A	B	C	D
Cross Sectional Area (km^2)	10	20	30	40
Spreading rate (mm/year)	150	20	100	50
Temperature (°C)	1300	1400	1500	1600

Question 47:
Assuming that the trends in this table can be reliably extrapolated, at which temperature would the crust volume formed in a year be expected to be 0 km^3?
A. 1,200°C B. 1,400°C C. 1,600°C D. 1,800°C E. 2,000°C

Question 48:

If the temperature at Location A increased by 50%, what would be the spreading rate?

A. 25 mm/year
B. 50 mm/year
C. 100 mm/year
D. 150 mm/year
E. 225 mm/year

Question 49:

What volume of crust is formed in a year at Location B?

A. 400 m^3
B. 400°C km^3
C. 40,000 km^3
D. 400,000 m^3
E. 560,000°C km^3

Question 50:

If the spreading rates of Locations A and C were exchanged, what would be the ratio of crust volume formed at the two locations each year (to 1 decimal place)?

A. 1:1.0
B. 1:3.3
C. 1:4.5
D. 1:5.6
E. 1:6.0

Question 51:

If the same crustal volume was produced in the same amount of time at 2 locations, E with temperature 1300°C and F with temperature 1450°C, how many percent faster/slower was the spreading rate at location E than F?

A. 250% faster
B. 25% slower
C. 400% faster
D. 40% slower
E. 500% faster

Question 52:

If the temperature at Location D was decreased by 10%, what would be the crustal volume formed in 3 years?

A. 2,000 m^3
B. 2,000 °C km^3
C. 3,200 km^3
D. 3,200,000 m^3
E. 3,600,000,000,000,000 mm^3

SET 13

A new drug to treat vision problems in diabetics is tested on volunteers. It is also tested on control groups of diabetics without vision problems and healthy volunteers with or without vision problems. Some volunteers are given one inactive placebo pill which they are told is the drug. There are the same number of people in each group testing either the drug or placebo, as indicated below.

The table below shows the number of volunteers in Groups A-D who self-reported improved vision and their measured average accuracy reading letters before and after taking the drug or a placebo.

	Group A		Group B		Group C		Group D	
	Drug	Placebo	Drug	Placebo	Drug	Placebo	Drug	Placebo
Number Improved	15	9	8	6	9	7	7	8
Accuracy Before (%)	27	27	60	60	29	29	68	68
Accuracy After (%)	36	31	66	61	31	32	70	70

Group A: 50 diabetics with vision problems (25 in each group)
Group B: 46 diabetics without vision problems (23 in each group)
Group C: 44 healthy volunteers with vision problems (22 in each group)
Group D: 48 healthy volunteers without vision problems (24 in each group)

Question 53:
What is the average percentage of participants who self-report vision improvements after receiving an inactive pill to the nearest percent?
A. 26% B. 31% C. 32% D. 33% E. 36%

Question 54:
By what ratio is visual accuracy in reading letters increased by the drug in diabetics with poor sight relative to healthy volunteers with poor sight (to 2 decimal places)?
A. 1:0.78 B. 3.50:1 C. 4.21:1 D. 4.50:1 E. 4.83:1

Question 55:
If there are 10 women in Group A and their average accuracy was 45% after receiving the drug, what was the average accuracy of the men in the group after receiving the drug?
A. 16% B. 27% C. 30% D. 36% E. 41%

Question 56:
If the general population has 100 000 diabetics with vision problems, how many of these people would be expected to self-report improvements in their vision because of the effects of the drug?
A. 24,000 people
B. 32,000 people
C. 36,000 people
D. 60,000 people
E. 96,000 people

Question 57:
When the drug dose was doubled, the placebo groups showed no change in numbers or accuracy, but the number of Group A volunteers who reported improved vision jumped to 18. Assuming that drug effectiveness is dose dependent, what percent of volunteers in Group A taking the drug would be expected to self-report improved vision if the dose was tripled?
A. 54.0%
B. 72.0%
C. 84.0%
D. 90.0%
E. 100.0%

Question 58:
Which of the following statements is supported by the data in the table?
A. The placebo is more effective than the drug.
B. The drug acts to improve vision in diabetics and healthy volunteers.
C. Volunteers who see well are more motivated to improve vision than those with vision problems.
D. Thinking you have taken a drug to improve vision improves your vision.
E. The data are inconclusive.

SET 14

Dave weighs 200 pounds and has a Basal Metabolic Rate (BMR) of 2000 calories. Elizabeth weighs 140 pounds and has a BMR of 1500 calories. The table below shows the calorific value of the foods they eat:

	Cereal	Sandwich	Apple	Chocolate	Lasagne	Chicken	Vegetables
Calories	400	500	100	350	700	250	200

To lose one pound of fat requires a 3500-calorie deficit, obtained by eating fewer calories than the BMR or burning calories by exercising. Running burns 5 calories per hour per pound you weigh at any running speed.

Cycling burns calories according to the following relationship, where M is mph cycling speed:

Calories burned per mile = 50 calories + (5 calories x (M-10))

Question 59:

Dave wants his workout to take one hour on a 5-mile track. What is the maximum number of calories he can burn by running or cycling?

A. Burn 125 calories running

B. Burn 125 calories cycling

C. Burn 1,000 calories running

D. Burn 1,000 calories cycling

E. Burn 1,250 calories running

Question 60:

Dave doesn't want to eat less than his BMR and can only run for 30 minutes a day, but cycles 20 miles every day in an hour. How long will it take him to lose 10 pounds?

A. 5 days B. 7 days C. 10 days D. 14 days E. 30 days

Question 61:

Elizabeth and Dave both want to lose 10% of their body weight without dieting or cycling. What is the ratio of minutes a day Elizabeth would have to run to those Dave would have to run to achieve their goal at the same time to 1 decimal place?

A. 1:0.5 B. 1:0.7 C. 1:1.0 D. 1:1.4 E. 1:2.0

Question 62:

If Elizabeth eats cereal for breakfast, a sandwich for lunch, chicken and vegetables for dinner and does no exercise, in how many full days will she have reached her goal of 10% weight-loss?

A. 327 days B. 354 days C. 372 days D. 416 days E. 435 days

Question 63:

If Elizabeth also began cycling 10 miles in 1 hour every day, how much faster would she reach her goal than in question 62?

A. 1.00 B. 2.50 C. 3.00 D. 3.33 E. 4.33

Question 64:

Elizabeth eats one chocolate every day, 3 times as much chicken as chocolate, and twice as much cereal as chicken. If she exchanged these foods with 3 different foods in the table in the same proportions (i.e. 1:3:6), what is the ratio of her rate of weight change before and after the switch, assuming she is trying to lose the most weight she can?

A. 1:1 B. 1:2 C. 1:5 D. 2:1 E. 5:1

SET 15

Visitors to an amusement park pay for food, rides and games with coupons. Coupons can be bought individually for £1 each or in multipacks at a discounted price. A £70 wristband gives free entry and access to all rides (but not games or food) without using coupons. The table below shows the cost in coupons for each activity:

	Entrance	Roller-coaster	Fun House	Swings	Carnival Games	Candy Floss
All Day	10	4	2	3	1	2
Night	5	3	2	2	1	2

Question 65:

Susan buys a 20 coupon multi-pack at 10% off single coupon price. She rides the rollercoaster five times at night. What percent off did she get on the first rollercoaster ride compared to buying single day tickets (to 1 decimal place)?

A. 10.0% B. 22.5% C. 25.0% D. 32.5% E. 33.3%

Question 66:

One weekend the single coupon prices are raised 20%. Greg wants to ride the rollercoaster 10 times, buy 3 candy floss, play a carnival game, go through the fun house 2 times and ride the swings during the day. What is the ratio of the cost with a wristband to the cost without a wristband to 2 decimal places?

A. 1:0.93 B. 1:0.98 C. 1:1.02 D. 1:1.10 E. 1:1.12

Question 67:

Andy went to the amusement park one night. He rode the rollercoaster 50% more times than he rode the swings and rode the swings 20% more times than he played carnival games. He used a whole number of coupons that were cheaper than getting a wristband. How much did Andy pay?

A. £31 B. £44 C. £49 D. £56 E. £70

Question 68:

Anna and James each spent one pound less than the cost of a wristband on single coupons one day at the amusement park. Anna went on the rollercoaster for half of her rides and the fun house for the rest. James went on the swings every odd ride and into the fun house every even ride. Neither of them went on any other rides or bought any food. What is the ratio of the number of rides Anna went on to the number James went on?

A. 1:0.78 B. 1:0.81 C. 1:1.23 D. 1:1.28 E. 1:2.56

Question 69:

A 10-weekend season pass covers all costs in the park and is available for £1,000. Erik goes to the park one day every weekend and buys a wristband each time. On the first weekend he buys one candyfloss, and the next four weekends increases the number of candyfloss he buys by 100%, relative to the previous weekend. The four weekends after that he increases the number of candyfloss he buys by 50% each weekend, relative to the previous weekend. On the 10th weekend he is sick of candyfloss and buys none. What is the ratio of the cost without and with a season pass (to 2 decimal places)?

A. 0.7:1 B. 0.92:1 C. 1:0.92 D. 1:1.15 E. 1.15:1

SET 16

The table shows the prices a pizzeria charges for their pizza:

	Italian		Pan Pizza		
Type	Cheese	Toppings	Cheese	Topping	Stuffed Crust
Price Small	£6.00	+50p/topping	£10.00	+50p/topping	+£1.00
Price Medium	£8.00	+£1.00/topping	£12.00	+£1.00/topping	+£1.50
Price Large	£10.00	+£1.50/topping	£14.00	+£2.00/topping	+£2.00

The pizzeria also offers three discount deals: 20% off orders from £20 – £29.99, 30% off orders from £30 – £49.99, and 50% off orders over £50. Small pizzas have 6 slices, medium pizzas have 8 slices, and large pizzas have 10 slices.

Question 70:

Josh gets 2 large stuffed-crust 2-topping pan pizzas, 1 medium 3-topping Italian pizza and 3 small cheese pan pizzas. How much does he pay?

A. £31.00 B. £40.50 C. £52.50 D. £81.00 E. £96.00

Question 71:

Janet bought cheese pan pizzas for the cheapest cost per slice and got £35 off as a discount. How many slices did she buy?

A. 35 B. 48 C. 50 D. 64 E. 70

Question 72:

Joey bought some plain cheese pizzas for a total price of £60 post-discount. All the plain cheese pizzas were the same. What is the price of the one type of pizza he could NOT have bought?

A. £6.00 B. £8.00 C. £10.00 D. £12.00 E. £14.00

Question 73:

Lea always buys 30 slices of cheese pan pizza with 2 toppings and stuffed crust. What is the ratio of the cost of buying all large to all small pizzas (to 2 decimal places)?

A. 1:0.50 B. 1:0.75 C. 1:0.80 D. 1:1.00 E. 1:1.25

Question 74:

Kate and two friends each order cheese pan pizzas (with no toppings) and get 30% off their order. They ordered the pizzas to pay the smallest price which gets this discount, but ended up with 25% more slices than they could eat. How many slices did they manage to eat?

A. 16 B. 18 C. 20 D. 25 E. 32

SET 17

Sarah has three journalist jobs she splits her time across. The table shows a breakdown of what she earns at each job. Her salary is composed of a fixed starter wage she earns for showing up and an hourly wage on top of that. Her hourly wage increases in each job the more hours she works at that job. She must pay for her own travel expenses. Each travel cost occurs once per job she completes, and is not affected by the length of the job in hours.

	Travel Cost	Fixed Starter Wage	Hourly Wage	Average Job Length	Hourly Wage Growth
Job A	£5	£10	£10 per hour	2 hours	£5 per 50 worked
Job B	-	£5	£15 per hour	1 hours	£10 per 100 worked
Job C	£10	£5	£20 per hour	4 hours	£5 per 100 worked

Question 75:

If Sarah works for 1 hour at each job, what will be the ratio of the earnings expressed as [Job A Earnings:Job B Earnings:Job C Earnings] (to 2 decimal places)?

A. : 0.75 : 1.00 B. : 1.00 : 0.75 C. : 1.25 : 1.00 D. : 1.33 : 0.75 E. : 1.33 : 1.00

Question 76:

Sarah worked 25 2-hour jobs, 4 1-hour jobs and 1 4-hour job for Job A in her first month. How much did she earn?

A. £625.00 B. £730.00 C. £770.00 D. £980.00 E. £1,020.00

Question 77:

Sarah can work 50 2-hour jobs per month. For which single job should she work these hours to earn the most from 2-hour jobs at the end of the month?

A. Job A
B. Job B
C. Job C
D. A and B are the same
E. B and C are the same

Question 78:

Sarah pays 10% income tax if her monthly salary exceeds £1275. How many hours should she work in her first month for Job C, if all jobs are the average job length, to earn the highest amount possible whilst not paying tax, to the nearest half-hour?

A. 60.0 hours B. 62.5 hours C. 65.0 hours D. 68.0 hours E. 75.0 hours

Question 79:

At the start of her third month, Sarah has worked 200 hours at Job C. She works 100 hours at average job length this month. How much of her month's earnings go to 10% income tax?

A. £150.00 B. £187.50 C. £200.00 D. £287.50 E. £300.00

Question 80:

Job B wants her to work a minimum of 50 hours a month for them, and Job A and Job C require that she works at least the same hours for them as she does at any other jobs she has, or no hours at all. Assuming all jobs are the average job length, which arrangement would give her maximum earnings in her first 100-hour work month?

A. 50 hours for B and 50 hours for A
B. 50 hours for B and 50 hours for C
C. 50 hours for A and 50 hours for C
D. 100 hours for B
E. None of the above

SET 18

The table below shows the number of cars passing a toll booth going into the town centre and how many passengers in each, including the drivers. It also shows the number of passengers who got off at the town's central underground station each day.

	Mon	Tue	Wed	Thu	Fri	Sat
Number of cars	1,517	1,632	987	1,465	2,024	478
Total car passengers (including drivers)	1,873	2,421	1,116	2,101	2,822	1,339
Underground passengers	2,346	1,798	3,103	2,118	1,397	576

Question 81:

Taking the underground costs £5. On Wednesdays this fare is reduced 15% and it is cheaper for some drivers to leave the car at home. How much more revenue is generated on Wednesday than the next highest grossing day?

A. £1,457.75
B. £3,537.25
C. £5,275.75
D. £11,730.00
E. £13,187.75

Question 82:

On weekdays, what is the ratio of the average number of people being driven (not driving) in cars to the average number of people riding on the underground (to 2 decimal places)?

A. 1:0.25
B. 1:0.78
C. 1:3.97
D. 1:7.60
E. 1:9.60

Question 83:

What is the ratio of the average number of people per car on Tuesday compared to Saturday?

A. 1:0.67
B. 1:0.85
C. 1:1.27
D. 1:1.33
E. 1:1.89

Question 84:

What is the ratio of the number of Underground passengers on Monday compared to that on Saturday?

A. 1:0.13
B. 1:0.25
C. 1:0.40
D. 1:1.50
E. 1:4.08

Question 85:

The tollbooths charge £4 per car and an additional £1 per passenger (including the driver). 80% of this payment is tax. How much tax is paid at the tollbooths next week from Monday-Friday if there are 4,219 commuters everyday split in the ratio of 2 : 1.7 : 1 (in the format of underground passenger : car passenger (including driver) : car ratio)?

A. £1,938.45
B. £4,219.00
C. £4,560.50
D. £5,198.40
E. £6,498.96

SET 19

Music practice rooms are available seven days a week, with each day being split into three sessions: morning (8am-2pm), day (2pm-8pm) and night (8pm-2am). The table below gives the prices for the hourly rental of the music practice rooms. Some information is missing. The two sessions' column indicates the hourly charge if two sessions are booked on the same day.

Type of room	Deposit	Cost per Hour			
		1-2 hours (night session)	3-6 hours (night session)	Two sessions	All day
Basic (no piano)	£10.00	-	-	£11.00	£8.00
Standard (upright piano)	£25.00	£20.00	£18.00	£16.00	£12.00
Superior (baby grand piano)	£50.00	£30.00	£26.00	£22.00	£16.50
Deluxe (grand piano)	-	£45.00	£38.00	£30.00	£20.00

NB: All prices above include VAT (25%).

Question 86:

The hourly rate for a day session is 10% more expensive than a night session. What is the total cost, excluding the deposit, for 3 hours in the Superior room during a day session?

A. £59.40 B. £70.20 C. £78.00 D. £84.18 E. £85.80

Question 87:

The total cost for two 6-hour sessions in the Deluxe room is £460. How much is the deposit?

A. £64 B. £75 C. £82 D. £100 E. £136

Question 88:

Mike books a Basic room and a Standard room for a full night session. The total cost is £221 including deposit. What is the hourly rate for a full night session in a Basic room?

A. £12.50 B. £13.00 C. £15.00 D. £16.83 E. £18.83

Question 89:

The hourly rate for a morning session up to 6hrs is 5% cheaper than a night session. The deposit remains the same. A Superior room is booked for 90 minutes one morning, all costs paid up front. How much is paid at the start of the session? (Assume half hours can be booked at half the hourly rate).

A. £97.25 B. £92.75 C. £95.00 D. £90.50 E. £90.25

Question 90:

A Basic room is booked for 18hrs each day for three full weeks. What is the total cost of this excluding VAT and deposit?

A. £1,935.36 B. £2,419.20 C. £2,459.52 D. £3,024.00 E. £3,074.40

SET 20

A group of 180 people took part in a perception study and were asked to count how many differences they could spot between two similar pieces of short video footage. The results are given below

		Age (years)					
		10 to 16	16 to 22	22 to 34	34 to 48	48 to 65	65+
Differences correctly spotted	<5	9	10	10	16	15	19
	5 to 10	7	12	9	8	8	5
	11 to 15	11	8	6	2	8	9
	15+	3	2	0	1	2	0

Question 91:

What percentage of people under the age of 22 spotted more than 10 differences?

A. 31.3% B. 33.3% C. 38.7% D. 46.7% E. 63.2%

Question 92:

75% of the results for the people who spotted 5 to 10 differences correctly were removed from the study. What percentage of the remaining people aged 16-22 spotted more than 15 differences?

A. 6.3% B. 6.9% C. 8.5% D. 8.7% E. 9.4%

Question 93:

25% of people who correctly spotted over 10 differences, also *incorrectly* spotted over 10 differences. How many people was this?

A. 11 B. 12 C. 13 D. 14 E. 15

Question 94:

10,000 people aged 48 or older take this test. Using the data, estimate how many spotted fewer than five differences to the nearest 50.

A. 2,300 B. 2,900 C. 4,500 D. 5,100 E. 5,200

Question 95:

The test is repeated with the same population. The number of 16-34 year olds who spot 11-15 differences increases by 50%. All other age groups experience no change. What is the new ratio between 16-34 year olds and the total number of people in the other age groups who spot 11-15 differences?

A. 1:3 B. 4:17 C. 14:44 D. 14:51 E. 21:51

SET 21

The pie chart below shows the favourite sports of some high school students. Every student plays only their favourite sport in games lessons. The school has 1300 students, with an exact 50:50 split between boys and girls.

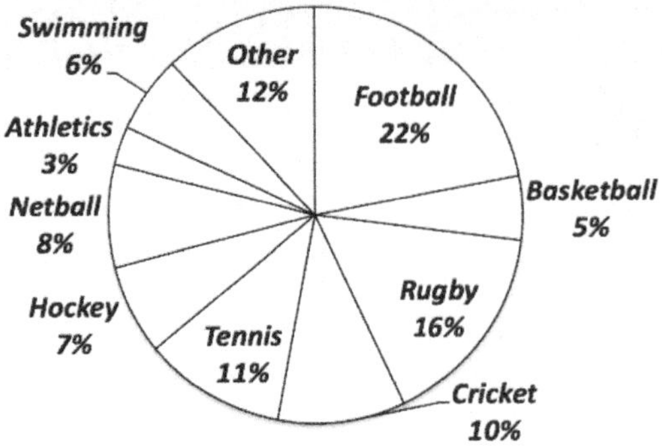

Question 96:

What is the difference between the number of boys that play football and the number that play netball in games lessons?

A. 90 B. 91 C. 104 D. 180 E. 286

Question 97:

The senior football teams are picked from the two most senior years – a total of 350 students. Only those whose favourite sport is football play. At least 11 people are needed per team. What is the maximum number of teams that could be made? Assume that the values given in the chart are representative of these years.

A. 4 B. 5 C. 6 D. 7 E. 8

Question 98:

All those whose favourite sport is basketball are boys and all those whose favourite sport is netball are girls. 80% of the basketball boys are invited to play netball. What proportion of the netball-playing population do they then make?

A. 17% B. 25% C. 33% D. 42% E. 50%

Question 99:

One quarter of students in the *Other* category have a favourite sport which is a ball sport. In the whole school, how many students have a favourite sport which is a ball sport?

A. 39 B. 117 C. 572 D. 1,066 E. 1,183

Question 100:

Only boys play cricket. Only girls play hockey. The gender split for tennis follows that of the school as a whole. How many more boys play cricket or tennis than girls play hockey or tennis?

A. 39 B. 58 C. 59 D. 111 E. 112

SET 22

The number of apples picked by a company per year is given below, along with the quality of the apples. 30% of edible apples are sold as they come. Passable apples and the remaining edible apples are processed into cider. Apples which are No Good are not used for human consumption and are instead discarded for animal food.

	1998	1999	2000	2001	2002	2003
Edible	1,100,547	1,398,663	1,563,327	1,443,599	1,763,870	1,931,784
Passable	2,983,411	2,691,553	3,008,941	2,790,456	2,651,399	2,439,012
No Good	400,001	391,747	398,014	568,440	494,309	571,221

Question 101:

What is the percentage increase in the number of apples used for human consumption from 1998 to 2003?

A. 7% B. 10% C. 22% D. 76% E. 93%

Question 102:

What percentage of all No Good apples was produced in the year most apples could not be used for humans?

A. 11.6% B. 11.8% C. 13.9% D. 19.9% E. 20.2%

Question 103:

2004 saw a three-fold increase on 2003 in the number of No Good apples. The total number of apples fit for consumption remained the same. What was the difference in number between processed and No Good apples in 2004 to the nearest apple?

A. 2,077,598 B. 2,224,675 C. 2,478,954 D. 2,675,133 E. 2,765,131

Question 104:

The next six-year period saw an overall 20% increase on the period 1998-2003 in the total number of edible apples picked. How many were sold as they came between 2004 and 2009?

A. 3,588,698 B. 3,321,646 C. 3,312,644 D. 2,392,465 E. 2,208,430

Question 105:

Generally, 20 apples give 1 litre of cider. Given that 2004 saw the same number of apples fit for human consumption as 2003, roughly how many litres of cider were produced in 2004?

A. 122,000 l B. 189,600 l C. 215,400 l D. 247,100 l E. 988,400 l

SET 23

Jen tracks her daily jogs using an app which gives her data on her performance. It tells her that her average speed is 5 mph.

Conversion factor: 1 mile = 1.6 km.

Question 106:

On wet days, Jen's average speed decreases by 8%. How many kilometres does she cover in 40 minutes?

A. 3.1 km B. 3.3 km C. 4.9 km D. 5.3 km E. 7.4 km

Question 107:

Jen begins training for a marathon (26 miles). She starts off by trying to complete a marathon over the space of four equally long jogs. Estimate how long each jog is. Assume dry conditions.

A. 42 minutes
B. 46 minutes
C. 1 hour 18 minutes
D. 1 hour 25 minutes
E. 1 hour 30 minutes

Question 108:

After starting marathon training, her average speed decreases to her old wet speed; her average wet speed remaining 8% slower than this. Estimate, therefore, how long it would take her to cover 12km in the rain. 1 hour 38 minutes

A. 1 hour 46 minutes
B. 2 hours 17 minutes
C. 2 hours 37 minutes
D. 2 hours 50 minutes

Question 109:

After bringing her average speeds back to their original values, Jen starts a new regime. She goes on four jogs, each being 50% further than the last. Her first jog is 4km long. How long does the final jog take in dry conditions?

A. 1 hour 8 minutes
B. 1 hour 41 minutes
C. 1 hour 50 minutes
D. 2 hours 9 minutes
E. 2 hours 42 minutes

Question 110:

Lots of training later, Jen completes the marathon in a time of 3hrs 42mins on a dry day. What is the percentage increase in Jen's dry average speed during the marathon compared to her original one?

A. 7%
B. 12%
C. 41%
D. 52%
E. 53%

SET 24

The table below gives the prices per person per week for different luxury holiday accommodations with different swimming facilities. Some types of accommodation offer a choice between swimming facilities. Some information is missing. Additional days are charged at 1/7 of the weekly cost.

	Studio	Apartment	Villa	Palazzo
No pool	£50.00	£70.00	£95.00	£155.00
Shared pool	£60.00	£80.00	-	-
Private pool	-	£100.00	-	£325.00
Beachfront	-	-	£220.00	£480.00

Question 111:

Villas are available with a private pool, and currently they are on sale: 20% off the standard price, where the standard price sits halfway between that of an apartment with a private pool and a palazzo with a private pool. How much would this cost for two people for one week?

A. £323
B. £332
C. £340
D. £415
E. £664

Question 112:

A group of twelve rents out a beachfront palazzo for four weeks. A booking fee is required from each member of the group, in this case charged at 10% of the weekly cost per person. What is the total cost of the booking?

A. £23,040
B. £23,161
C. £23,616
D. £25,344
E. £25,614

Question 113:

A couple rents an apartment with a shared pool for 20 days. The total cost is £492.89. How much is the booking fee?

A. £35.55 B. £35.57 C. £35.75 D. £37.55 E. £37.75

Question 114:

A family of four stays at a beachfront villa for two weeks, with no booking fee. Due to a complaint, they are refunded 20% of the standard charge. How much does the family pay?

A. £1,408 B. £1,760 C. £1,920 D. £2,340 E. £2,620

Question 115:

A company hires three palazzi with private pools for a week for the grand total of £19,500. The booking fee is 10% of the total cost. Assuming each palazzo has the same number of people staying in it, how many people are there in each palazzo?

A. 18 B. 20 C. 22 D. 54 E. 60

SET 25

FastFoodCo is a fast-food take-away that delivers directly to customers' homes. Delivery rates are £3.00 for orders less than £10, £1.50 for orders from £10–15 and free for orders over £15. Below is a selection from their menu (delivery and food prices exclude 20% VAT, which is payable on all orders). VAT is added after delivery and any discounts have been taken into account.

Item	Cost
Green Curry	£3.95
Chicken Curry	£2.95
Noodles	£2.95
Chicken Tikka	£4.95
Vegetarian Curry	£3.95

Question 116:

John orders a green curry, noodles and a vegetarian curry. What is the total price?

A. £16.62 B. £14.82 C. £14.52 D. £12.35

Question 117:

Katy orders 3 noodles, 2 chicken tikkas and a green curry. What is her total price?

A. £22.44 B. £25.67 C. £27.24 D. £29.04

Question 118:

John orders 2 noodles and a vegetarian curry. What is his total price?

A. £15.42 B. £14.24 C. £13.62 D. £12.14

Question 119:

Katy orders a green curry, 3 noodles and a vegetarian curry. What is her total?

A. £21.89 B. £20.10 C. £18.52 D. £18.09

Question 120:
A final 'two for the price of one' offer is applied for noodles. John orders 4 noodles, 2 chicken tikkas and a green curry. What is his total?
A. £18.20 B. £21.33 C. £22.51 D. £23.70

SET 26
The graph below shows the first quarter profits (in GBP) of four suppliers of prescription medicine.

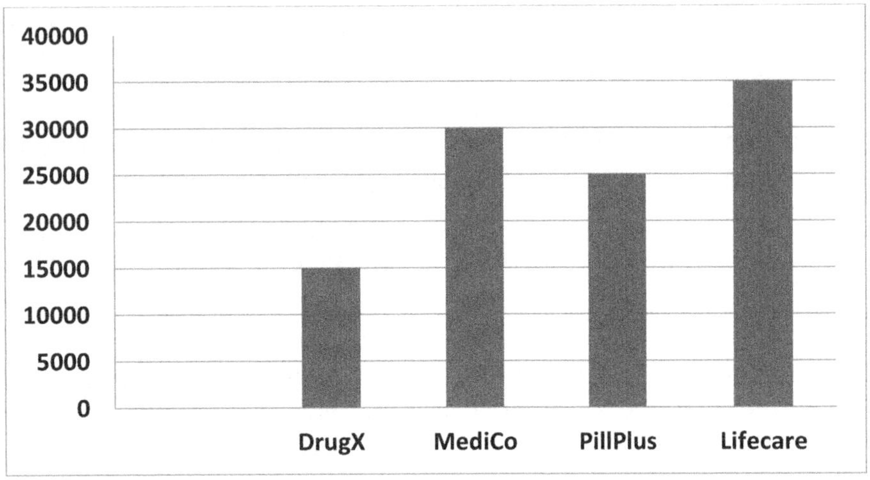

Question 121:
What percentage of total first quarter profits were earned by MediCo?
A. 26.6% B. 28.6% C. 30.4% D. 33.3%

Question 122:
What percentage of the total first quarter profit is from MediCo and Lifecare combined?
A. 56.8% B. 59.5% C. 61.9% D. 62.3%

Question 123:
PillPlus offers a 10% discount on all products in the second quarter. As a result, their sales increase and profit increases by 15%. Assuming that the profits of all other suppliers remain constant into the second quarter, what percentage of the total second quarter profits did PillPlus make?
A. 16.4% B. 23.8% C. 26.4% D. 27.3%

Question 124:
During the third quarter, all profits fall by 10% from second quarter values. Lifecare then buys DrugX. Assume this question follows on from Question 123. What percentage of the third quarter profits was made by Lifecare?
A. 46.0% B. 46.6% C. 47.9% D. 48.2%

Question 125:
Production costs are increased in the fourth quarter, resulting in all profits falling by a further 5%, despite an increase in sales. The information given in question 124 still applies. How much money does Lifecare make in this quarter?
A. £41,800 B. £42,750 C. £43,490 D. £47,002

SET 27

The chart below shows the cost of a variety of cars and optional extras. All prices are excluding 20% VAT, which must be paid by all customers.

Model	Price	Leather Seats	Sound System	Easy-Park Technology
Racer	£15,000	£395	£195	£395
Stuntman	£12,500	£345	£145	£295
Saloon	£21,500	£495	£245	£445
Pod	£18,000	£445	£395	£495

Question 126:

What is the total cost of the Stuntman (with all optional extras)?

A. £15,942 B. £15,904 C. £15,894 D. £15,616

Question 127:

What is the price difference between the Saloon and the Pod (both with all optional extras)?

A. £3,900 B. £4,020 C. £4,040 D. £4,100

Question 128:

What is the difference in price between the Racer (with no optional extras) and the Stuntman (with all optional extras)?

A. £2,040 B. £2,048 C. £2,058 D. £2,142

Question 129:

There is a 10% discount on the Racer and all its optional extras. What is the difference in price between the Pod (with no optional extras) and the Racer (with all optional extras)?

A. £4,236.20 B. £4,285.50 C. £4,336.20 D. £4,438.40

Question 130:

A final offer on the Saloon is 20% off, including all options. What is the difference in final price between the Saloon with Leather seats and Easy-Park technology and the Pod with only basic features?

A. £18.60 B. £37.20 C. £48.30 D. £57.60

SET 28

The graph below shows the total amount of CO_2 (in Tonnes) emitted by the country Aissur in each year from 2000 onwards.

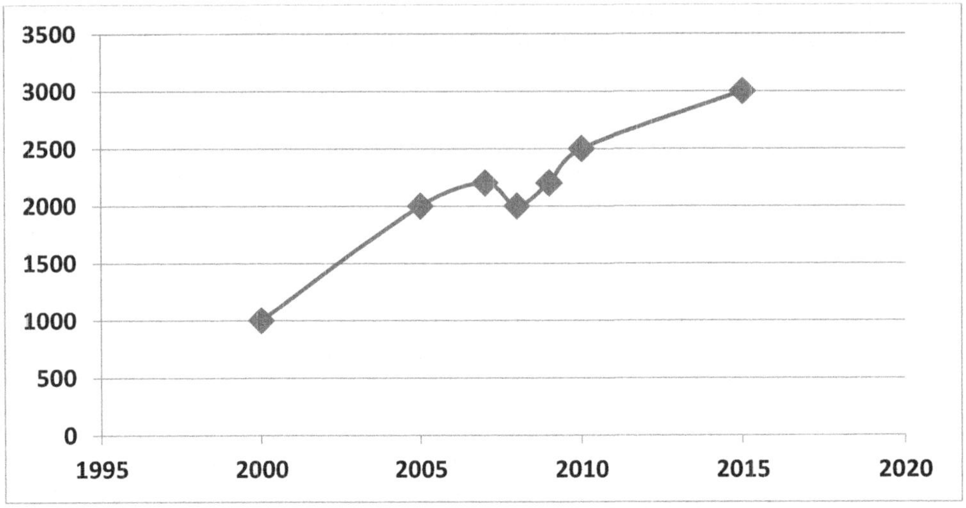

Question 131:

What was the rate of increase of CO_2 emissions between 2000 and 2005?

A. 250 Tonnes/year B. 225 Tonnes/year C. 200 Tonnes/year D. 100 Tonnes/year

Question 132:

The economic crash of 2008 caused global CO_2 emissions to decrease due to a decrease in industrial output. How much less CO_2 was emitted in the year 2010 compared to if emissions had continued to rise at the same rate seen from 2000 to 2005.

A. 500 Tonnes B. 750 Tonnes C. 1,000 Tonnes D. 2,500 Tonnes

Question 133:

What is the percentage increase in CO_2 emissions from 2005 to 2015?

A. 25% B. 33% C. 50% D. 150%

In 2015, the government of Aissur voted on a new energy bill. The bill seeks to reduce the rate of CO_2 increase over the past 5 years by 50% over the next 5 years, and keep the increase at this level thereafter.

Question 134:

If the new energy bill voted on in 2015 is successful in meeting its aims, how much CO_2 will be saved by the end of 2020 relative to the 2010–2015 trend continuing?

A. 200 Tonnes B. 250 Tonnes C. 500 Tonnes D. 750 Tonnes

Question 135:

What will the total CO_2 be in 2020 according to this new act?

A. 2,750 Tonnes B. 3,000 Tonnes C. 3,250 Tonnes D. 3,500 Tonnes

SET 29

The chart below shows the price per item for different styles of printing. The price is lower when larger orders are made, as shown in the table.

Type	1	10+	100+
Single sided black & white	£0.10	£0.07	£0.05
Single sided colour	£0.25	£0.20	£0.15
Double sided black & white	£0.15	£0.12	£0.10
Double sided colour	£0.45	£0.30	£0.25

Question 136:

What is the price per job of 74 single sided black & white sheets?

A. £3.70 B. £5.18 C. £5.24 D. £7.40

Question 137:

How many double-sided colour sheets can you buy for £100?

A. 222 B. 333 C. 400 D. 425

A 10% discount is offered for orders above 50 units, applying to the whole order. All other offers still apply.

Question 138:

What is the price of 150 units of double sided black & white?

A. £13.50 B. £15.50 C. £16.20 D. £20.25

Question 139:

Compared to buying 150 double sided black & white sheets individually, how many sheets worth (at the standard price for 1 sheet) is saved by buying in one transaction at the discounted price?

A. 65 sheets B. 60 sheets C. 53 sheets D. 50 Sheets

Question 140:

What is the total cost of an order of double-sided pages, with 227 requiring black and white printing and 34 requiring colour printing?

A. £22.38 B. £29.61 C. £32.90 D. £34.32

SET 30

4 groups of 300 volunteers take part in a clinical trial for a new drug, which is aimed at reducing the effects of asthma. The responses received are recorded below.

Group	Positive	Negative	No Effect
1	75%	20%	5%
2	65%	30%	5%
3	70%	15%	15%
4	55%	25%	20%

Question 141:
How many people reacted positively overall?
A. 135 B. 265 C. 523 D. 795

Question 142:
How many more people reacted negatively from set 2 compared to set 3?
A. 15 B. 33 C. 45 D. 56

Question 143:
What proportion of those tested overall reacted negatively (to the nearest whole number)?
A. 21% B. 23% C. 26% D. 28%

After modifications to the drug, a new survey of 300 volunteers was taken. The results of this are shown below:

Group	Positive	Negative	No Effect
5	82%	15%	3%

Question 144:
What was the percentage increase in the success rate (i.e. the percentage of people reacting positively) in the 5th group compared to the first 4 groups?
A. 7.81% B. 15.75% C. 17.93% D. 23.77%

Question 145:
Across all groups, including group 5, how many people reacted negatively to the drug?
A. 275 B. 315 C. 355 D. 380

SET 31
The graph below shows the total number of views for two rival local television dramas, The Last Chase and The Final Frontier, across the 4 yearly quarters in 2014.

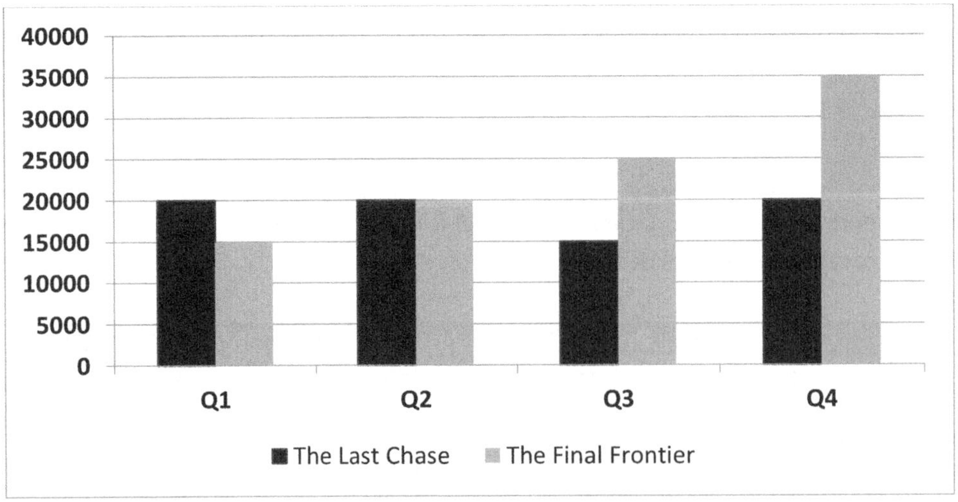

Question 146:
What is the difference between the total number of views of the Final Frontier and The Last Chase during 2014?
A. 10,000 B. 15,000 C. 20,000 D. 25,000

Question 147:
Broadcasters earn £2,500 from advertisements per 1,000 views. What is the difference in money earned through advertising between the two shows in 2014?
A. £45,000 B. £50,000 C. £55,000 D. £60,000

Question 148:
If the number of views of The Final Frontier continues to increase at same rate it did from Q1 – Q3 of 2014, how many views will it have during the final quarter of year 2015?
A. 50,000 B. 55,000 C. 60,000 D. 65,000

Question 149:
If the number of views of The Final Frontier continues to increase at same rate it did from Q1 – Q3 of 2014, how many views will it have in 2015 in total?
A. 180,000 B. 190,000 C. 200,000 D. 250,000

Question 150:
Under different circumstances, at the end of the third quarter of 2014, the broadcasters decide to terminate The Last Chase. As a result, half of The Last Chase's views instead transfer to The Final Frontier. How many views will The Final Frontier have at the end of the final quarter of 2014 under these circumstances?
A. 25,000 B. 35,000 C. 37,500 D. 45,000

SET 32
The table below shows the average time, in minutes, spent waiting for GP appointments by patients, according to a series of surveys from 2014. On average, 20% of patients who wait between 11 and 30 minutes and 40% of those who wait for more than 30 minutes register a complaint during a customer satisfaction survey. No patients who waited for 10 minutes or less registered complaints.

	0-10	11-30	31+	Survey size
England	60%	30%	10%	100,000
Scotland	55%	25%	20%	50,000
Wales	50%	25%	25%	25,000
Northern Ireland	60%	25%	15%	25,000

Question 151:
How many patients waited for a half an hour or less for an appointment in Scotland?
A. 12,500 B. 27,500 C. 40,000 D. 45,000

Question 152:
What percentage of patients across the UK waited for more than half an hour for an appointment?
A. 10% B. 15% C. 20% D. 25%

Question 153:
How many complaints are received from this survey at the end of the year?
A. 20,250 B. 21,500 C. 23,000 D. 24,250

Question 154:
What proportion of patients complained about waiting times by the end of the 2014 survey?
A. 12.1% B. 11.5% C. 11.0% D. 10.7%

Question 155:
In January 2015, the government announced a target to reduce the number of patients waiting for longer than 30 minutes for an appointment by 50%, and by 25% for those waiting between 11-30 minutes. Proportionally, what will be the decrease in the number of complaints recorded by an identical survey at the end of 2015, if all targets are met?
A. 40% B. 38% C. 36% D. 34%

SET 33
The graph below shows the price of crude oil in US Dollars during 2014:

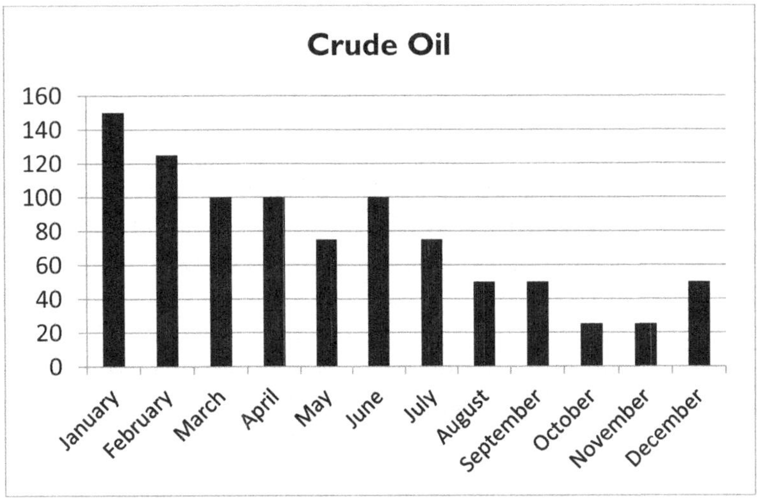

The total oil production, in millions of barrels per day, is shown on the graph below:

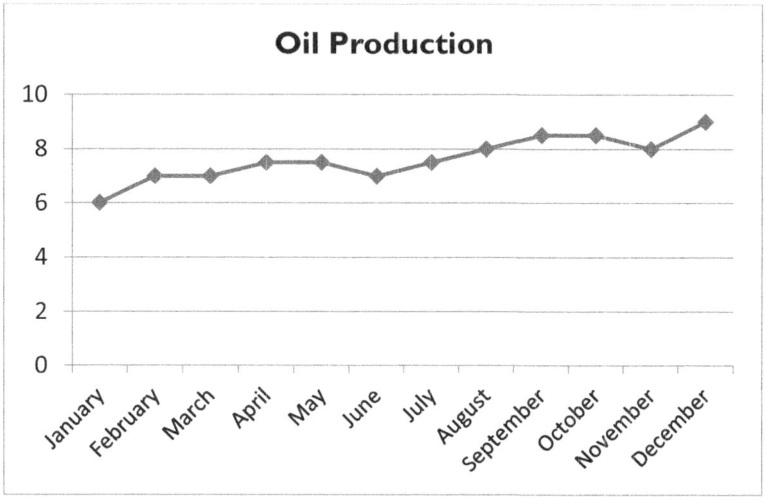

Question 156:
At what rate did the price of oil fall between January and March of 2014?
A. $16.70 per month
B. $20.00 per month
C. $22.70 per month
D. $25.00 per month

Question 157:
What was approximate total oil production in 2014?
A. 1,750 million barrels
B. 2,146 million barrels
C. 2,300 million barrels
D. 2,700 million barrels

Question 158:
How much did oil sales total in July 2014? Assume that all that is produced is sold.
A. $0.56 billion
B. $16.9 billion
C. $17.4 billion
D. $21.1 billion

Question 159:
On average, the price of extraction and production of oil makes up 40% of the total price. The rest of the price is profit. How much profit was made from oil sales during June 2014? Assume that all that is produced is sold.
A. $8.4 billion
B. $12.6 billion
C. $13.0 billion
D. $21.0 billion

Question 160:
Profit from oil extraction is 60% of the total sale price. This profit is split between the oil companies and nation producing the oil in a ratio of 5:2. Of the oil company profits, 30% are used for corporation tax in the companies' home countries. Given that the overall sales value was $204 billion over the year, how much corporation tax was paid in 2014 (to 2 decimal places).
A. $26.23 billion
B. $36.74 billion
C. $43.71 billion
D. $67.57 billion

SET 34

The chart below shows the severity of asthma amongst a sample of 5 groups of 50 people of different ages. The average cost of asthma inhalers per patient is £50 per year. The population of the United Kingdom averaged 50 million during the period of interest. Children aged 0-5 years made up 7% of the population and children aged 5-10 years made up 10% of the population.

Children below the age of 10 who suffer from mild asthma have a half chance of developing respiratory problems in adult life. This figure is 90% for children below the age of 10 who suffer severe asthma. Children without asthma will not develop respiratory problems.

A review into doctors' practices concluded that between 1990 and 1995, 35% of mild asthma diagnoses of children between 0-10 were incorrect.

Age	No Asthma	Mild	Severe
0-5	80%	15%	5%
5-10	75%	20%	5%
10-21	85%	12%	3%
21-30	95%	3%	2%
30+	95%	4%	1%

Question 161:

How many people surveyed suffer from asthma?

A. 25 B. 35 C. 45 D. 55

Question 162:

What is the proportion of children (aged 0–10) surveyed who are likely to develop respiratory problems?

A. 13.00% B. 13.25% C. 13.50% D. 14.25%

Question 163:

How many 0-10 year olds from the survey have been incorrectly diagnosed with asthma?

A. 6.1% B. 6.9% C. 7.4% D. 8.0%

Question 164:

What proportion of children below the age of 10 who were correctly diagnosed with asthma will develop respiratory problems?

A. 9% B. 10% C. 11% D. 12%

Question 165:

How much money was wasted on mistakenly prescribing medication to children who were wrongly diagnosed with asthma from 1990 to 1995?

A. £133 million B. £157 million C. £187 million D. £255 million

SET 35

The following table shows data related to equity shares issued by five public sector companies on 1 March 2015.

Company	Number of equity shares (million)	Current market price Per share (£)	Percentage of equity share held by UK government
A	10	60	75%
B	20	50	50%
C	30	40	33.33%
D	40	30	25%
E	50	20	12.5%

Question 166:

If the government disinvested 50% of its stake in A at current market price, what (in £) is the amount of revenue generated by the government through the disinvestment?

A. 375 million B. 325 million C. 275 million D. 225 million

Question 167:

If the government disinvested 25% of its stake in B at current market price, what (in £) is the amount of revenue generated by the government through the disinvestment?

A. 125 million B. 150 million C. 175 million D. 200 million

Question 168:

The government disinvested its entire stake in C at a price of £35 per share. What would have been the additional revenue generated by the government had it done the given disinvestment at the given market price?

A. £25 million B. £50 million C. £75 million D. £100 million

Question 169:

If the share price of D fell to £25 on 2 March 2015, then what was the decline in the total value of D's shares held by the government from that of the previous day?

A. £25 million B. £50 million C. £75 million D. £100 million

Question 170:

If the share price of E rose to £25 on 2 March 2015, then what was the increase in the total value of E's shares held by the government over that of the previous day (in £)?

A. £30.25 million B. £30.75 million C. £31.25 million D. £31.75 million

Question 171:

Which of the following will fetch higher revenue for government?

A. Redeeming all its stock from company A.
B. Redeeming all its stock from company B.
C. Both of the above will fetch the same value.
D. None of the above.

SET 36

The table below shows the production of some agricultural crops in Harvestland in the years 2011-12 and the targets that were earlier set for that growing season.

Crop	Targeted production For 2011-12 (tonnes)	Actual production for 2011-12 (tonnes)	% Increase in production from 2010-11
Food grains	120	100	25
Oil seeds	60	50	25
Sugarcane	50	40	10
Cotton	40	30	20
Jute	25	20	25

Question 172:

The production of food grain (in tonnes) in 2010-11 was:

A. 40 B. 60 C. 80 D. 100

Question 173:

What was the difference in targeted production in 2011-12 and actual production in 2010-11 for oil seeds (in tonnes)?

A. 10 B. 20 C. 30 D. 40

Question 174:

How much more sugarcane should have been produced in order to meet the target in 2011-12 (in tonnes)?

A. 5 B. 10 C. 15 D. 20

Question 175:

What was the combined production of Cotton and Jute in year 2010-11 (in tonnes)?

A. 11 B. 21 C. 31 D. 41

Question 176:

How much more food grain was produced than oil seeds in 2010-11 (in tonnes)?

A. 10 B. 20 C. 30 D. 40

Question 177:

Cotton constituted what percentage of total crops in year 2011-12?

A. 10 B. 12.5 C. 15 D. 17.5

SET 37

The table given below shows the sales volume of four products A, B, C and D manufactured by a company from January to April in the year 2014.

	January	February	March	April
Product A	9,500	10,250	10,500	11,000
Product B	6,500	7,000	7,250	7,500
Product C	3,500	3,750	4,000	4,250
Product D	2,500	3,100	3,500	4,000

Question 178:

In February, sale of product B constituted what percentage of total sales of all 4 products put together?

A. 26% B. 27% C. 28% D. 29%

Question 179:

Which of the following products recorded maximum percentage increase from March to April?

A. Product A B. Product B C. Product C D. Product D

Question 180:

In May 2014, the sales of product C witnessed an increase of 20% over the previous month. The sales of D were the same as those of C. What was the percentage increase in the sales of D in May relative to April?

A. 22.5% B. 25.0% C. 27.5% D. 30.0%

Question 181:

By what percentage did the combined sales of product A and product C increase from January to April?

A. 17.0% B. 17.1% C. 17.2% D. 17.3%

Question 182:

Assume a different scenario – May 2015 witnessed a 20% growth in sales for products A and B, and a 30% growth in sales for products C and D over April values. What was the total sales value in May for all the products combined?

A. 32,925 B. 33,925 C. 34,925 D. 35,925

Question 183:

Assume a different scenario – May 2015 witnessed a 20% growth in sales of product A and 10% growth in sales for the other 3 products (B, C and D). Sales of A constituted what percentage of total sales in May 2015?

A. 40.25% B. 41.25% C. 42.25% D. 43.24%

SET 38

A courier company uses three modes of transportation for delivering consignments – Road, Rail and Air. The following table shows the percentage distribution of the total number of consignments delivered, the revenue generated and the cost incurred, across the three modes of transportation in 2014.

Mode of transportation	Number of consignments (%)	Revenue (%)	Cost (%)
Rail	30	35	25
Road	45	20	25
Air	25	45	50

Question: 184

In 2012, the profit made by Courier Company was 30% of the total revenue. The company made a profit of £2.5 million. What was the total revenue?

A. £3.6 million B. £7.2 million C. £8.3 million D. £25 million

Question 185:

In 2014, the cost per consignment was the lowest through which method?

A. Rail B. Road C. Air D. Equal between road and rail

Question 186:

In 2014, the cost per consignment through rail was £5 and the revenue per consignment through rail was £20. What was the ratio of the total revenue through rail to the total cost through rail? Assume the number of consignments is equal to that given in the table.

A. 4:1 B. 5:1 C. 6:1 D. 7:1

Question 187:

In 2013, the total costs of the company are £54,000. What is the total cost of air transportation in the year 2013?

A. £13,500 B. £17,000 C. £27,000 D. £32,000

Question 188:

In 2014, if the total number of consignments delivered was 17,145 then what was total number of consignments delivered using rail and road?

A. 11,670 B. 11,974 C. 12,463 D. 12,859

SET 39

The following table provides partial information about the composition of three different alloys – A, B and C. Each of these alloys contains five different elements: Zinc, Tin, Lead, Copper and Nickel (and no other substances). An alloy, Alloy G, the composition of which is not given in the table, contains alloys A, B, C in the ratio 2:1:3. It is also known that in Alloy G, there is Tin, Lead and Copper present in equal quantities.

Alloy	Zinc	Tin	Lead	Copper	Nickel
A	10%	40%			10%
B	25%	15%	50%	5%	5%
C	15%		20%		35%

Question 189:

Find the percentage of Lead in alloy A.

A. 8.33% B. 4.16% C. 2.70% D. 2.08%

Question 190:

Find the percentage of Tin in alloy C.

A. 31.3% B. 15.8% C. 10.6% D. 7.9%

Question 191:

An alloy X contains A, B and C in equal proportion. What is the percentage of Zinc in this alloy?

A. 12.50% B. 16.67% C. 25.00% D. 33.33%

Question 192:

Find the percentage of Tin and Copper combined in alloy C.

A. 15% B. 20% C. 25% D. 30%

Question 193:

Find the percentage of Tin in alloy G.

A. 11.11% B. 21.11% C. 31.11% D. 41.11%

Question 194:

How many elements have exactly the same concentration in Alloy G?

A. One B. Two C. Three D. Four

SET 40

The following table chart represents the number of people in the USA surveyed by CNN-Time in an opinion poll for "***The most influential person of the year 2001***". The number of people surveyed is 11,500.

Response	Percentage
Voted in favour of George Bush	39
Voted in favour of Donald Rumsfield	5
Voted in favour of Robert Guiliani	4
Voted in favour of Bill Clinton	2
Voted in favour of Lady Politicians	17
Non-respondents	33
Total	**100**

Question 195:

How many people voted in favour of Hillary Clinton, who received 60% of total votes polled for lady politicians?

A. 1,173 B. 1,223 C. 1,253 D. 1,273

Question 196:

If everyone who voted in favour of Robert Guiliani is a citizen of New York, then out of all the people surveyed, the number of citizens from New York is:

A. 460 B. 960 C. 1,040 D. Cannot be determined

Question 197:

Out of the respondents, 20% are not US citizens. Given that only US citizens voted for George Bush, determine the percentage of US citizens who voted in favour of Bush.

A. 42.8% B. 45.3% C. 46.6% D. 48.8%

Question 198:

Out of the total people surveyed, 40% are employees of the Federal Government and out of these 10% are in favour of Rumsfield. Find the number of people who are in favour of Rumsfield but are NOT employees of the Federal Government.

A. 105 B. 110 C. 115 D. 120

Question 199:

A mid-year survey has also been done on the same group of people, in which 16% of people were in favour of Bill Clinton. Find the decrease in the number of people who voted in favour of Bill Clinton from mid-year survey to the actual survey.

A. 1,210 B. 1,410 C. 1,610 D. 1,810

Question 200:

A mid-year survey has also been done on the same group of people. In that survey 40% of the people were in favour of Bush. Find the decrease in the number of people who voted in favour of Bush from mid-year survey to the actual survey.

A. 115 B. 230 C. 460 D. 920

SET 41

Shop A sells merchandised mugs and also offers to print flyers at the prices shown below:

Number of flyers	Colour printing	Black and white printing
0-9	20p	5p
10-99	10p	4p
100+	5p	2p

Number of mugs	Basic mug cost per mug	Medium mug cost per mug	Premium mug cost per mug	Cost for logo/picture per mug
0-49	20p	30p	50p	5p
50-99	15p	26p	45p	4p
100-499	10p	20p	34p	3p
500+	7p	10p	20p	2p

Question 201:

Before Christmas, the shop offers an extra 15% discount. Customer A decides to buy 5 premium mugs and 4 basic mugs with a unique picture printed on the basic mugs. How much will this cost?

A. £2.50 B. £2.59 C. £2.76 D. £2.81 E. £2.98

Question 202:

Customer B needs 750 premium mugs, 130 basic mugs and 80 flyers after Christmas. She wants a logo printed on the basic mugs. She wants black and white flyers. To the nearest pound, how much will she have to pay?

A. £160 B. £170 C. £172 D. £388 E. £395

Question 203:

Customer C wants to spend £250. How many medium mugs with a logo can she buy with this money if she also wants to buy 50 colour flyers?

A. 1200 B. 1225 C. 2041 D. 2452 E. 2500

Question 204:

The price of extra logo printed on the mug decreased by 1p, the price of premium mug decreased by 2p and the price of colour flyer decreased by 1p across all quantities in 2015. In percentage terms, how much cheaper would have been to order 70 medium mugs with logo and 150 colour flyers in 2015 instead of 2014?

A. 4% B. 5% C. 7% D. 8% E. 11%

Question 205:

The shop made a profit of £325,750 in 2015. This was a compound average growth rate of 1.2% between 2012 and 2015. What was the profit in 2012?

A. £188,513
B. £231,862
C. £314,299
D. £318,071
E. £362,059

SET 42

In St. Mary College, all students must have at least one device to interact with digital, interactive study materials. There are thirty students who have all three gadgets: smartphone, tablet and laptop.

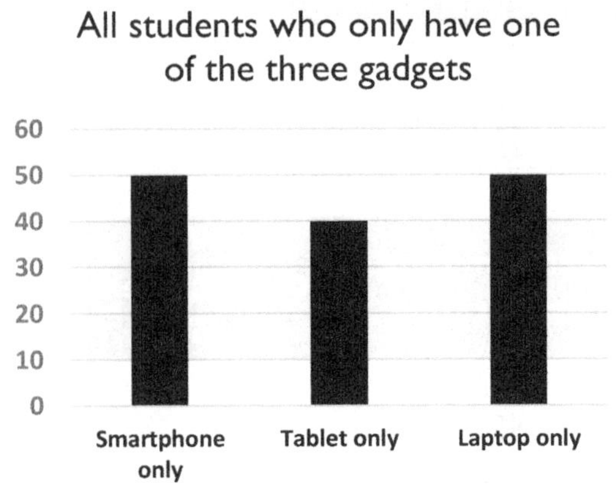

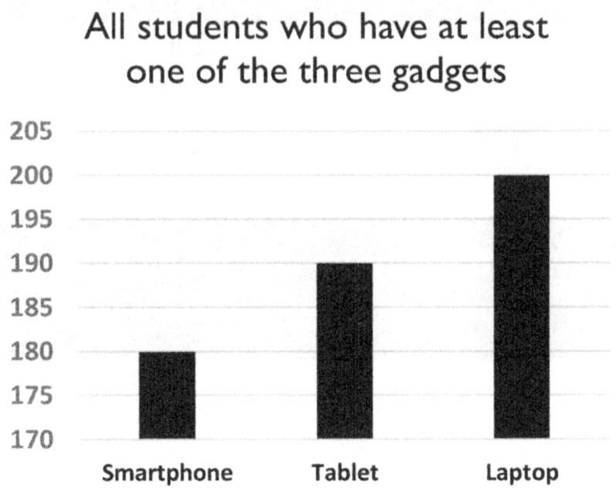

Question 206:

How many students are studying at St. Mary College in total?

A. 325 B. 340 C. 345 D. 350 E. 360

Question 207:

How many students have both a tablet and smartphone but no laptop?

A. 40 B. 45 C. 50 D. 55 E. 65

Question 208:

How many more students have a smartphone, than both a tablet and laptop?

A. 80 B. 85 C. 95 D. 100 E. 80

Question 209:

What percentage of all students have both a smartphone and a laptop?

A. 20.5% B. 23.1% C. 23.5% D. 25.4% E. 25.9%

Question 210:

Five more students come to St. Mary College. Three of the students have both a smartphone and a tablet. Two of the students have a smartphone only. What percentage of all students in the college have a smartphone now?

A. 34% B. 45% C. 54% D. 55% E. 60%

SET 43

Train Timetable [Cambridge to London Liverpool Street]

Cambridge	6.45	7.00	7.10	Then every 20 minutes	23.10
Whittlesford Parkway	7.25	7.40	7.50	Then every 20 minutes	23.50
Audley End	7.35	7.50	8.00	Then every 20 minutes	00.00
Bishops Stortford	7.42	7.57	8.07	Then every 20 minutes	00.07
Sawbridgeworth	7.53	8.08	8.18	Then every 20 minutes	00.18
Tottenham Hale	8.03	8.18	8.28	Then every 20 minutes	00.28
Liverpool Street	8.14	8.29	8.39	Then every 20 minutes	00.39

Question 211:

How many trains leave from Cambridge Station going to Liverpool Street between 2pm and 6.15pm?

A. 10 B. 12 C. 15 D. 18 E. 20

Question 212:

At 2.45pm, Antonia is at Sawbridgeworth station waiting for the next train to London Liverpool Street. What is the earliest time can she expect to arrive at Liverpool Street?

A. 3.01pm B. 3.09pm C. 3.19pm D. 3.31pm E. 3.51pm

Question 213:

How many trains run from Cambridge Station to Liverpool Street all day?

A. 46 B. 47 C. 50 D. 51 E. 56

Question 214:

It is 3pm and Mark wants to take the next train from Cambridge Station to Tottenham Hale for a 1-hour meeting straight at the station. What is the earliest time that Mark could schedule the meeting?

A. 4.25pm B. 4.28pm C. 4.45pm D. 4.55pm E. 5.02pm

Question 215:

If the distance between Audley End and Bishops Stortford is 10.5 miles. What is the speed of the train?

A. 60 miles/hour
B. 70 miles/hour
C. 80 miles/hour
D. 90 miles/hour
E. 100 miles/hour

SET 44

The list of the longest rivers in the UK by length in 2014.

River	Length (miles)	Drainage Area (square mile)	Average Discharge (m^3/s)
River Severn	220	4,409	61.17
River Thames	215	4,994	65.8
River Trent	185	4,029	84
River Great Ouse	143	3,236	15.7
River Wye	134	1,597	3.4
River Ure	129	560	2.4
River Tay	117	431	2.3

Question 216:

What is the total length of the five longest rivers in the UK?

A. 897 B. 905 C. 1026 D. 1143 E. 1234

Question 217:

In 2015, the drainage area of the River Thames increased by 1345.5 square miles. In percentage terms, how much did the drainage area of the seven longest rivers in England increase in 2015 if the other rivers the same?

A. 2% B. 7% C. 17% D. 93% E. 97%

Question 218:

In percentage terms, how much bigger was the drainage area of the River Thames than the River Wye in 2014?

A. 213% B. 276% C. 313% D. 345% E. 425%

Question 219:

What was the difference in length between the two rivers with the highest and lowest average discharge?

A. 68 miles B. 91 miles C. 117 miles D. 185 miles E. 213 miles

Question 220:

What was the average drainage area of the six longest rivers in England in 2014?

A. 2750 B. 3138 C. 3210 D. 3455 E. 4235

SET 45

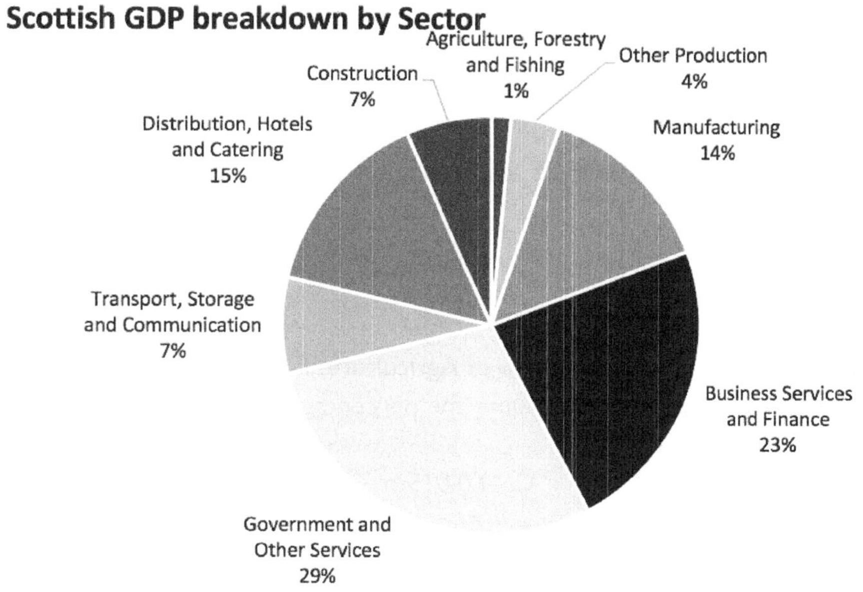

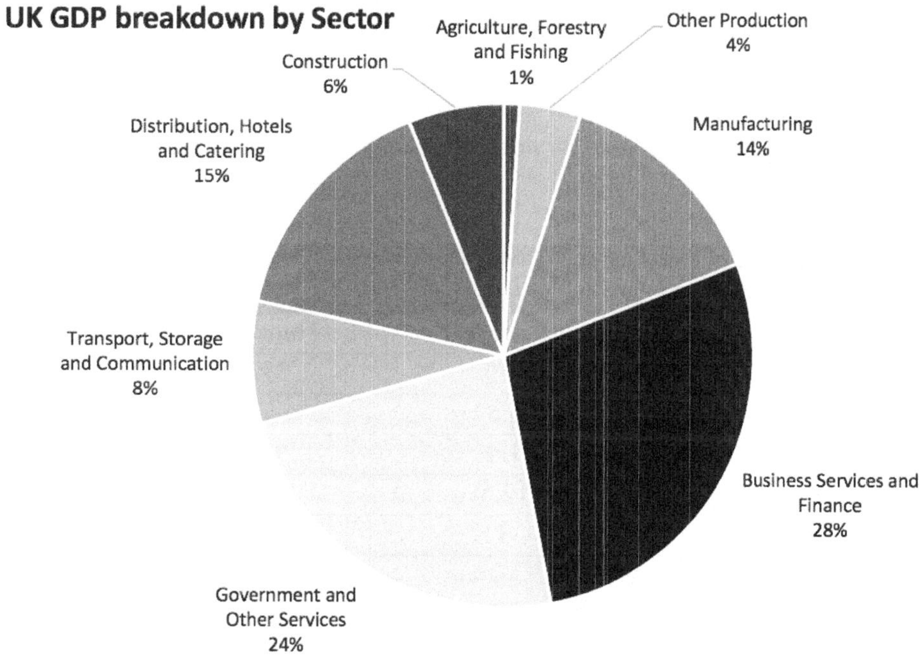

Question 221:

Which industry has the largest contribution to Scottish GDP?

A. Agriculture, Forestry and Fishing
B. Construction
C. Government and Other Services
D. Manufacturing
E. Other Production

Question 222:
In 2015, UK GDP increased by 5% overall to 4.2tn pounds. How much was the UK GDP in 2014?

A. 3.9tn B. 4.0tn C. 4.1tn D. 4.2tn E. 4.4tn

Question 223:
How much bigger is the contribution of Business Services and Finance to total UK GDP than the contribution of Manufacturing to Scottish GDP?

A. 3% B. 4% C. 5% D. 7% E. 14%

Question 224:
Scottish GDP was £1.2tn in 2014. What is the share of Agriculture, Forestry and Fishing in Scottish GDP in 2015 if there was an overall increase in GDP by 3%? Assume the percentage share of GDP for Agriculture, Forestry and Fishing does not change from 2014 to 2015.

A. £0.007tn B. £0.012tn C. £0.015tn D. £0.022tn E. £1.11tn

Question 225:
What are the top three contributing sectors to UK GDP?

A. Agriculture, Forestry and Fishing; Manufacturing; Construction
B. Government and Other Services; Manufacturing; Construction
C. Business Services and Finance; Government and Other Services; Manufacturing
D. Distribution, Hotels and Catering; Business Services and Finance; Government and Other Services
E. Distribution, Hotels and Catering; Business Services and Finance; Manufacturing

SET 46

Top-5 TV Shows	Viewers (millions)		% people watching show in Year 2	
	Year 1	Year 2	Females	Males
The Voice	3.4	4.1	5%	2%
Britain's Got Talent	5.2	5.6	4.5%	4%
Big Brother	1.3	1.4	9%	15%
Geordie shore	9.2	12.5	21%	19%
Fresh Meat	5	3	19%	5%

Question 226:
In percentage terms, how much did the most-watched TV show increase in the number of viewers between year 1 and year 2?

A. 29% B. 33% C. 36% D. 41% E. 42%

Question 227:
How many more viewers did The Voice and Britain's Got Talent have together in year 2 than in year 1?

A. 0.1 million B. 0.2 million C. 0.5 million D. 0.7 million E. 1.1 million

Question 228

Which is the least-watched TV show by males in year 2?

A. Big Brother
C. The Voice
E. Can't tell
B. Fresh Meat
D. Britain's Got Talent

Question 229:

In percentage terms, what was the total increase in the number of viewers across all TV shows from year 1 to year 2?

A. 5% B. 10% C. 15% D. 20% E. 25%

Question 230:

If the total population of females in year 2 was 30 million, how many males watched Geordie Shore in year 2?

A. 1.75 million
C. 2.9 million
E. 6.3 million
B. 2.38 million
D. 6.2 million

SET 47

Mobile Phone Plans

	Basic Plan Charges		**Premium Plan Charges**	
	Included minutes	**Cost per additional minute**	**Included minutes**	**Cost per additional minute**
Text Messages	250 free texts	15p per text	500 free texts	22p per text
Standard Calls	50	4p	75	6p
Mobiles (same network)	150	9p	500	15p
Mobiles (other networks)	100	15p	250	25p

Monthly fee for basic and premium plan fees: £45.29 and £47.89 respectively.

Question 231:

Each month, Claire sends 300 text messages and makes 75 mobile calls in the same network, each is one minute on average. Which plan would be cheaper for Claire and by how much per month?

A. Basic plan by £4.90
D. Premium plan by £4.90
B. Basic plan by £5.90
E. Premium plan by £5.90
C. Premium plan by £3.90

Question 232:

Adam wants to spend maximum £60 per month on a mobile plan. Excluding any included minutes, what is the maximum number of additional minutes he can use if he has the premium plan?

A. 105 minutes
C. 201 minutes
E. 283 minutes
B. 145 minutes
D. 245 minutes

Question 233:
All basic plan charges increase by 1p; the basic plan fee remains unchanged. Andrew sends 45 texts and uses 125 minutes in the same network and 325 minutes in other networks on average. How much is he worse off?

A. 0p B. 75p C. £1.55 D. £2.05 E. £2.25

Question 234:
Daisy does not send any text messages ever. She makes 800 minutes of calls in the same network. Which plan would be cheaper for Daisy and by how much?

A. Basic plan by £2.10
B. Premium plan by £5.75
C. Premium plan by £9.33
D. Premium plan by £10.90
E. Premium plan by £11.89

Question 235:
Kevin sends only text messages, 450 per month on average. If there were a 15% price increase in the monthly fee for both basic and premium plans, how much would Kevin save by changing to premium plan now?

A. £23.43 B. £25.01 C. £27.01 D. £27.10 E. £28.91

SET 48

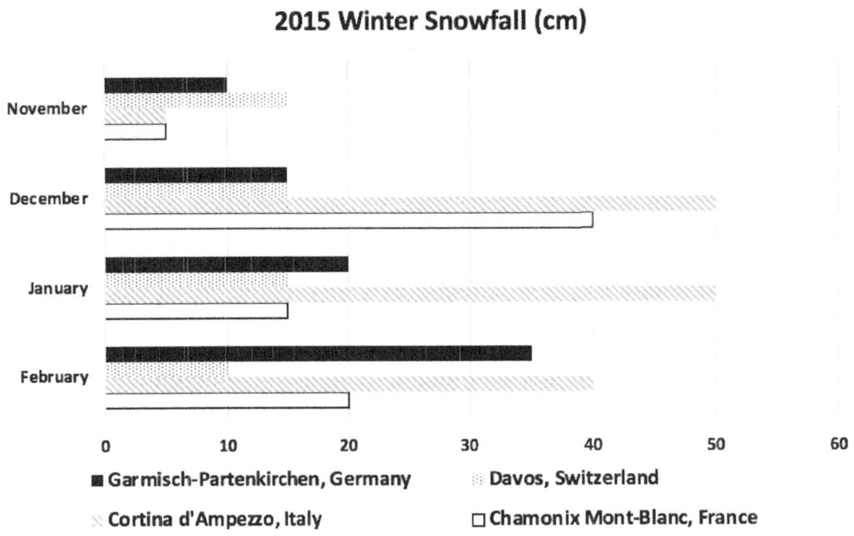

Question 236:
What was the mean monthly snowfall in cm across Davos and Chamonix Mont-Blanc during winter in 2015?

A. 12.325 cm B. 16.875 cm C. 19.738 cm D. 26.842 cm E. 43.123 cm

Question 237:
During Winter 2015, where was the average monthly snowfall the highest?

A. Davos
B. Chamonix Mont-Blanc
C. Cortina d'Ampezzo
D. Garmisch Partenkirchen
E. Can't tell

Question 238:
In percentage terms, how much more snow fell in December than in February overall?

A. 8% B. 12% C. 14% D. 20% E. 22%

Question 239:
In November 2014, 30cm snow fell in the four areas together. In percentage terms, how much more snow fell in November 2015 in the four areas together?

A. 5% B. 17% C. 19% D. 24% E. 29%

Question 240:
How much snow fell in Cortina d' Ampezzo and Garmisch Partenkirchen in November and February together?

A. 20 cm B. 30 cm C. 60 cm D. 90 cm E. 145 cm

SET 49
Please find below Kevin's expenses for December 2015.

Date	Client	Detail of expense	Cost
01.12.15	HSBC	Mileage to and from presentation in Cambridge	£16.80
01.12.15	Soros Fund Management	Single ticket - Train journey to meeting in London	£15.40
13.12.15	HSBC	Breakfast with client	£35.90
16.12.15	Black Rock	Return ticket – Train journey to meeting in London	£20.00
20.12.15	MKB	Lunch with client	£49.50

Mileage paid at £0.25 per mile for the first 100 miles each month and £0.10 thereafter

Question 241:
The greatest proportion of December expenses related to which client?

A. HSBC
B. Soros Fund Management
C. Black Rock
D. MKB
E. Can't Tell

Question 242:
What is the total expense in December?

A. £121.50 B. £137.60 C. £142.45 D. £146.50 E. £210.40

Question 243:
In percentage terms, how much more did Kevin spend on meals than on train tickets?

A. 35% B. 41% C. 59% D. 149% E. 141%

Question 244:
How many miles did Kevin travel by his car in December?

A. 50.5 miles
B. 67.2 miles
C. 67.9 miles
D. 78.4 miles
E. 112.6 miles

Question 245:
The company decides to change its policy from 2016 and only 75% of travel expenses and 90% of accommodation and meal expenses will be reimbursed. How much money would Kevin have lost in December if the new policy had been implemented already in 2015?

A. £8.54 B. £14.22 C. £13.05 D. £21.59 E. £39.15

SET 50

The table below shows the cost of jet ski renting. There are four different jet skis: Alpha, Beta, Gamma and Delta. The deposit is non-refundable.

Type	Deposit	Cost per hour	Total cost for first hour
Alpha	---	£30	£50
Beta	£20	£90	£110
Gamma	£25	£115	£140
Delta	£100	£150	£250

Question 246:

How much is the deposit for Alpha jet ski?

A. £20 B. £30 C. £40 D. £50 E. £60

Question 247:

What is the difference between the total cost of renting a Beta and a Gamma jet ski for 6 hours each?

A. £150 B. £155 C. £200 D. £205 E. £215

Question 248:

Aron has £500 for jet ski renting. Which jet skis can he afford to rent for an hour?

A. Alpha only
B. Alpha and Beta and Gamma
C. Alpha and Beta and Gamma and Delta
D. Beta only
E. Gamma only

Question 249:

Andrew and Thomas want to rent Alpha and Gamma jet ski for three hours. How much will they pay in total?

A. £360 B. £480 C. £660 D. £690 E. £960

Question 250:

If the deposit for Delta jet ski is increased by 5% on Sundays, what will be the total cost of renting a Delta jet ski for 8 hours on a Sunday?

A. £990 B. £1200 C. £1305 D. £1605 E. £1900

SET 51

Flight tickets to various regions from the UK

	In The Air	Good Fly	Take Me There	Around the World
North America	250£	290£	560$	360 €
South America	190£	275£	370$	300 €
Europe	80£	100£	210$	110 €
East Asia	290£	280£	570$	400 €
Australia	290£	300£	610$	450 €

Assumed exchange rate is 1£ = 2$ = 1.5€

Question 251:

What is the price of the cheapest offer to East Asia in pounds (£)?

A. £238 B. £252 C. £267 D. £276 E. £280

Question 252:

On average how much more expensive is it to choose a non-European destination with Good Fly than to choose a European one (rounded up to one digit)?

A. £185.2 B. £186.3 C. £186.9 D. £189.8 E. £191.0

Question 253:

Take Me There decides to offer a 50$ discount on every travel to the Americas. In percentages, how much more expensive is the discounted ticket to North America than the original price offered by In The Air?

A. 2% B. 4% C. 5% D. 7% E. 11%

Question 254:

Around The World only sells 10 tickets to Australia and 5 tickets to South America. Good Fly only sells 25 tickets to Europe and 12 tickets to Australia.

Rounded to two decimals, what is the difference between the total revenues of these two companies, in percentage of the higher revenue?

A. 33.33% B. 34.86% C. 34.43% D. 35.35% E. 36.36%

Question 255:

The £ to $ exchange rate changes in a way that £1 = $2.5. In pounds, what is the difference between the original and the new ticket price of Take Me There to Australia?

A. £55 B. £58 C. £61 D. £64 E. £75

SET 52

Indian GDP

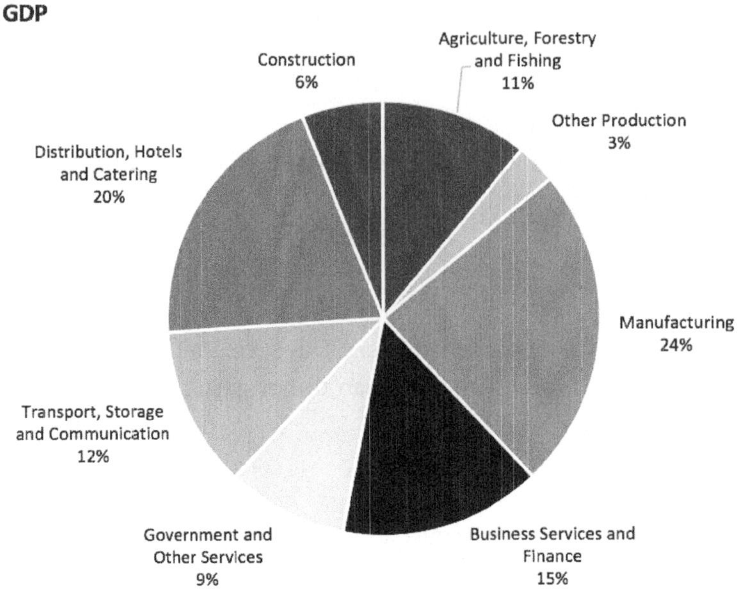

UK GDP

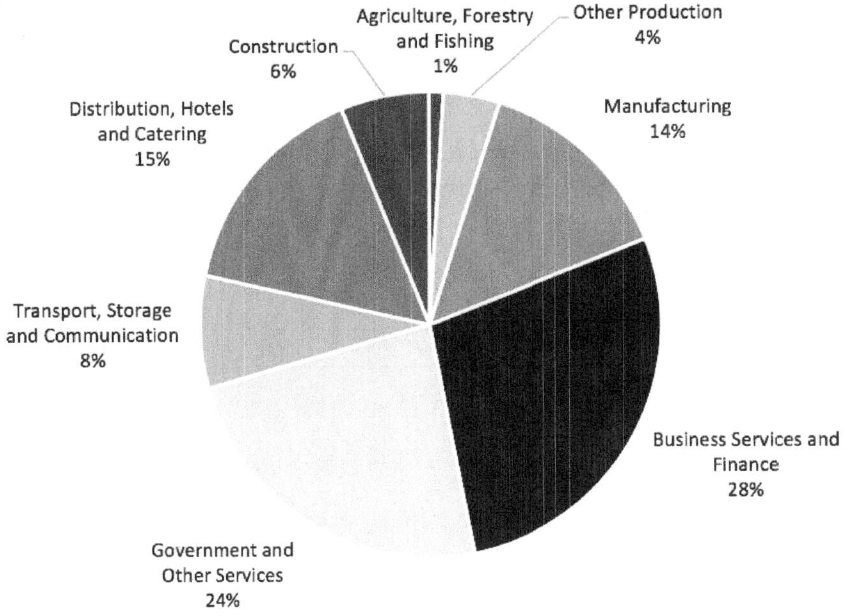

Question 256:

Which industry has the largest contribution to Indian GDP?

A. Agriculture, Forestry and Fishing
B. Construction
C. Government and Other Services
D. Manufacturing
E. Other Production

Question 257:

Expressing 'Government and Other Services' as a percentage of 'Business Services and Finance', what is the difference between these ratios in India and the UK?

A. 10%
B. 12%
C. 26%
D. 34%
E. 67%

Question 258:

What are the top three contributing sectors to Indian GDP?

A. Business Services Finance; Distribution, Hotels and Catering; Manufacturing
B. Agriculture, Forestry and Fishing; Business Services Finance; Manufacturing
C. Distribution, Hotels and Catering; Government and Other Services; Business Services and Finance
D. Construction; Manufacturing; Transportation, Storage and Communication
E. Distribution, Hotels and Catering

Question 259:

If the Indian GDP was £2 trillion and the UK GDP was £4.2 trillion in 2014. How much more did the bottom two performing sectors contribute to the UK GDP than to the Indian GDP?

A. £10 Billion B. £15 Billion C. £21 Billion D. £30 Billion E. £40 Billion

Question 260:

If the Indian GDP was £2 trillion and the UK GDP was £4.2 trillion in 2014. In monetary terms which sector was the largest?

A. Business Services and Finance in the India with £400 Billion
B. Business Services and Finance in the UK with £400 Billion
C. Manufacturing in India with £1.176 trillion
D. Business Services and Finance in the UK with £1.176 trillion
E. Business Services and Finance in the UK with £2 trillion

SET 53

The table below shows the average value of 1 Japanese Yen (JPY).

	2010	2011	2012	2013
GBP	0.021	0.020	0.019	0.022
USD	0.010	0.013	0.013	0.015
EUR	0.015	0.016	0.015	0.015
CAD	0.123	0.115	0.119	0.125

Question 261:

How much USD could you get for 1500 Yen in 2011?

A. USD 19.50 B. USD 21.00 C. USD 21.90 D. USD 25.50 E. USD 100.50

Question 262:

What was the GBP/USD average exchange rate in 2013 based on the information available?

A. 0.85 B. 0.92 C. 1.26 D. 1.47 E. 1.54

Question 263:

In percentage terms, what was the increase in JPY/CAD exchange rate between 2011 and 2012?

A. 3.5% B. 3.9% C. 4.5% D. 5.1% E. 11.5%

Question 264:

How much more JPY would I have received for USD 1300 in 2010 than in 2013?

A. JPY 43,333
B. JPY 45,000
C. JPY 45,225
D. JPY 46,310
E. JPY 47,450

Question 265:

Which exchange rate has been the least volatile between 2010 and 2013?

A. CAD
B. USD
C. EUR
D. JPY
E. GBP

SET 54

The table below shows changes in car use and population in four American cities between 2009 and 2014.

		Boston	Chicago	Denver	El Monte
2009	**Population**	4 million	3.5 million	2 million	0.8 million
	Number of cars	235,675	345,526	231,456	54,000
2014	**Population**	4.4 million	3.3 million	2.1 million	1.5 million
	Number of cars	542,000	350,685	249,990	62,044

Question 266:

In which city was the population growth the largest between 2009 and 2014?

A. Boston
B. Chicago
C. Denver
D. El Monte

Question 267:

In which city was the growth in the number of cars used the largest between 2009 and 2014?

A. Boston
B. Chicago
C. Denver
D. El Monte

Question 268:

In which city was the number of cars per person the lowest in 2014?

A. Boston
B. Chicago
C. Denver
D. El Monte

Question 269:

In which city was the change in the number of cars per person the largest between 2009 and 2014?

A. Boston
B. Chicago
C. Denver
D. El Monte

Question 270:

What is the difference between the number of cars per person in 2009 and 2014 in Boston?

A. 0.0064
B. 0.035
C. 0.054
D. 0.064

SET 55

The table shows the change in tax rates and bands from tax year 2014-15 to 2015-16.
A family is made up of Adam, Lewis, Courtney and Bruno.

Income Tax Bands	2014-15 Rate	2015-16 Rate	2014-15 (GBP)	2015-16 (GBP)
Starting rate	15%	10%	≤ 2,450	≤ 2,730
Basic rate	25%	25%	2,450 < to ≥33,500	2,731 < to ≥ 37,000
Higher rate	40%	40%	33,500 <	37,000 <

Question 271:
Adam earned £37,000 in 2014-15. How much income was deducted from his salary during that year?

A. £4560
B. £6730
C. £8129.50
D. £9110.75
E. £9530

Question 272:
Bruno and Lewis each have a part-time job at a local pub, and each earned £7,000 per year in 2014-15. What is the difference between their annual incomes after income tax has been deducted?

A. £0
B. £50
C. £176
D. £450
E. £745

Question 273:
Courtney received £42,000 in the tax year 2014-15. What was her average monthly income tax deduction?

A. £878.98
B. £898.98
C. £910.15
D. £960.83
E. £1024.58

Question 274:
Adam earned a performance bonus of £4,000 in 2014-15, increasing his salary from £37,000 to £41.000. By how much did his income tax change from what it would have been for this year without the performance bonus?

A. £1200
B. £1600
C. £1800
D. £2100
E. £3400

Question 275:
How much did the starting rate upper bound change from 2014-15 to 2015-16?

A. £80 decrease
B. £150 decrease
C. £280 decrease
D. £150 increase
E. £280 increase

SET 56

The table below shows the annual summary for performance evaluation of four partners at a management consulting firm. The bonus earned is calculated by multiplying the total sales by the bonus rate.

Partner	Projects Acquired (No.)	Total Sales	Bonus	Customer Satisfaction Rate
Adam	**5**	£45,000,000	**1%**	**97%**
John	**2**	£150,453,000	**5%**	**90%**
Richard	**3**	£180,000,000	**4%**	**75%**
Daniel	**7**	£654,150,000	**10%**	**25%**

Question 276:

Who received the highest bonus?

A. Adam
B. John
C. Richard
D. Daniel
E. Can't Tell

Question 277:

What is the average sales per project generated by Daniel?

A. £83,755,000
B. £93,450,000
C. £96,345,000
D. £99,950,000
E. £100,145,000

Question 278:

How much bonus did Richard and Adam receive together?

A. £5,500,000
B. £6,000,000
C. £6,350,000
D. £7,250,000
E. £7,650,000

Question 279:

Whose customer satisfaction rate was the highest?

A. Adam
B. John
C. Richard
D. Daniel
E. Can't Tell

Question 280:

How much was the total sales generated by the four partners together?

A. £1,029,603,000
B. £1,135,150,000
C. £1,529,540,000
D. £1,529,110,000
E. £2,130,042,000

SET 57

The table below shows the daily share price movements of four UK companies:

Name	Current Share Price (in pence)	Percentage Change from Previous Day	High	Low	Volume
HSBC	25.432	-0.03%	27.000	25.123	7,345,321
BP	286.123	+4.5%	286.456	284.567	4,431,748
GSK	134.432	+0.13%	142.511	131.678	1,125,469
British Land	54.923	+1.11%	54.934	54.914	4,999,432

Market Capitalisation is calculated as: number of shares outstanding (volume) multiplied by share price.

Question 281:

What was the share price of GSK yesterday?

A. £132.873
B. £134.157
C. £134.257
D. £134.345
E. £135.012

Question 282:

What was difference between the daily highest and lowest price of British Land?

A. £0
B. £0.01
C. £0.02
D. £0.025
E. £0.3

Question 283:

What was the market capitalisation of HSBC yesterday assuming that the volume is unchanged?

A. £186,250,178.618
B. £186,350,178.618
C. £186,450,178.618
D. £186,650,178.618
E. £186,862,262.351

Question 284:

Which company's actual share price changed the most from yesterday?

A. HSBC
B. British Land
C. BP
D. GSK
E. Can't Tell

Question 285:

What is the difference between the latest market capitalisation of BP and British Land?

A. 993,441,229.268
B. 993,941,234.268
C. 994,114,112.268
D. 994,241,299.268
E. 1,113,345,891.268

SET 58

The table below is a summary of students who signed up for the following courses at St. Mary Grammar School. Students can take more than one course.

Courses	Women	Men
Psychology	10	6
Maths	8	7
Physics	10	15
Programming	4	5
Literature	12	8
History	7	7

Question 286:

For which course is the ratio of women and men most similar to that of Psychology?

A. Mathematics
B. Physics
C. Programming
D. Literature
E. History

Question 287:

For which course is the ratio of women and men most similar to that of Physics?

A. Mathematics
B. Psychology
C. Programming
D. Literature
E. History

Question 288:

What is the total number of women in St. Mary Grammar School?

A. 34
B. 51
C. 64
D. 145
E. Can't tell

Question 289:

What is the total proportion of women to men?

A. 0.25
B. 0.5
C. 0.96
D. 1
E. Can't tell

Question 290:

If three new students arrive at St. Mary Grammar School and they are all women studying Psychology. What is the change in the ratio of women to men studying Psychology?

A. 0.1
B. 0.3
C. 0.5
D. 0.7
E. 1.2

SET 59

This graph below shows the employment statistics (in percentages) of the men and women living in the UK in September 2015. A person is considered being in employment if they are shown as employed, self-employed, or 'employed other'.

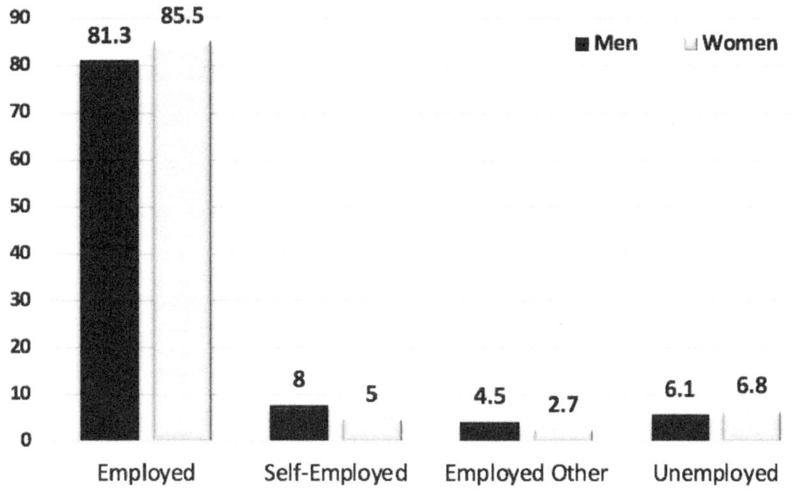

Question 291:

The difference between the percentage of women and men in employment is:

A. 0.6 B. 0.7 C. 1.2 D. 3.2 E. 4.2

Question 292:

The proportion of men to women self-employed or unemployed is:

A. 0.1 B. 0.5 C. 0.9 D. 1.2 E. 1.7

Question 293:

If there are overall 21 million women in employment in the UK how many women are self-employed?

A. 0.59 million
B. 0.86 million
C. 0.93 million
D. 1.07 million
E. 1.13 million

Question 294:

If there are 31 million men and 32 million women living in the UK, how many more women are unemployed than men?

A. 285,000
B. 423,000
C. 659,500
D. 735,000
E. 810,000

Question 295:

What is the proportion of employed to unemployed women in the UK?

A. 2.87 B. 5.43 C. 8.51 D. 13.7 E. 15.9

SET 60

This chart shows the expenses of the Jones household for this month. Overall they spent 360 pounds.

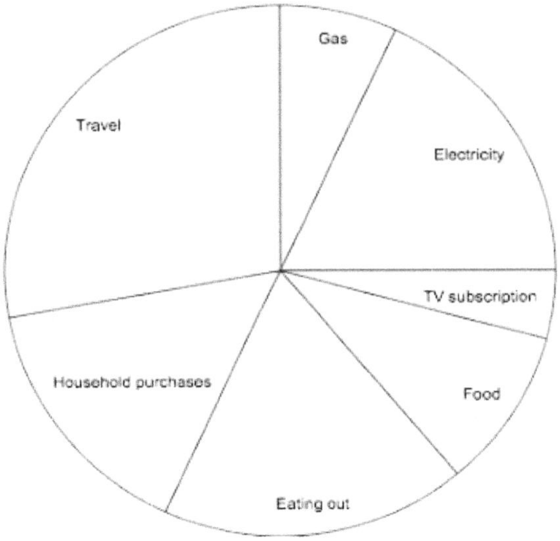

Question 296:

How much was their energy cost (electricity and gas) this month?

A. 65 pounds
B. 85 pounds
C. 90 pounds
D. 155 pounds
E. 200 pounds

Question 297:

What is the ratio of household purchases, travel and gas costs to energy costs (electricity and gas)?

A. 0.5:1
B. 1:1
C. 1.5:1
D. 2:1
E. 3:1

Question 298:

Which cost item was the greatest this month?

A. Gas
B. Travel
C. Electricity
D. Household purchases
E. Energy

Question 299:

If the total cost of household purchases, travel and gas costs was 180 pounds. How much were the energy costs in total this month?

A. 80 pounds
B. 87.5 pounds
C. 89.5 pounds
D. 90 pounds
E. 95 pounds

Question 300:

Which was the smallest cost item this month?

A. Gas
B. Travel
C. Electricity
D. Household purchases
E. TV subscription

FOR THE FOLLOWING QUESTIONS – PAY ATTENTION TO THE INSTRUCTIONS PROVIDED, AND ANSWER EACH QUESTION INDIVIDUALLY.

Questions 301 to 303 are based on the following passage:

It has recently been questioned as to whether the recommended five fruit and vegetables a day is sufficient or if it would be more beneficial to eat 7 fruit and vegetable portions each day. A study at UCL looked at the fruit and vegetables eating habits of 65,000 people in England. Analysis of the data showed that eating more portions was beneficial and vegetables seemed to have a greater protective effect than fruit. The study however did not distinguish whether vegetables themselves have a greater protective effect, or whether these people tend to eat an overall healthier diet. A meta-analysis carried out by researchers across the world complied data from 16 studies which encompassed over 800,000 participants, of whom 56,423 had died.

They found a decline in death of around 5% from all causes for each additional portion of fruit or vegetables eaten, however they recorded no further decline for people who ate over 5 portions. Rates of cardiovascular disease, heart disease or stroke, were shown to decline 4% for each portion up to five, whereas the number of portions of fruit and vegetables eaten seemed to have little impact on cancer rates. The data from these studies points in a similar direction, that eating as much fruit and vegetables a day is preferable, but that five portions is sufficient to have a significant impact on reduction in mortality. Further studies need to look into the slight discrepancies, particularly why the English study found vegetables more protective, and if any specific cancers may be affected by fruit and vegetables even if the general cancer rates more greatly depend on other lifestyle factors.

Question 301:

Which of the following statements is correct?

A. The UCL study found no additional reduction in mortality in those who eat 7 rather than 5 portions of fruit and vegetables a day.
B. People who eat more fruit and vegetables are assumed to have an overall healthier diet which is what gives them the beneficial effect.
C. The meta analysis found fruit and vegetables are more protective against cancer than cardiovascular disease
D. The English study showed fruit had more protective effects than vegetables.
E. The meta-analysis found no additional reduction in mortality in those who eat 7 rather than 5 portions of fruit and vegetables a day.
F. The meta-analysis suggests people who eat 7 portions would have a 10% lower risk of death from any cause than those who eat 5 portions.
G. Fruit and vegetables are not protective against any specific cancers.

Question 302:

If rates of death were found to be 1% lower in the UCL study than the meta-analysis, approximately how many people died in the UCL study?

A. 3,000 B. 3,200 C. 3,900 D. 4,550 E. 5,200

Question 303:

Which statement does the article **MOST** agree with?

A. Eating more fruit and vegetables does not particularly lower the risk of any specific cancers.
B. The UCL research suggests that the guideline should be 7 fruit and vegetables a day for England.
C. The results found by the UCL study and the meta-analysis were contradictory.
D. Many don't eat enough vegetables due to cost and taste.
E. Fruit and vegetables are only protective against cardiovascular disease.
F. The UCL study and meta-analysis use a similar sample of participants.
G. People should aim to eat 7 portions of fruit and vegetables a day.

Questions 304-306 relate to the following table regarding average alcohol consumption in 2010.

Country	Total	Recorded Consumption	Unrecorded consumption	Beer (%)	Wine (%)	Spirits (%)	Other (%)	2020 Consumption Projection
Belarus		14.4	3.2	17.3	5.2	46.6	30.9	17.1
Lithuania	15.4	12.9	2.5		7.8	34.1	11.6	16.2
Andorra	13.8		1.4	34.6		20.1	0	9.1
Grenada	12.5	11.9	0.7	29.3	4.3		0.2	10.4
Czech Republic	13	11.8	1.2	53.5	20.5	26	0	14.1
France	12.2	11.8		18.8	56.4	23.1	1.7	11.6
Russia		11.5	3.6	37.6	11.4	51	0	14.5
Ireland	11.9	11.4	0.5	48.1	26.1	18.7	7.7	10.9

NB: Some data is missing.

Question 304:

Which of the following countries had the highest total beer and wine consumption for 2010?

A. Belarus B. Lithuania C. Ireland D. France E. Andorra

Question 305:

Which country has the greatest difference for spirit consumption in 2010 and 2020 projection, assuming percentages stay the same?

A. Russia B. Belarus C. Lithuania D. Grenada E. Ireland

Question 306:

It was later found that some of the percentages of types of alcohol consumed had been mixed up. If the actual amount of beer consumed by each person in the Czech Republic was on average 4.9L, which country were the percentage figures mixed up with?

A. Lithuania
B. Grenada
C. Russia
D. France
E. Ireland
F. Belarus
G. Andorra

Questions 307-310 are based on the following information:

The table below shows the incidence of 6 different types of cancer in Australia:

	Prostate	Lung	Bowel	Bladder	Breast	Uterus
Men	40,000	25,000	20,000	8,000	1,000	0
Women	0	20,000	18,000	4,000	50,000	9,000

Question 307:

Supposing there are 10 million men and 10 million women in Australia, how many percentage points higher is the incidence of cancer amongst women than amongst men

A. 0.007 % B. 0.07 % C. 0.093 % D. 0.7 % E. 0.93 %

Question 308:

Now suppose there are 11.5 million men and 10 million women in Australia. Assuming all men are equally likely to get each type of cancer and all women are equally likely to get each type of cancer, how many of the types of cancer are you more likely to develop if you are a man than if you are a woman?

A. 1 B. 2 C. 3 D. 4

Question 309:

Suppose that prostate, bladder and breast cancer patients visit hospital 1 time during the first month of 2015 and patients for all other cancers visit hospital 2 times during the first month of 2015. 10% of cancer patients in Australia are in Sydney, and patients in Sydney are not more or less likely to have certain types of cancer than other patients.

How many hospital visits are made by patients in Sydney with these 6 cancers during the first month of 2015?

A. 10,300 B. 18,400 C. 19,500 D. 28,700 E. 195,000 F. 287,000

Question 310:

Which of the graphs correctly represents the combined proportion of men versus women with bladder cancer?

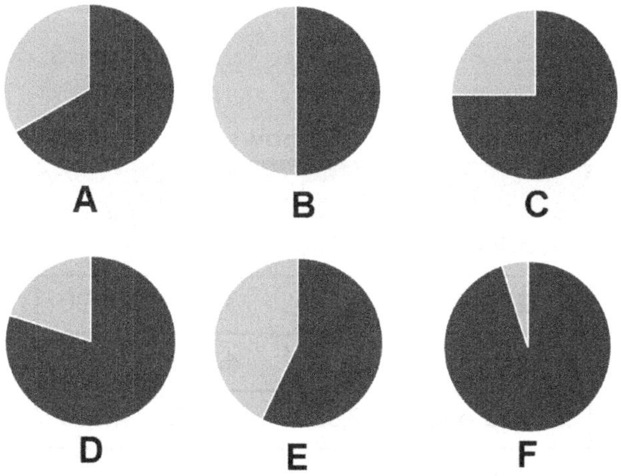

Questions 311 – 313 are based on the following information:

Units of alcohol are calculated by multiplying the alcohol percentage by the volume of liquid in litres, for example a 0.75 L bottle of wine which is 12% alcohol contains 9 units. 1 pint = 570 ml.

	Volume in bottle/barrel	Standard drinks per bottle/barrel	Percentage
Vodka	1250 ml	50	40%
Beer	10 pints	11.4	3%
Cocktail	750 ml	3	8%
Wine	750 ml	3.75	12.5%

Question 311:

Which standard drink has the most units of alcohol in?

A. Vodka B. Beer C. Cocktail D. Wine

Question 312:

Some guidance suggests the recommended maximum number of units of alcohol per week for women is 14. In a week, Hannah drinks 4 standard drinks of wine, 3 standard drinks of beer, 2 standard cocktails and 5 standard vodkas. This guidance states the recommended maximum number of units per week for men is 21. In a week, Mark drinks 2 standard drinks of wine, 6 standard drinks of beer, 3 standard cocktails and 10 standard vodkas.

Who has exceeded their recommended maximum number of units by more and by how many units more have they exceeded it by than the other person?

A. Hannah, by 1 unit
B. Hannah, by 0.5 units
C. Both by the same
D. Mark, by 0.5 units
E. Mark, by 1 unit

Question 313:

How many different combinations of drinks that total 4 units are there (the same combination in a different order doesn't count).

A. 2 B. 3 C. 4 D. 5 E. 6

Questions 314-316 relate to the table below which shows information about Greentown's population:

	Female	Male	Total
Under 20	1,930		
20-39	1,960	3,760	5,720
40-59		4,130	
60 and over	2,350	2,250	4,600
Total	11,430	12,890	24,320

Question 314:

How many males under 20 are there in Greentown?

A. 2,650 B. 2,700 C. 2,730 D. 2,750 E. 2,850

Question 315:

How many females aged 40-59 are there in Greentown?

A. Between 3,000 and 4,000

B. Between 4,000 and 5,000

C. Between 5,000 and 6,000

D. Between 6,000 and 7,000

Question 316:

Which is the approximate ratio of females:males in the age group that has the highest ratio of males:females?

A. 1.4:1 B. 1.9:1 C. 1:1.9 D. 1:1.4

Questions 317-319 relate to the follow graph:

The graph below shows the average temperatures in London (top trace) and Newcastle (bottom trace).

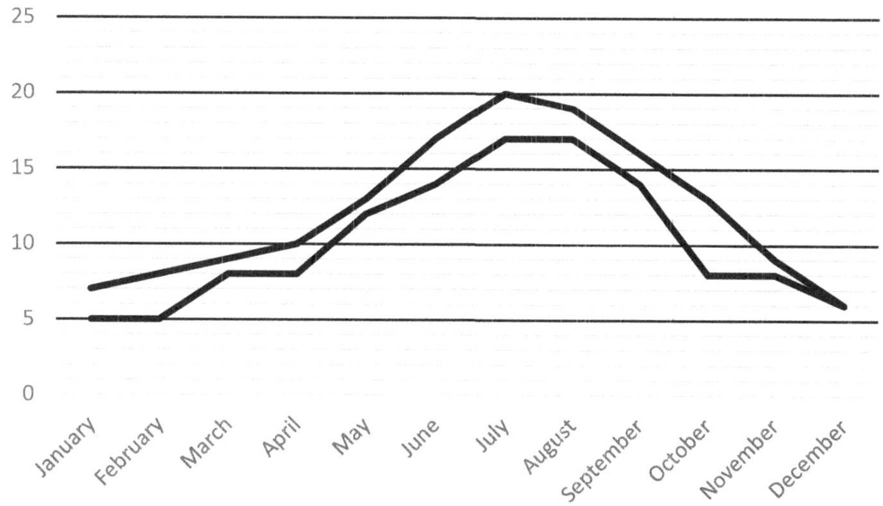

Question 317:

If the average monthly temperature is the same in every year, how many times during the period May 2007 to September 2013 inclusive is the average temperature the same in 2 consecutive months in Newcastle?

A. 20 B. 24 C. 25 D. 30

Question 318:

In how many months in the period specified in the previous question is the average temperature in London AND Newcastle lower than the previous month?

A. 19 B. 21 C. 25 D. 32

Question 319:

To the nearest 0.5 degrees Celcius, what is the average temperature difference between Newcastle and London?

A. 1.5°C B. 2°C C. 2.5 °C D. 3 °C

Questions 320-322 concern the following data:

The pie chart to the right shows sales of ice cream across the four quarters of a year from January to December. Sales are lowest in the month of February. From February they increase in every subsequent month until they get to the maximum sales and from that point they decrease in every subsequent month until the end of the year.

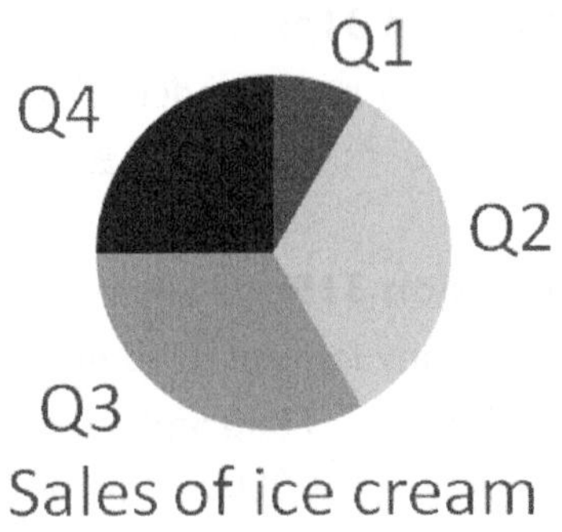

Question 320:

In which month are the sales highest?

A. June B. July C. August D. Cannot tell

Question 321:

If total sales of ice cream were £354,720 for the year, how much of this was taken during Q1?

A. 29,480 B. £29,560 C. £29,650 D. £29,720 E. £29,800

Question 322:

Assuming total sales revenue (i.e. before costs are taken off) is £180,000, and that each tub of ice cream is sold for £2 and costs the manufacturer £1.50 in total production and transportation costs, how much profit is made during Q2?

A. £15,000 B. £30,000 C. £45,000 D. £60,000

Question 323:

Data on the amount families spend on food per month to the nearest £100 was collected for families with 1, 2 and 3 children. The percentage of families with different spending sizes is displayed below:

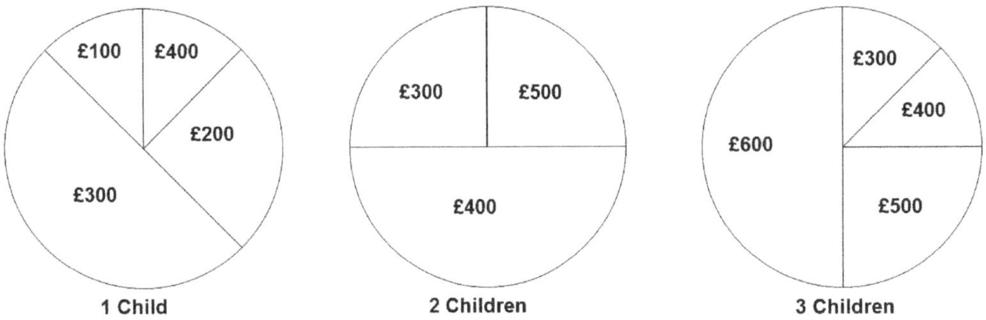

Which of the following statements is definitely true?

A. More families with 1 child than families with 2 children spent £300 a month on food.
B. The overall fraction of families spending £600 was 1/6.
C. All of the families with 2 children spent under £4000 on food per year.
D. The fraction of families with 1 child spending £400 on food per month is the same as the fraction of families with 3 children spending this amount.
E. The average amount spent on food by families with 2 children is £410 a month.

Questions 324-327 are based on the passage below:

A big secondary school recently realised that there were a large number of incidences of bullying occurring that were going unnoticed by teachers. It is possible that some believe bullying to be as much a part of student life as lessons and homework. In order to tackle the problem, the school emailed out a questionnaire to all students' parents and asked them to question their children about where they had experienced or seen bullying in school. Those children that answered yes were then asked if they had told their teachers about it, and asked why they did not if they had not. Those that had told their teacher were asked whether they had seen the teacher act upon the information and whether the bullying had stopped as a result.

Of the 2500 school students surveyed 2210 filled in the online questionnaire. The results were that, 1121 students, almost exactly half (50.7%) had seen bullying in school. Only 396 (35%) of these students told a teacher about the bullying. Of the students who told a teacher, 286 did not witness any action following sharing of the information and of those that did, 60% did not notice any direct action with the bully involved.

From those students who did not report the bullying, 146 gave the reason that they didn't think it was important. 427 cited fears of being found out. 212 students said they did not tell because they didn't think the teachers would do anything about it even if they did know. Assume that all the students who filled out the survey did so honestly.

Question 324:

To the nearest integer, what percentage of students did not respond?

A. 10% B. 12% C. 18% D. 8% E. 5%

Question 325:

If a student saw bullying occur and did not tell a teacher about it, what is the probability that the reasoning for this is that they thought it to be unimportant?

A. 0.1 B. 0.15 C. 0.2 D. 0.35 E. 0.13

Question 326:

After reporting the bullying, how many students saw the teacher act on the information directly with the bully?

A. 66 B. 44 C. 178 D. 104 E. 118

Question 327:

Which of the following does the questionnaire indicate is the best explanation for why students at the school did not report bullying?

A. Students do not think bullying happens at their school.
B. Students think the teachers will do nothing with the information.
C. Students think that bullying is a part of school life.
D. The student's were worried about others finding out.

Question 328:

The obesity epidemic is growing rapidly with reports of a three-fold rise in the period from 2007 to 2012. The rates of hospital admission have also been found to vary massively across different areas of England with the highest rates in the North-East (56 per 100,000 people), and the lowest rates in the East of England (12 per 100,000). During almost every year from 2001-12, there were around twice as many women admitted for obesity as men. The reason for this is however unclear and does not imply there are twice as many obese women as men.

What was the approximate number of admissions per 100 000 women in the North-East in 2011-12?

A. 18 B. 26 C. 37 D. 56 E. 62 F. 74

Question 329:

Health professionals are becoming increasingly worried by the decline in exercise being taken by both children and adults. Around only 40% of adults take the recommended amount of exercise which is 150 minutes per week. As well as falling rates of exercise, a shockingly low number of individuals eat five portions of fruit and vegetables a day. Figures for children aged 5-15 fell to only 16% for boys, and 20% for girls in 2011. Data for adults was only slightly better with 29% of women and 24% of men eating the recommended number of portions.

Using a figure of 8 million children between 5-15 years (equal ratio of girls to boys) in England in 2011, how many more girls than boys ate 5 portions of fruit and vegetables a day?

A. 80,000 B. 120,000 C. 160,000 D. 320,000 E. 640,000

Question 330:

The table below shows the leading causes of death in the UK.

WOMEN			MEN	
Rank	**Cause of Death**	**Number of Deaths**	**Cause of Death**	**Number of Deaths**
1	Dementia and Alzheimer's	31,850	Coronary Heart	37,797
2	Coronary Heart Disease	26,075	Lung Cancer	16,818
3	Stroke	20,706	Dementia and	15,262
4	Flu and Pneumonia	15,361	Lower Respiratory	15,021
5	Lower Respiratory Disease	14,927	Stroke	14,058
6	Lung Cancer	13,619	Flu and Pneumonia	11,426
7	Breast Cancer	10,144	Prostate Cancer	9,726
8	Colon Cancer	6,569	Colon Cancer	7,669
9	Urinary Infections	5,457	Lymphatic Cancer	6,311
10	Heart Failure	5,012	Liver Disease	4,661
	Total	**261,205**	**Total**	**245,585**

Using information from the table only, which of the following statements is correct?

A. More women died from cancers than men.
B. More than 30,000 women died due to respiratory causes.
C. Dementia and Alzheimer's is more common in women than men.
D. No cause of death is of the same ranking for both men and women.

Question 331:

The government has recently released a campaign leaflet saying that last year waiting times in NHS A&E departments decreased 20% compared to the year before. The opposition has criticised this statement, saying that there are several definitions which can be described as "waiting times", and the government's campaign leaflet does not make it clear what they mean by "waiting times in A&E".

The NHS watchdog has recently released the following figures describing different aspects of A&E departments, and the change from last year:

Assessment Criterion	2014	2013
Average time spent before being seen in A&E	1 hour	90 minutes
Average time between dialling 999 and receiving treatment in A&E	2 hours	3 hours
Number of people waiting for over 4 hours in A&E	3200	4000
Number of high-priority cases waiting longer than 1 hour	900	1000
Average waiting time for those seen in under 4 hours	50 minutes	40 minutes

Assuming these figures are correct, which criterion of assessment have the government described as "waiting times in A&E" on their campaign leaflet?

A. Number of people waiting for over 4 hours in A&E.
B. Number of people waiting for under 4 hours in A&E.
C. Number of high-priority cases waiting longer than 1 hour.
D. Average time spent before being seen in A&E.
E. Average time between dialling 999 and receiving treatment in A&E.
F. Average waiting time for those seen in less than 4 hours.

Questions 332– 334 refer to the following information:

The table below shows the final standings at the end of the season, after each team has played all the other teams twice each (once at home, once away). The teams are listed in order of how many points they got during the season. Teams get 3 points for a win, 1 point for a draw and 0 points for a loss. No team got the same number of points as another team. Some of the information in the table is missing.

Team	W	D	L
United	8	1	
Athletic	7		
City	7	2	
Town	1	4	
Rovers		0	9
Rangers		2	8

Question 332:

How many points did Rovers get?

A. 0 B. 3 C. 6 D. 9 E. More information needed.

Question 333:

How many games did Athletic lose?

A. 0 B. 1 C. 2 D. 3 E. More information needed.

Question 334:

How many more points did United get than Rangers?

A. 7 B. 15 C. 23 D. 25 E. More information needed.

Questions 335-337 use information from the graph recording A&E attendances and response times for NHS England from 2004 to 2014. Type 1 departments are major A&E units, type 2&3 are urgent care centres or minor injury units. The old target (2004 – June 2010) was 97.5%; the new target (July 2010 – 2015) is 95%.

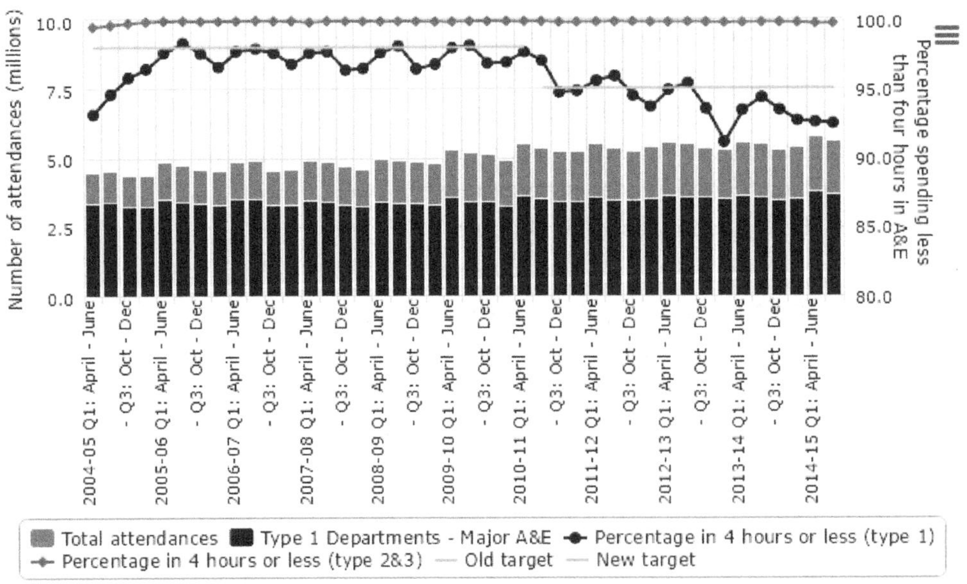

Question 335:

Which of the following statements is **FALSE**?

A. There has been an overall increase in total A&E attendances from 2004-2014.
B. The number of attendances in type I departments has been fairly constant from 2004-2014.
C. The new target of 4 hours waiting time has only been reached in two quarters by type I departments.
D. The change in attendances is largely due to an in increase people going to type 2&3 departments.

Question 336:

What percentage has the number of total attendances changed from QI 2004-5 to QI 2008-9?

A. +5%
B. –5%
C. +10%
D. –10%
E. +15%
F. –15%

Question 337:

If the new target was achieved by type I departments 4 times, in what percentage of the quarters was the target missed?

A. 25%
B. 60%
C. 75%
D. 90%

Questions 338-339 relate to the following data:

Ranjna is travelling from Manchester to Bali. She is required to make a stopover in Singapore for which he wants to allow at least 2 hours. It takes 14 hours to fly from Manchester to Singapore, and 2 hours from Singapore to Bali. The table below shows the departure times in local time [Manchester GMT, Singapore GMT + 8, Bali GMT + 8]:

Manchester to Singapore			Singapore to Bali			
Monday	**Wednesday**	**Thursday**	**Monday**	**Tuesday**	**Wednesday**	**Thursday**
08.00	09.30	02.30	13.00	00.00	15.30	13.00
10.45	14.00	08.30	15.30	07.30	18.00	16.00
13.30	18.00	12.30	21.00	08.30	20.30	19.00
15.00	20.00	19.00		12.00		

Question 338:

What is the latest flight Ranjna can take from Manchester to ensure she arrives at Bali Airport by Thursday 22:00?

A. 18:00 Tuesday
B. 14:00 Wednesday
C. 18:00 Wednesday
D. 20:00 Wednesday
E. 02:30 Thursday
F. 08:30 Thursday

Question 339:

Ranjna takes the 08:00 flight from Manchester to Singapore on Monday. She allows I hour to clear customs and collect her luggage at Bali Airport and another 45 minutes for the taxi to her hotel. At what time will she arrive at the hotel?

A. 16.45 Monday
B. 04:15 Tuesday
C. 10:30 Tuesday
D. 12:15 Tuesday
E. 12:30 Tuesday
F. 20:30 Tuesday

Question 340:

The graph below represents the percentage of adult smokers in the UK from 1974 to 2010. The top trace represents men and the bottom trace represents women. The middle trace is for both men and women.

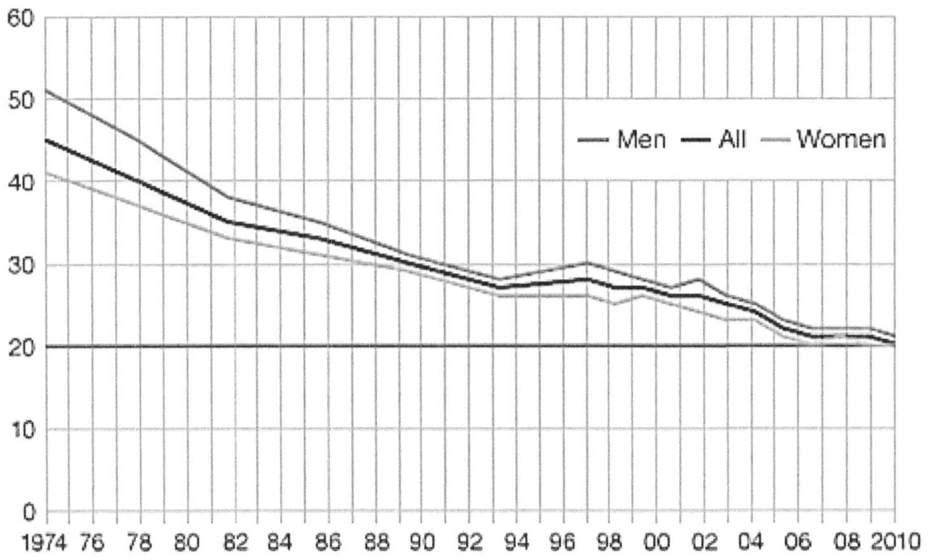

Which of the following statements can be concluded from the graph?

A. The 2007 smoking ban increased the rate in decline of smokers.
B. There has been a constant reduction in percentage of smoker since 1974.
C. The highest rate in decline in smoking for women was 2004-2006.
D. From 1974 to 2010, the smoking rate in men decreased by a half.
E. There has always been a significant difference between the smoking habits of men and women.

Question 341:

The name, age, height, weight and IQ of 11 people were recorded below in a table and a scatter plot. However, the axis labels were left out by mistake. Scale breaks are permitted.

Name	Age	Height (cm)	Weight (kg)	IQ
Alice	18	180	68	110
Ben	12	160	79	120
Camilla	14	170	62	100
David	25	145	98	108
Eliza	29	165	75	96
Rohan	15	190	92	111
George	20	172	88	104
Hannah	22	168	68	115
Ian	13	182	86	98
James	17	176	90	102
Katie	27	151	66	125

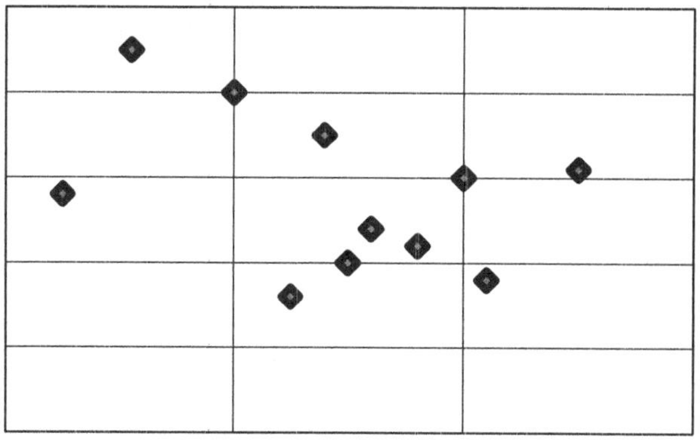

Which variants are possible for the X and Y axis?

	X axis	Y axis
A	Height	Weight
B	IQ	Height
C	Age	IQ
D	Height	IQ
E	Height	Age
F	IQ	Weight

Question 342:

A group of students looked at natural variation in height and arm span within their group and got the following results:

Name	Arm span (cm)	Height (cm)
Adam	175	168
Tom	188	175
Shiv	172	184
Mary	148	142
Alice	165	156
Sarah	166	168
Emily	159	160
Matthew	165	172
Michael	185	183

They then drew a scatter plot, but forgot to include names for each point. They also forgot to plot one student.

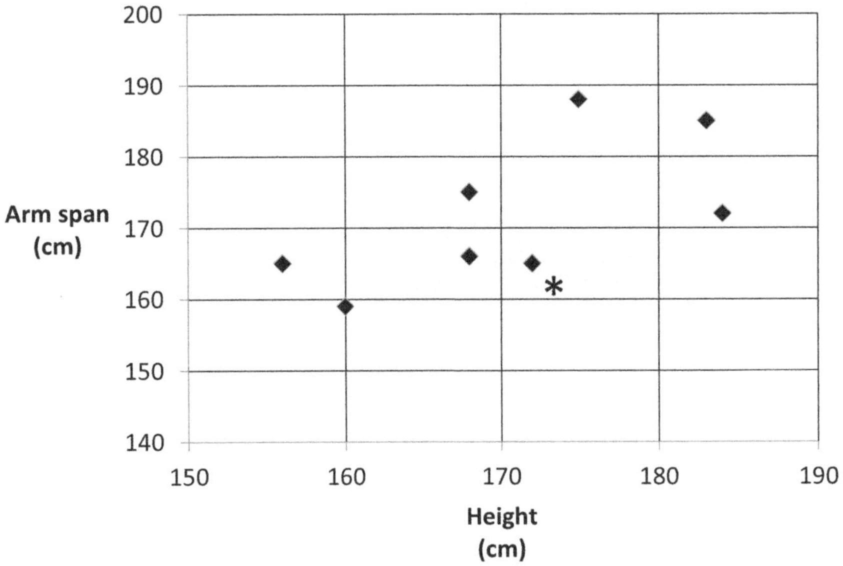

Which student is represented by the point marked with a *?

A. Alice
B. Sarah
C. Matthew
D. Adam
E. Emily
F. Michael

Questions 343 - 349 are based on the following information:

The rectangle represents women. The circle represents those that have children. The triangle represents those that work, and the square those that went to university.

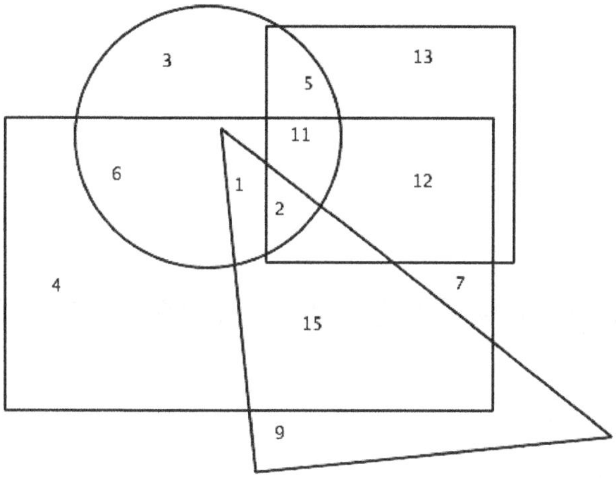

Question 343:

What is the number of non-working women who have children and who did not go to university?

A. 3 B. 5 C. 6 D. 7 E. 9

Question 344:

What is the total number of women who have children and work?

A. 1 B. 2 C. 3 D. 11 E. 14

Question 345:

How many women were surveyed in total?

A. 49
B. 51
C. 58
D. 67
E. 85
F. None of the above.

Question 346:

What is the number of people who went to university and had children?

A. 5
B. 11
C. 13
D. 16
E. 18
F. None of the above.

Question 347:

What is the total number of people who went to university, or have children but not both?

A. 18
B. 28
C. 35
D. 41
E. 53
F. None of the above.

Question 348:

The total number of men who went to university and had children was?

A. 3 B. 4 C. 5 D. 12 E. 13 F. 18

Question 349:

Which of the following people were not surveyed? Choose **TWO** options.

A. A non-working woman who went to university but did not have children.
B. A working man who went to university and has children.
C. A working woman who had children but did not go to university.
D. A non-working man who did not have children and did not go to university.
E. A working woman who went to university but did not have children.

Question 350:

Savers"R"Us is national chain of supermarkets. The price of several items in the supermarket is displayed below:

Item	Price
Beef roasting joint	£8.00
Chicken breast fillet	£6.00
Lamb shoulder	£7.00
Pork belly meat portion	£4.00
Sausages – 10 pack	£3.50

This week the supermarket has a sale on, with 50% off the normal price of all meat products. Alfred visits the supermarket during this sale and purchases a beef roasting joint, a 10 pack of sausages and a lamb shoulder, paying with a £20 note.

How much change does Alfred get?

A. £1.50
B. £5.00
C. £10.75
D. £11.75
E. £12.50
F. None of the above.

Question 351:

The local football league table is shown below, but the number of goals scored against Wilmslow is missing. Each team played the other teams in the league once at home and once away during the season.

Team Name	Points	Goals For	Goals Against
Sale	20	16	2
Wilmslow	16	11	?
Timperley	14	8	7
Altrincham	13	7	9
Mobberley	10	8	12
Hale	8	4	14

How many goals must Wilmslow have conceded?

A. 8
B. 9
C. 10
D. 11
E. 12
F. 14

Question 352:

The heights and weights of three women with BMI's 21, 22 and 23 were measured. If Julie and Lydia had different weights but the same height of 154 cm, and the weight of Emma, Lydia and Julie combined was 345 lbs, what was Emma's height?

A. 158 cm
B. 162 cm
C. 160 cm
D. 164 cm
E. 165 cm

		Weight (lbs)				
		100	**105**	**110**	**115**	**120**
Height (cm)	**152**	19	20	22	24	26
	154	18	19	21	23	25
	156	17	18	20	22	24
	158	15	17	19	21	23
	160	14	15	18	20	22
	162	13	14	17	19	21
	164	12	13	15	18	20
	166	11	12	14	17	19
	168	10	11	13	15	18
	170	9	10	12	14	17

Question 353:

The measurements for different types of fish appear below:

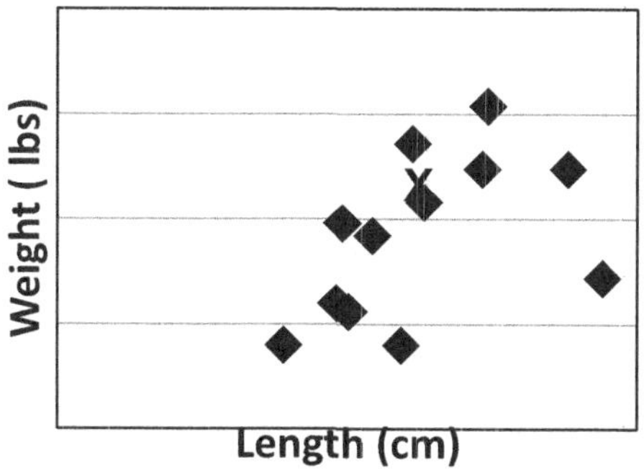

	Length (cm)	Weight (lbs)
Bluecup	78	40
Silverfinn	96	60
Starbug	98	98
Jawless	100	56
Lamprene	108	92
Scarfynne	118	40
Rayfish	122	136
Lobefin	126	108
Eringill	146	124
Whaler	148	154
Magic fish	176	124
Blondeye	188	72

Which fish is shown by the point marked **X**?

A. Silverfinn
B. Starbug
C. Lobefin
D. Blondeye
E. Eringill

SECTION 1 VISUAL THINKING QUESTIONS

For each of these sets, examine the shapes for each question and then mark whether they belong in Set A, Set B, or neither.

SET 1

Set A　　Set B

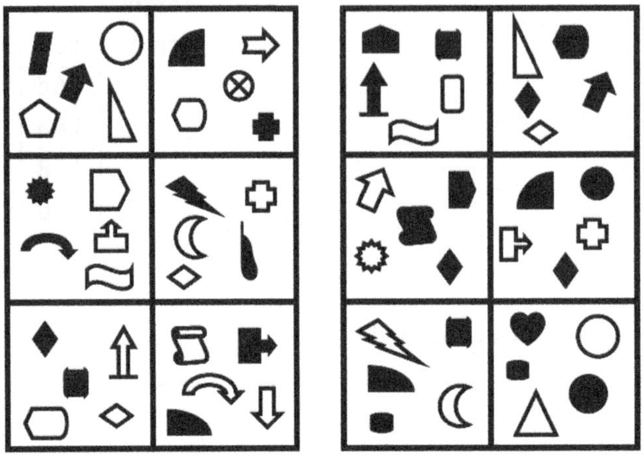

Questions 1-5

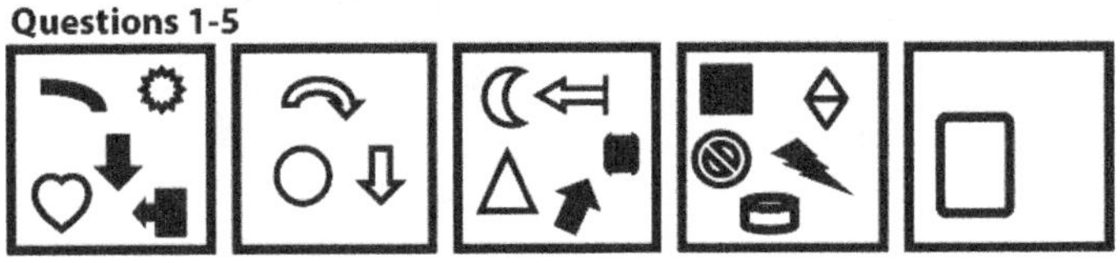

SET 2

Set A　　Set B

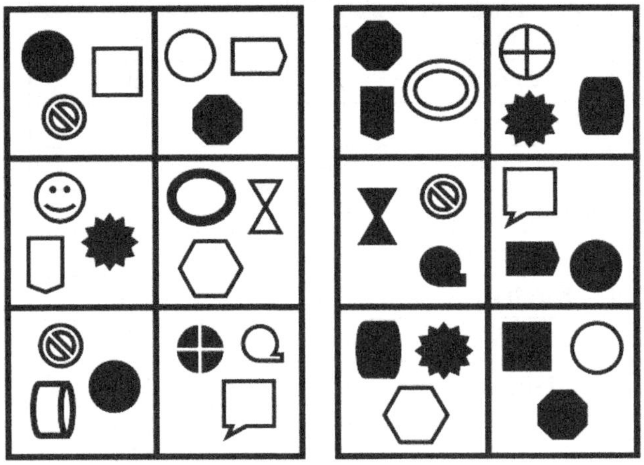

Questions 6-10

SET 3

Set A Set B

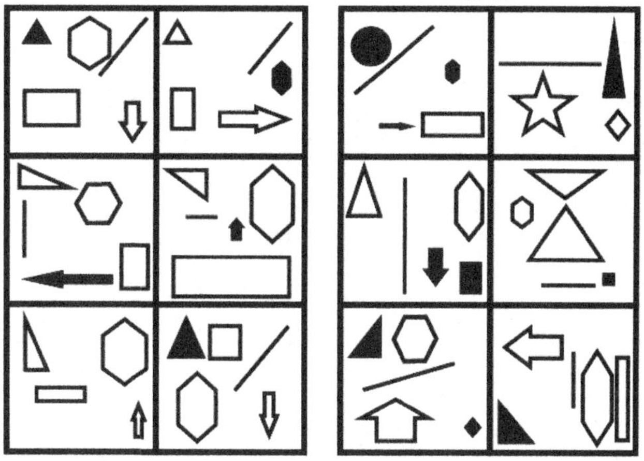

Questions 11-15

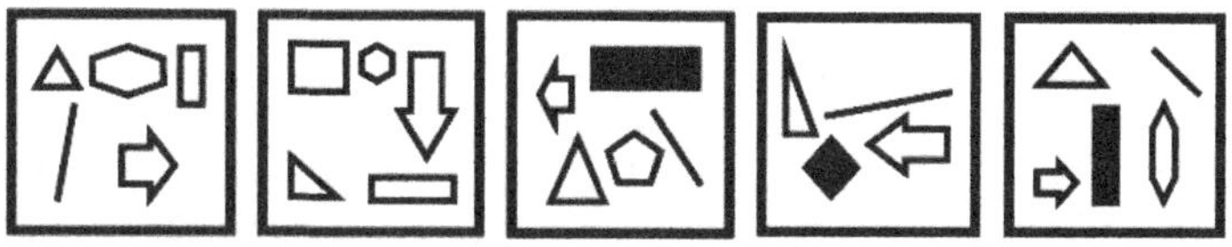

SET 4

Set A Set B

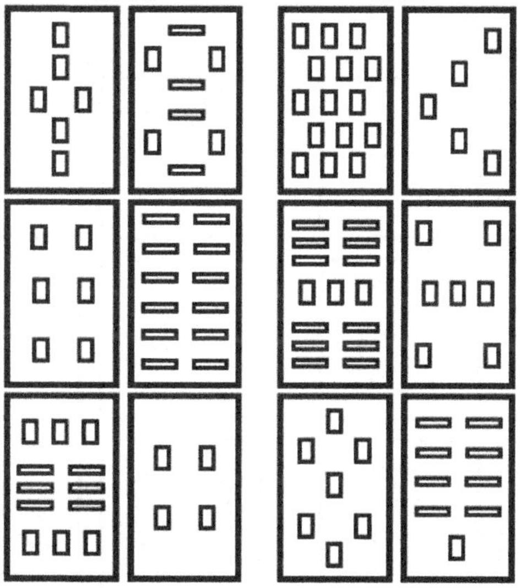

Questions 16-20

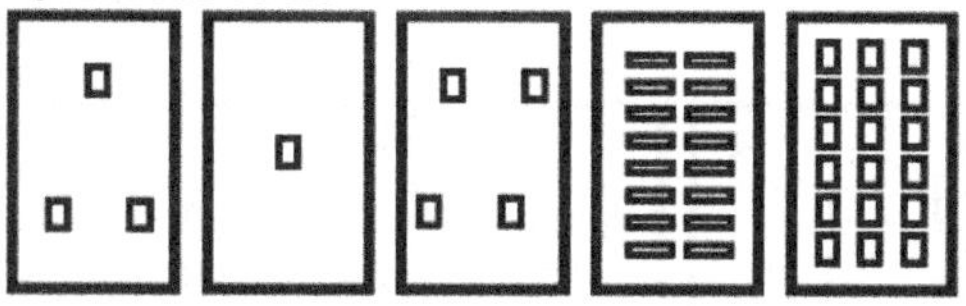

SET 5

Set A Set B

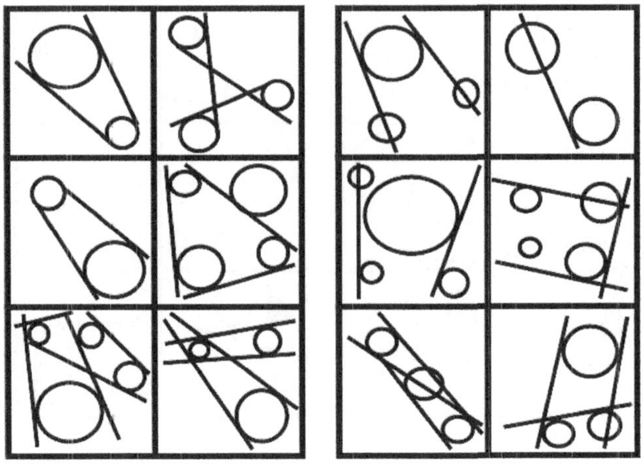

Questions 21-25

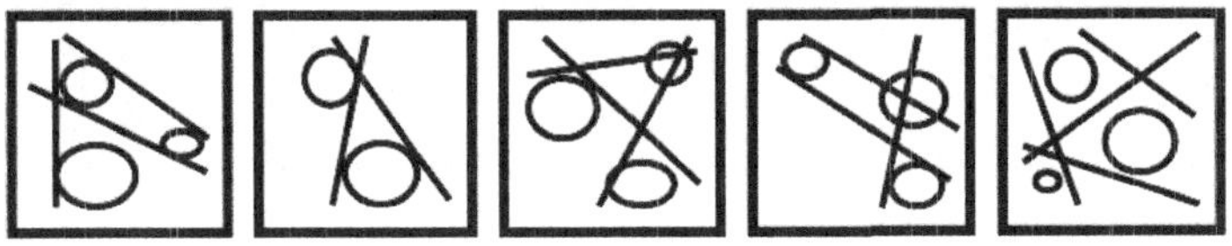

SET 6

Set A Set B

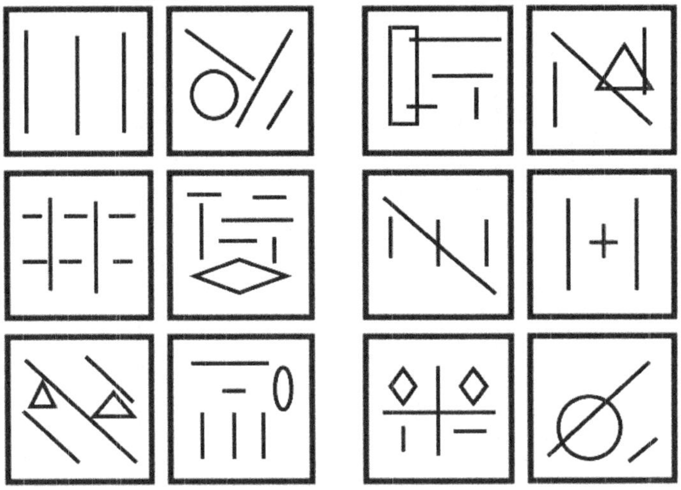

Questions 26-30

SET 7

Set A Set B

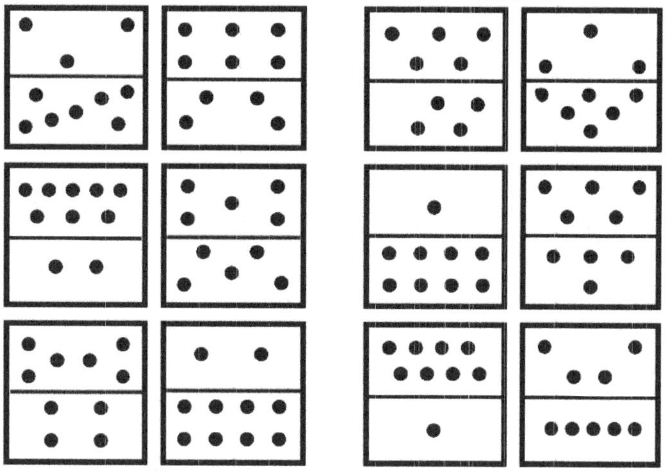

Questions 31-35

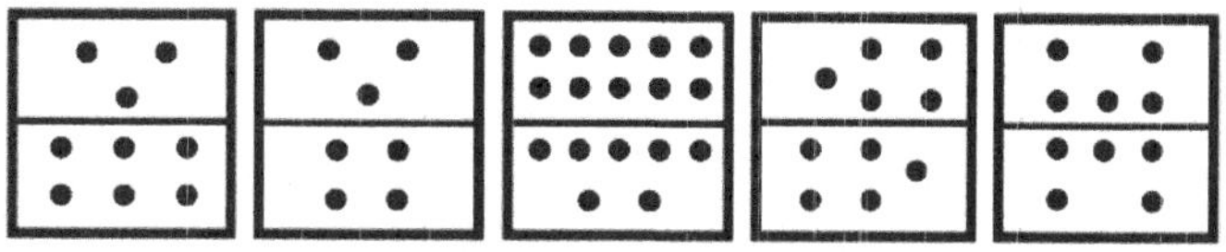

SET 8

Set A Set B

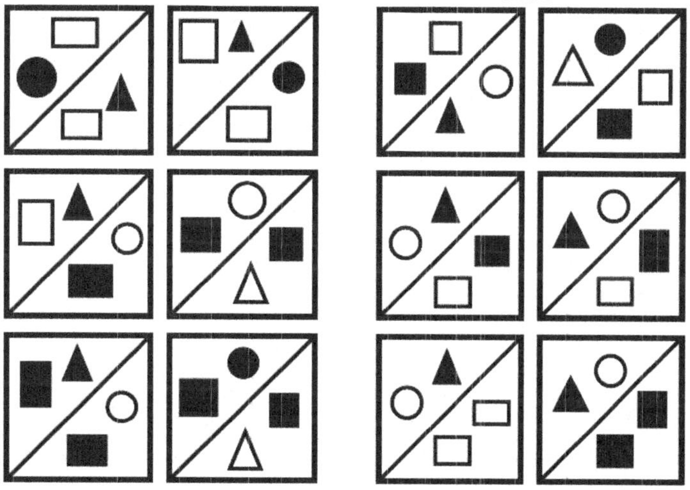

Questions 36-40

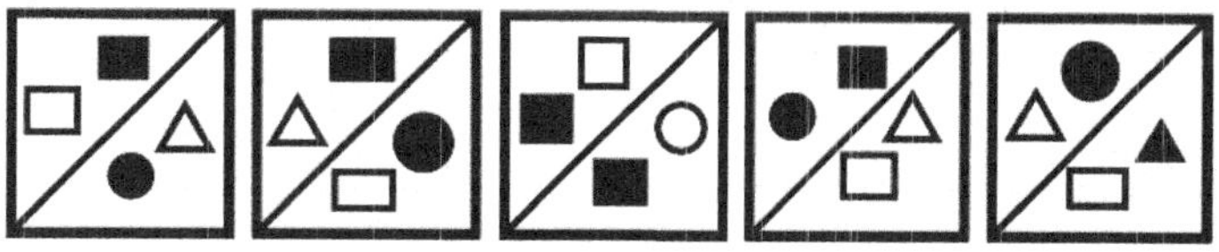

SET 9

Set A

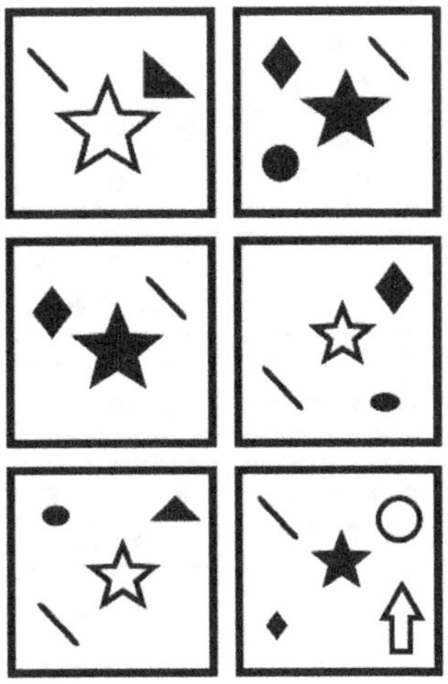

Set B

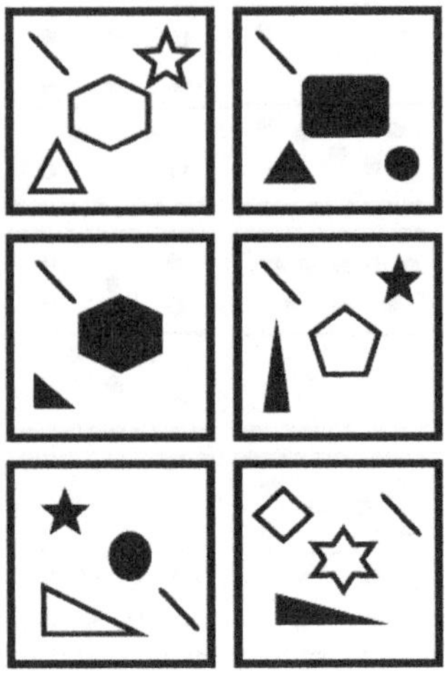

Questions 41-45

SET 10

Set A

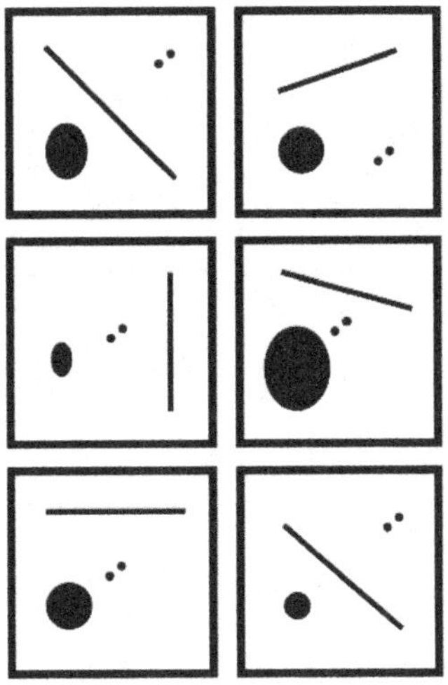

Set B

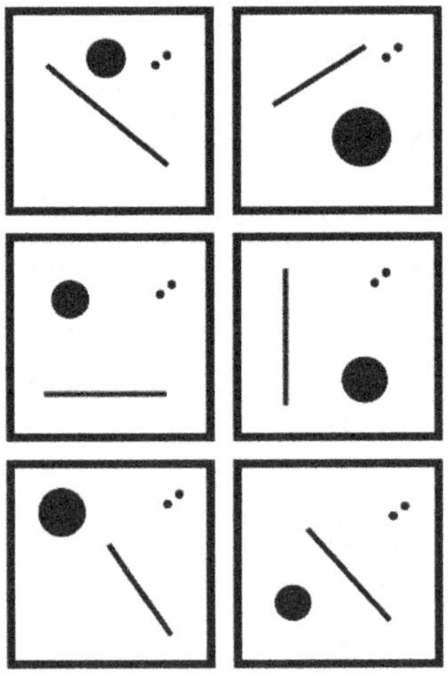

Questions 46-50

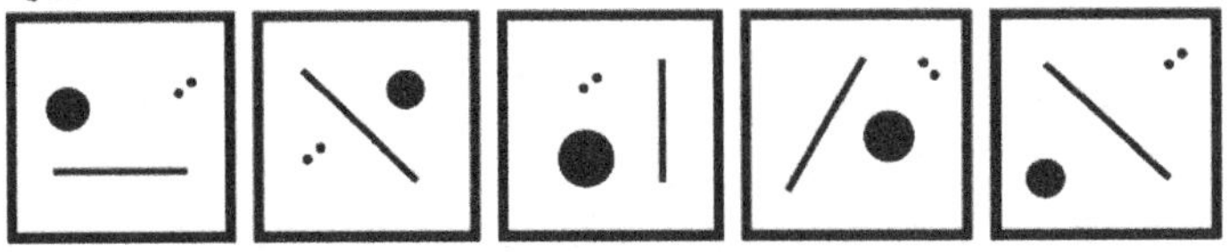

SET 11

Set A **Set B**

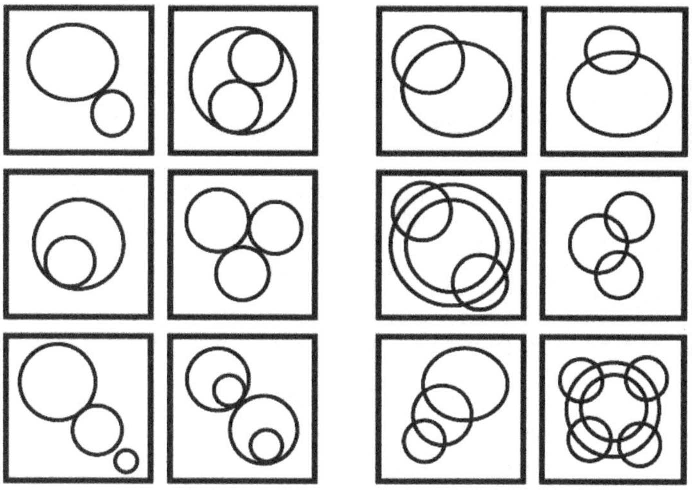

Questions 51-55

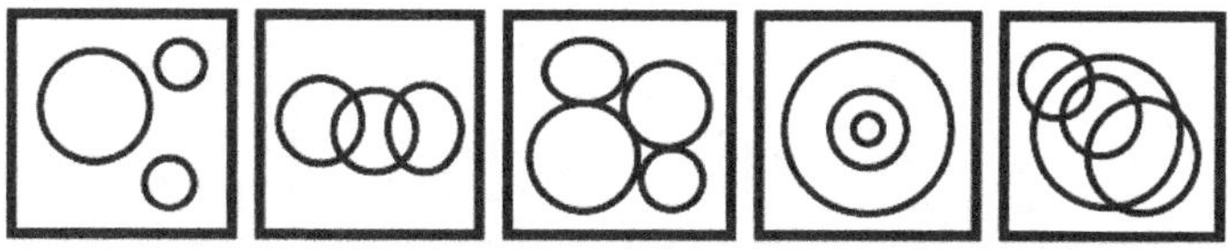

SET 12

Set A **Set B**

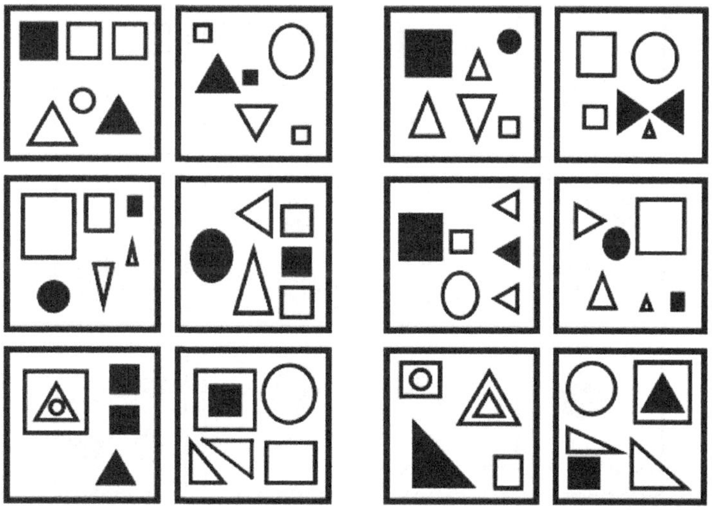

Questions 56-60

SET 13

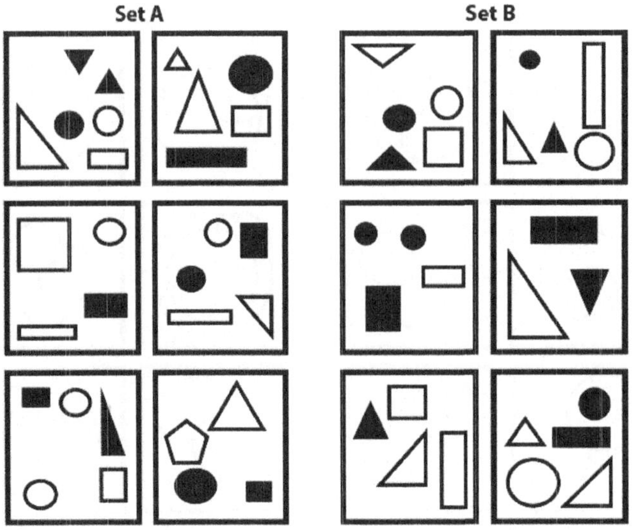

Questions 61-65

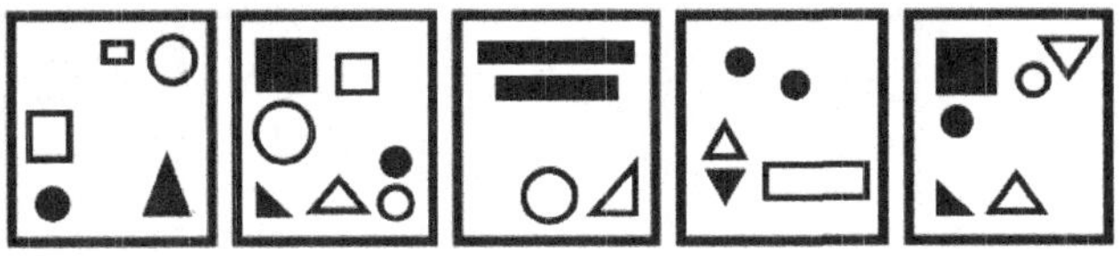

SET 14

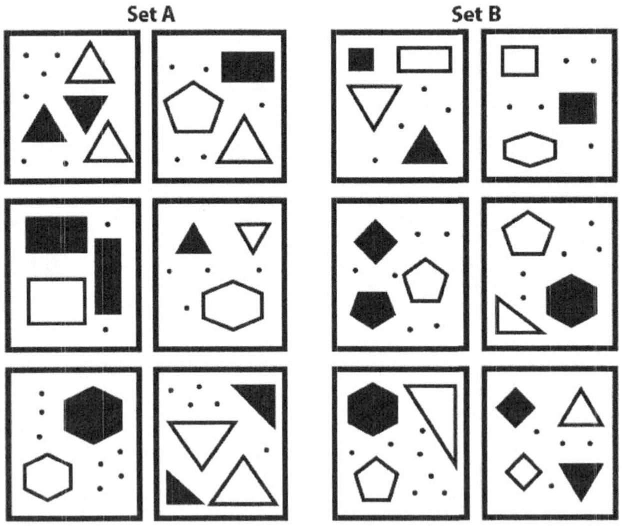

Questions 66-70

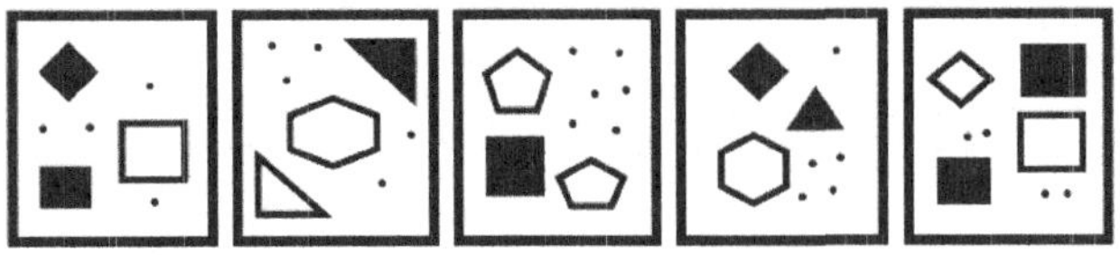

SET 15

Set A Set B

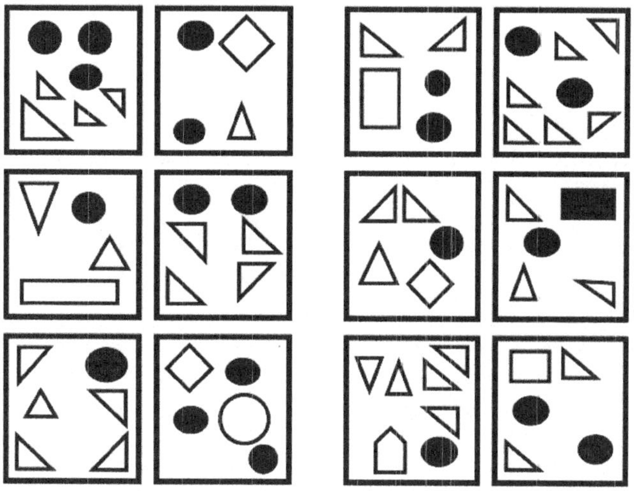

Questions 71-75

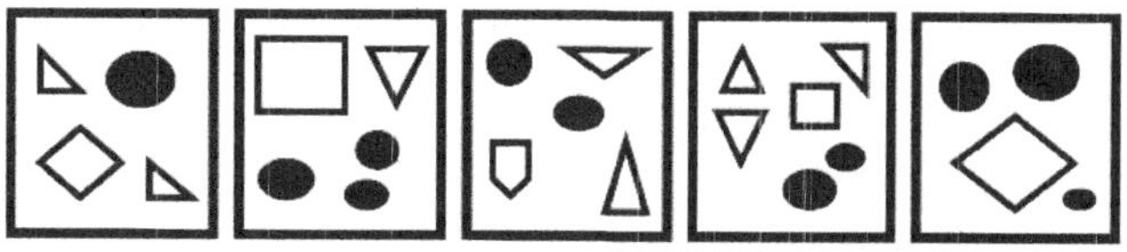

SET 16

Set A Set B

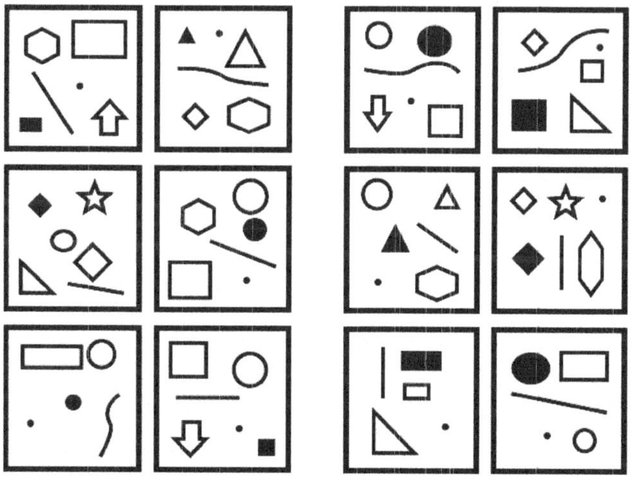

Questions 76-80

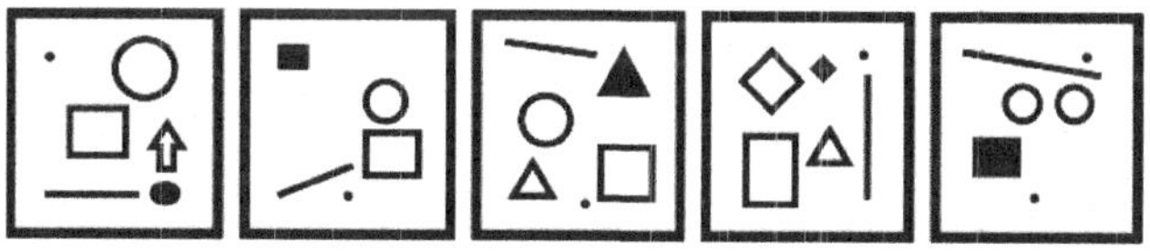

SET 17

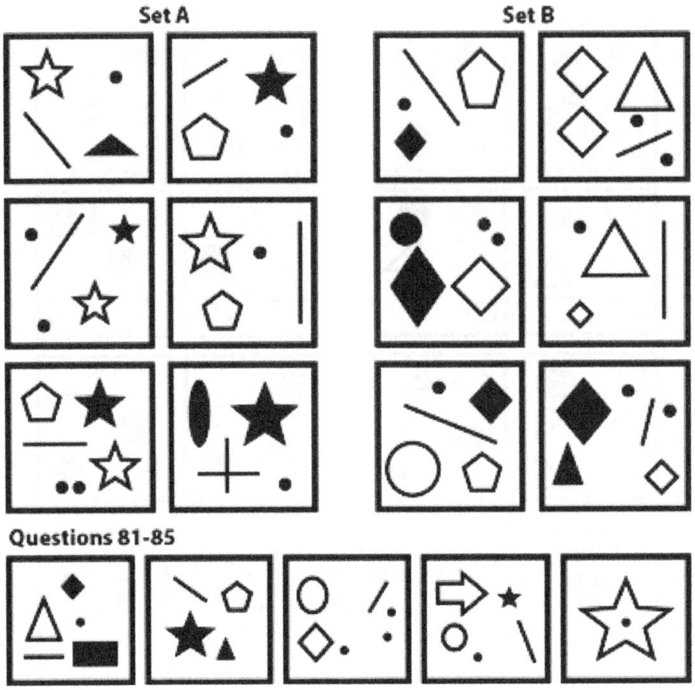

SET 18

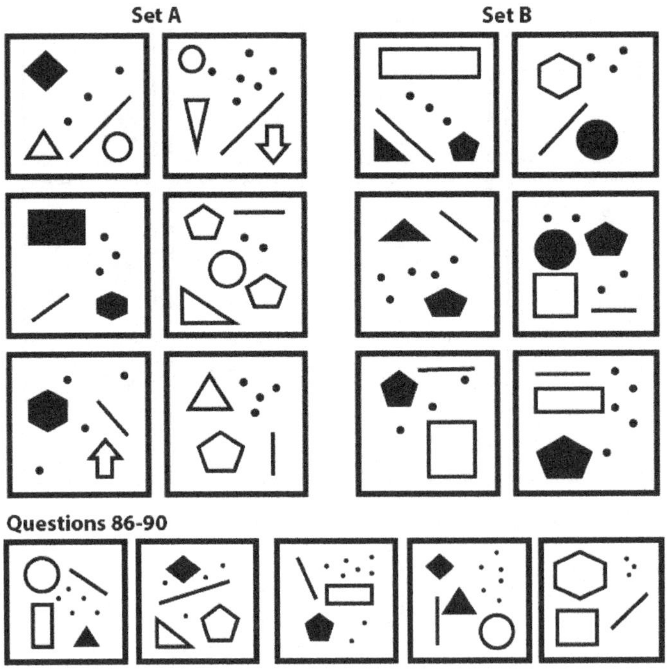

SET 19

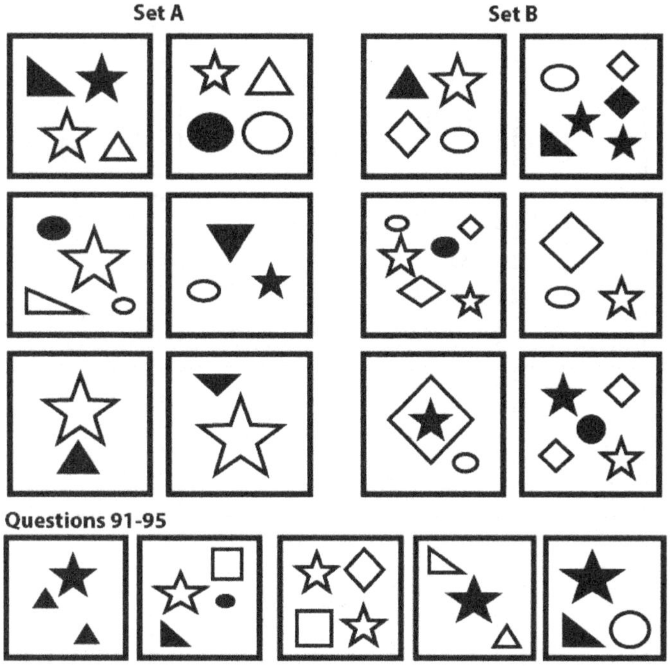

SET 20

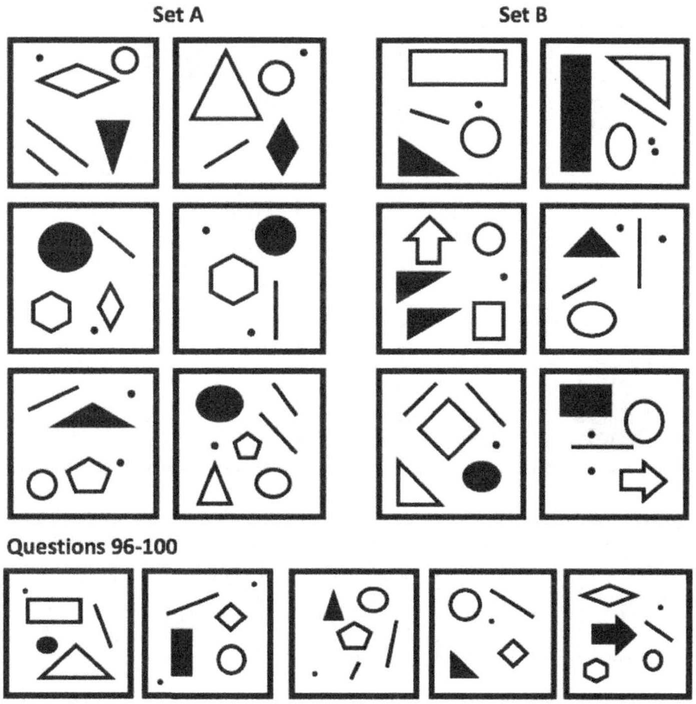

SET 21

Set A Set B

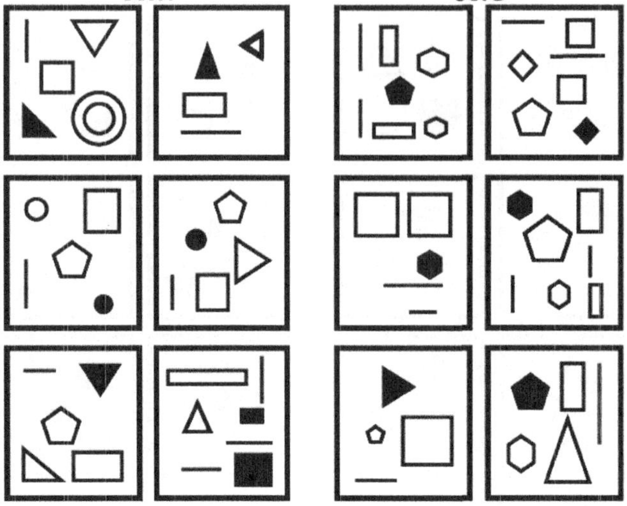

Questions 101-105

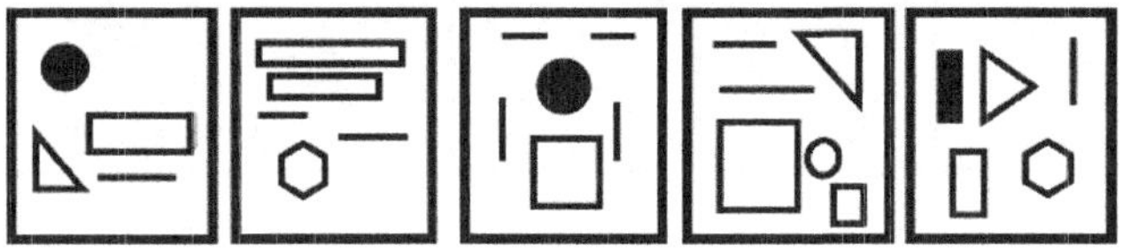

SET 22

Set A Set B

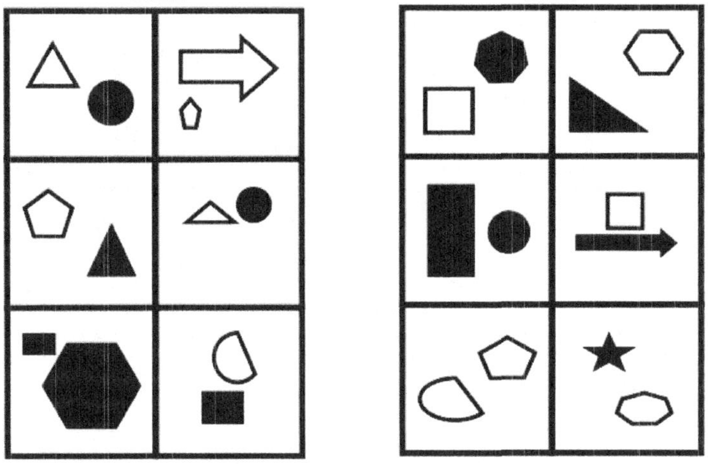

Questions 106-110

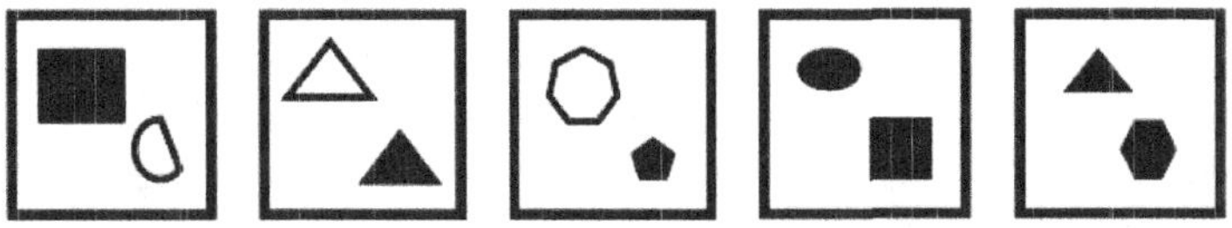

SET 23

Set A

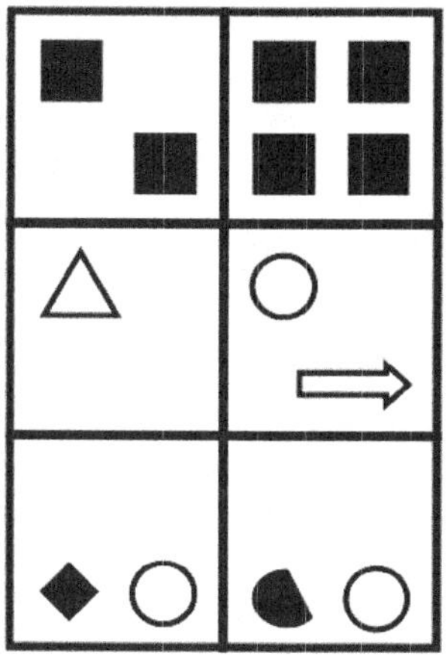

Set B

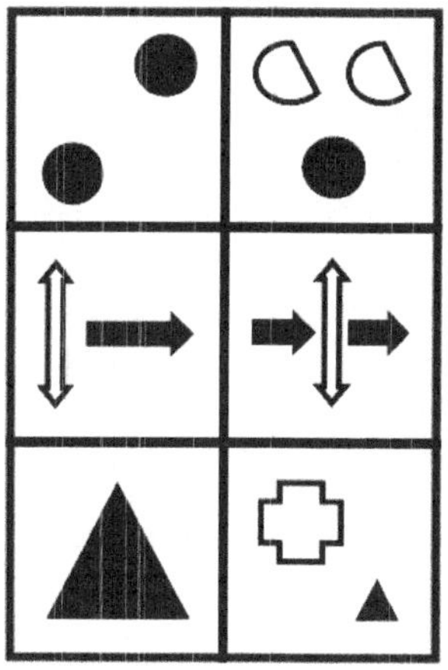

Questions 111-115

SET 24

Set A

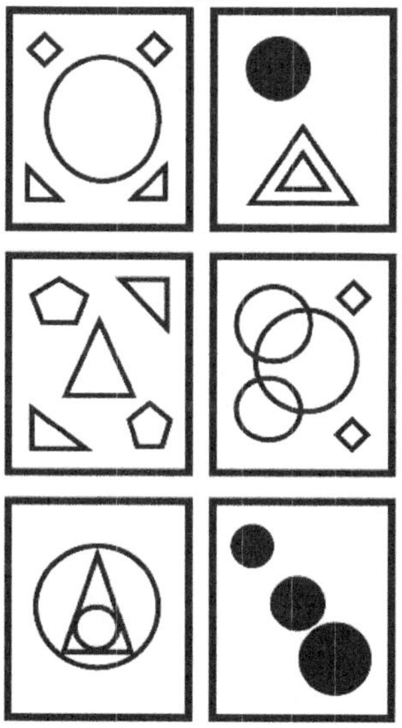

Set B

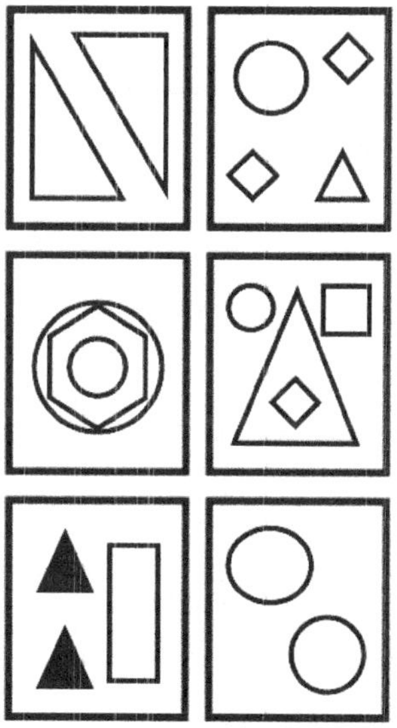

Questions 116-120

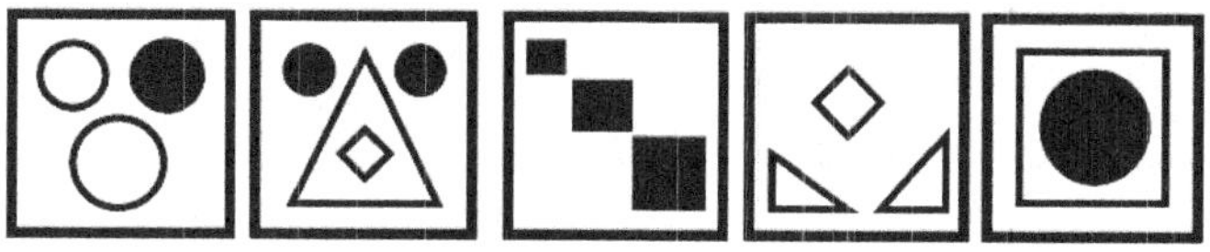

SET 25

Set A

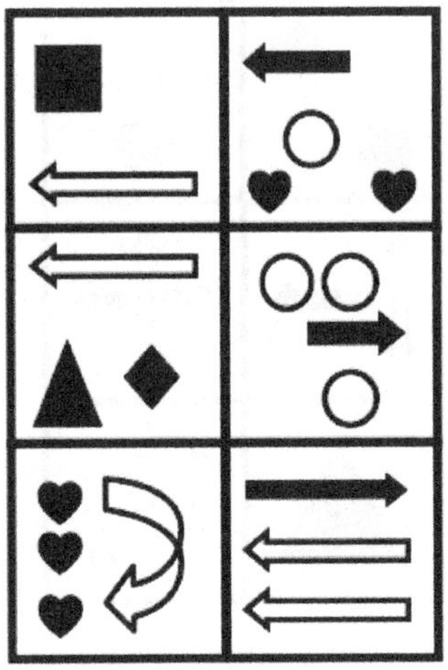

Set B

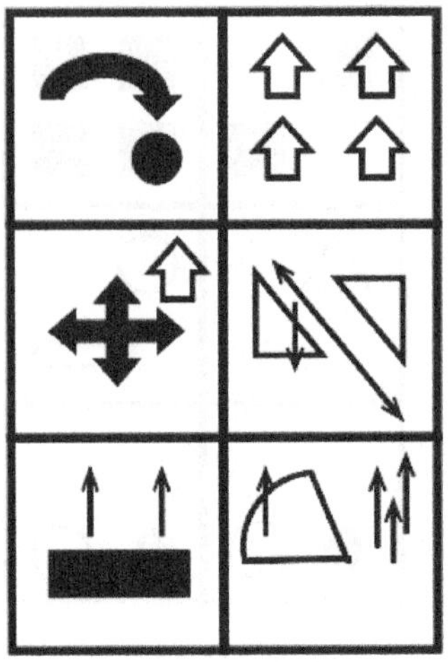

Questions 121-125

SET 26

Set A

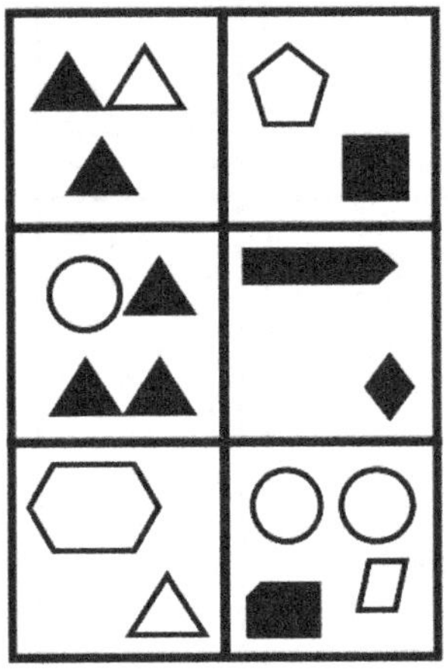

Set B

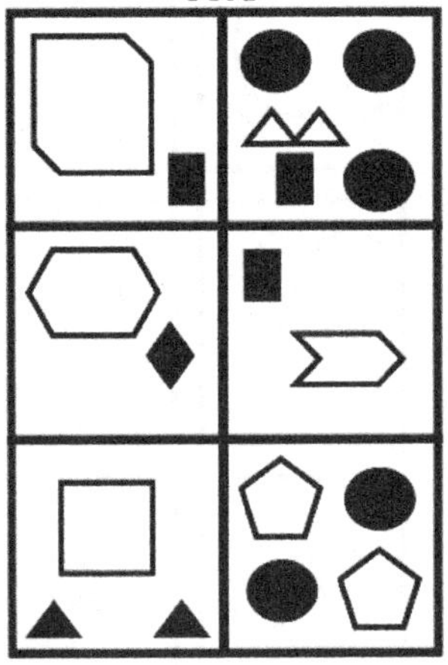

Questions 126-130

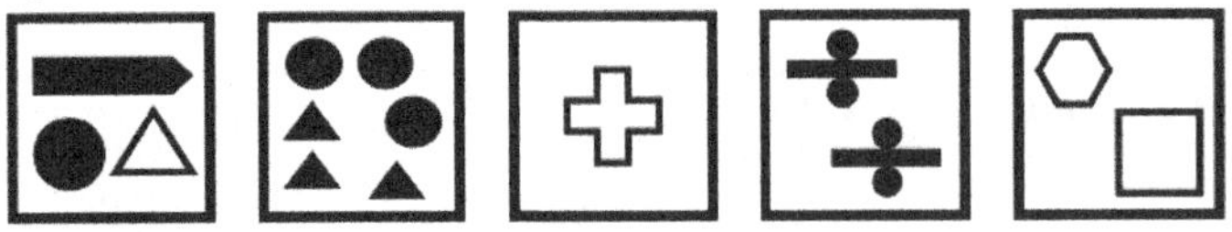

SET 27

Set A Set B

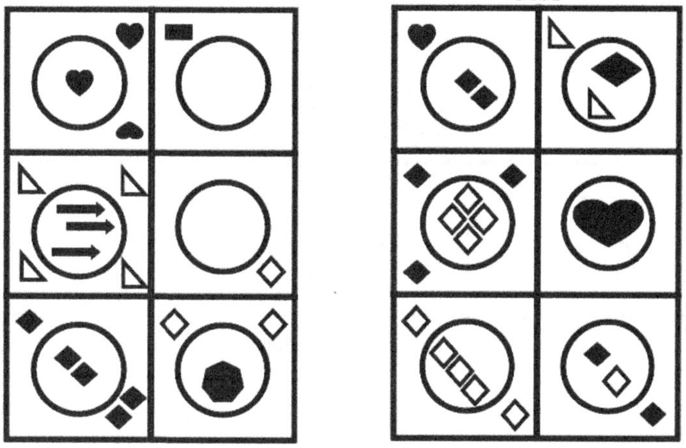

Questions 131-135

SET 28

Set A Set B

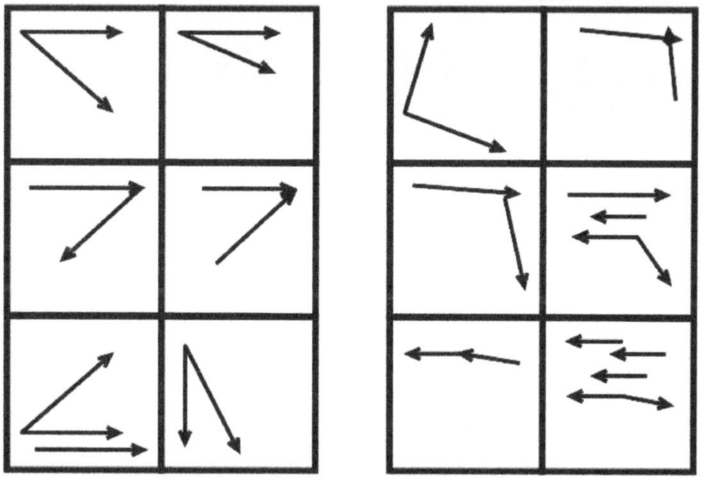

Questions 136-140

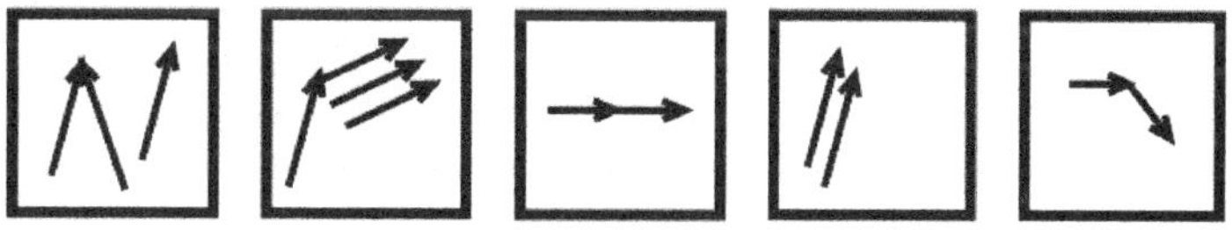

SET 29

Set A

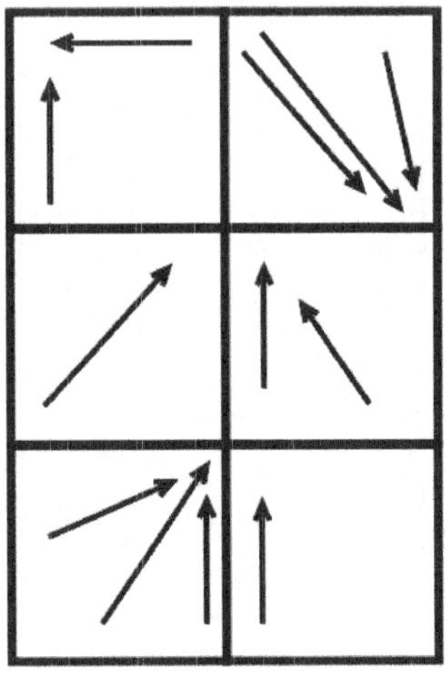

Set B

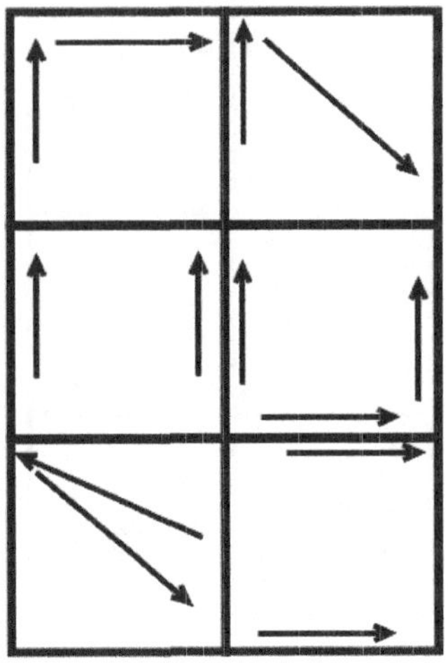

Questions 141-145

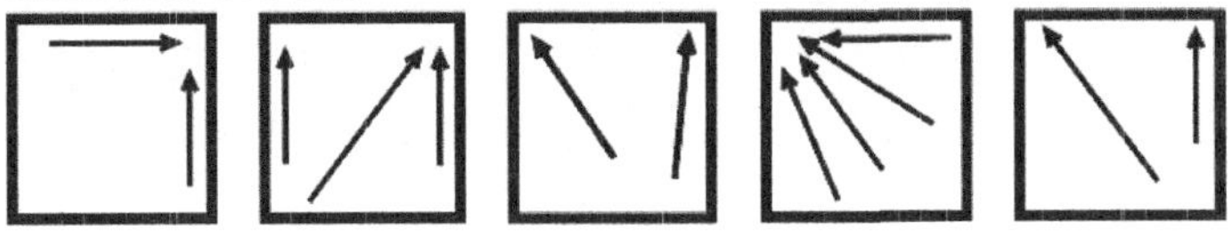

SET 30

Set A

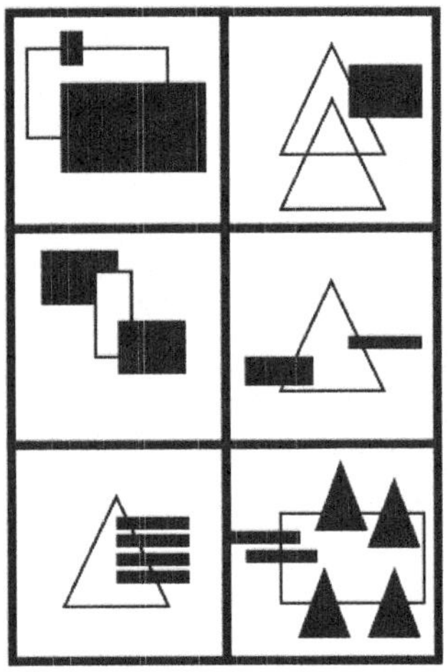

Set B

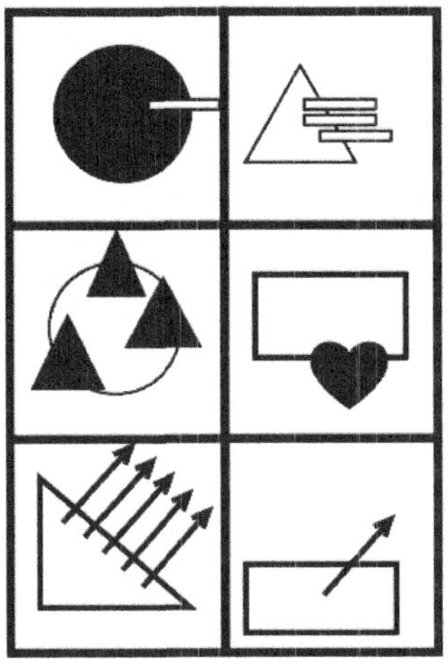

Questions 146-150

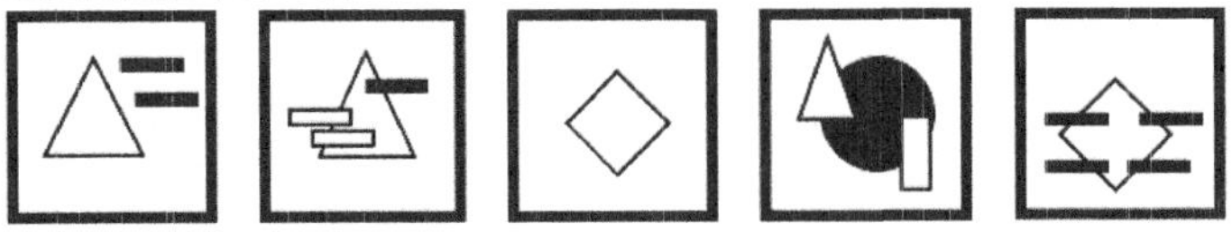

SET 31

Set A

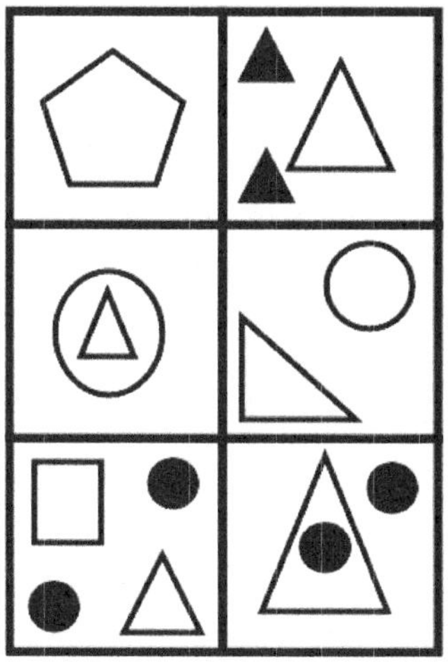

Set B

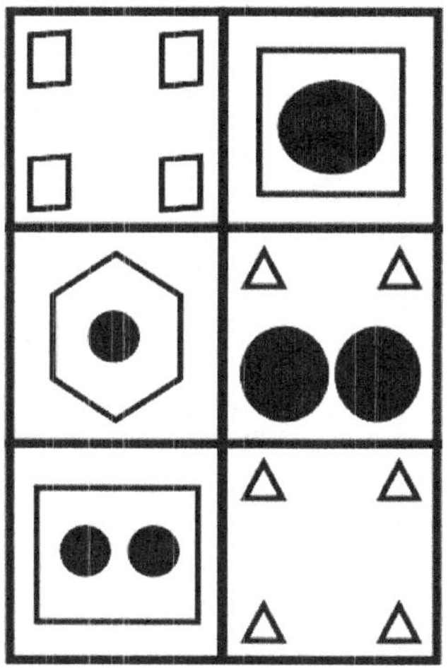

Questions 151-155

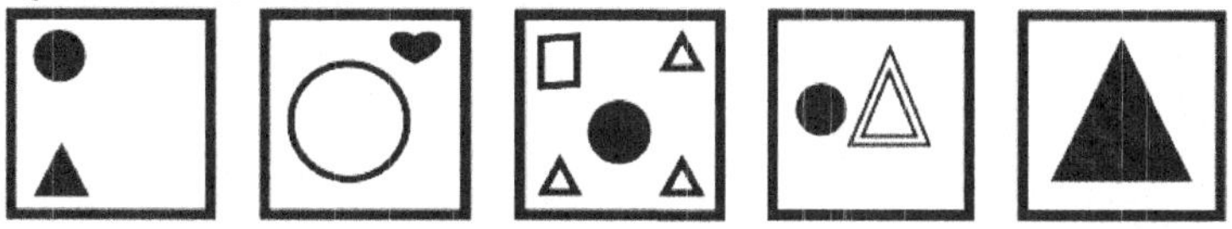

SET 32

Set A

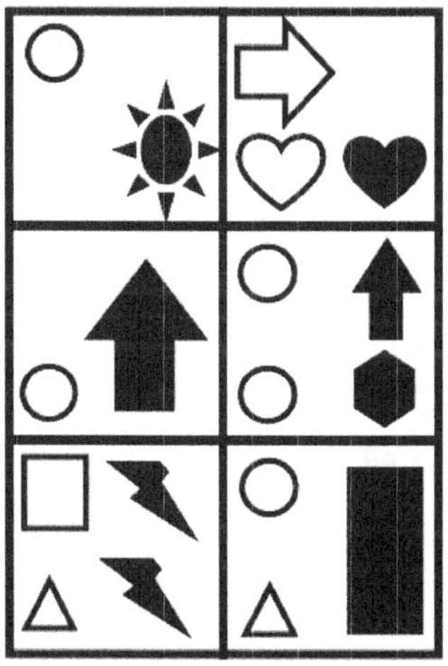

Set B

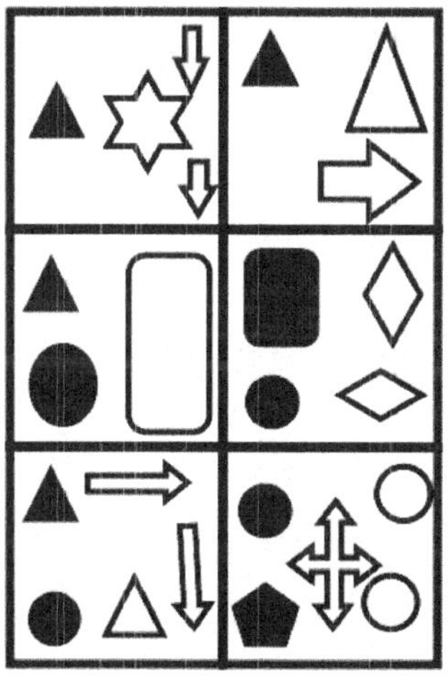

Questions 156-160

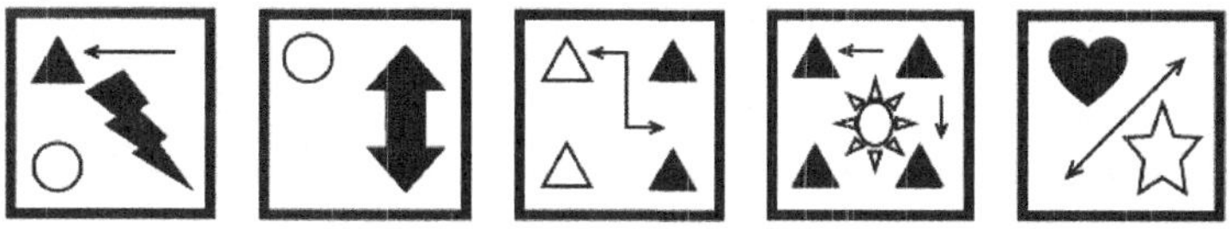

SET 33

Set A **Set B**

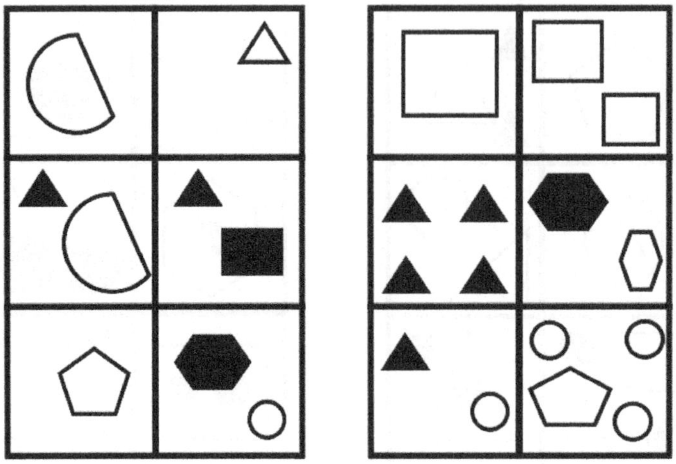

Questions 161-165

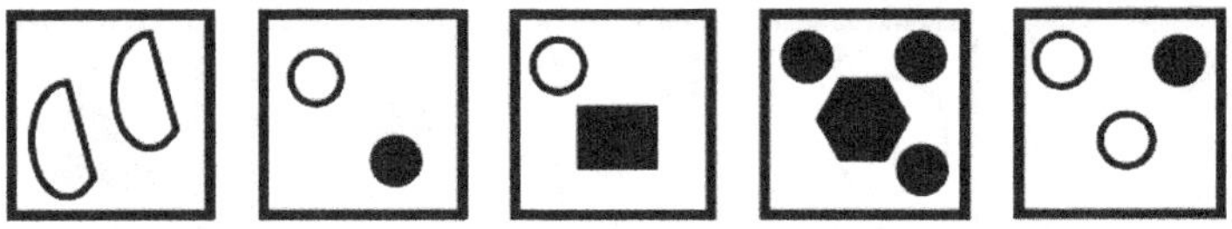

SET 34

Set A **Set B**

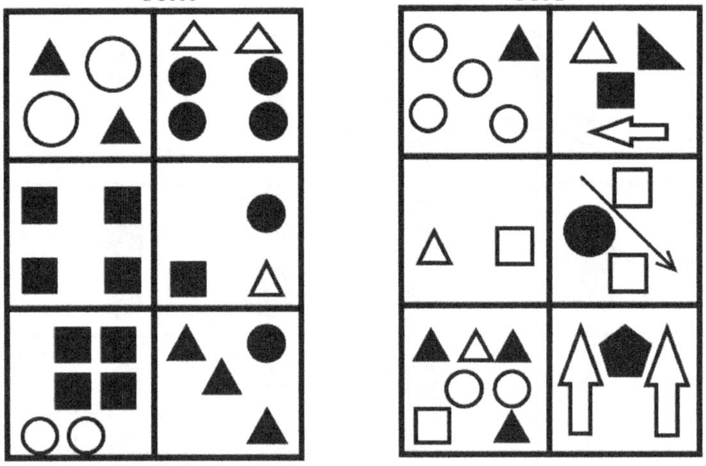

Questions 166-170

SET 35

Set A

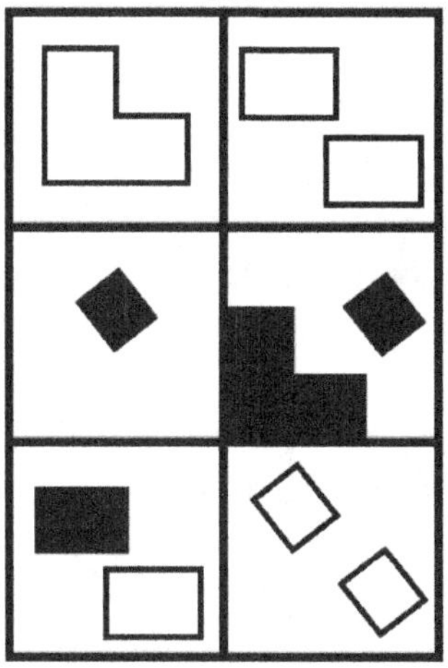

Set B

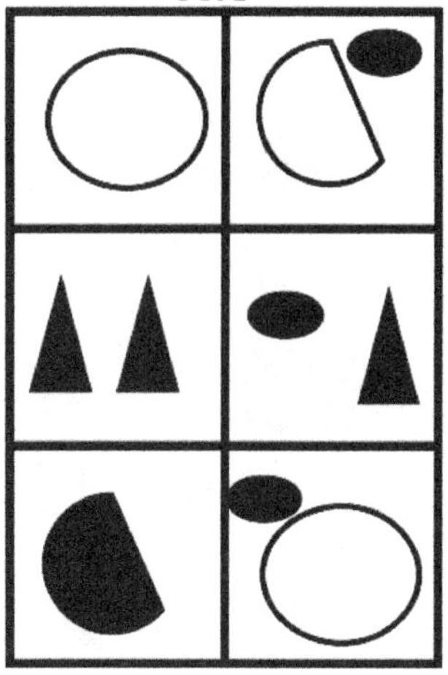

Questions 171-175

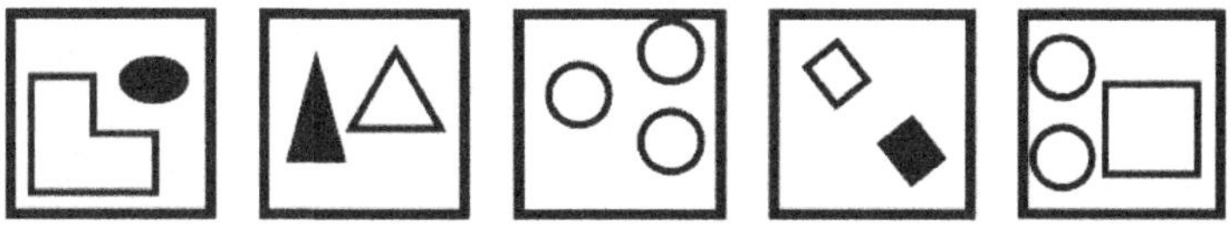

SET 36

Set A

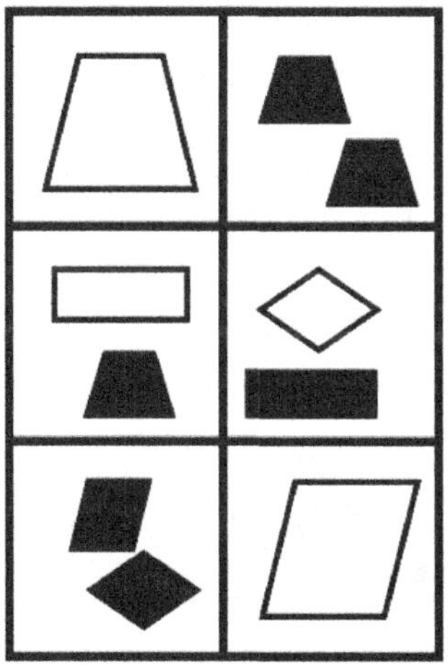

Set B

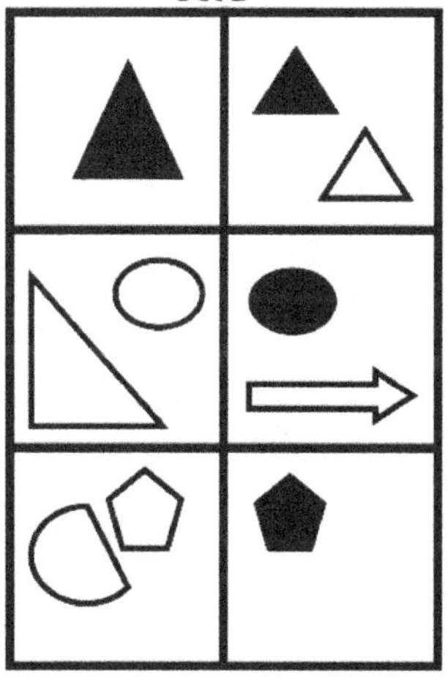

Questions 176-180

SET 37

Set A **Set B**

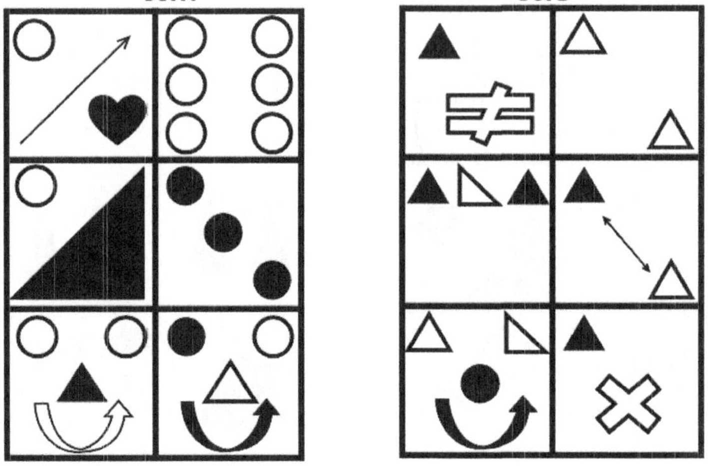

Questions 181-185

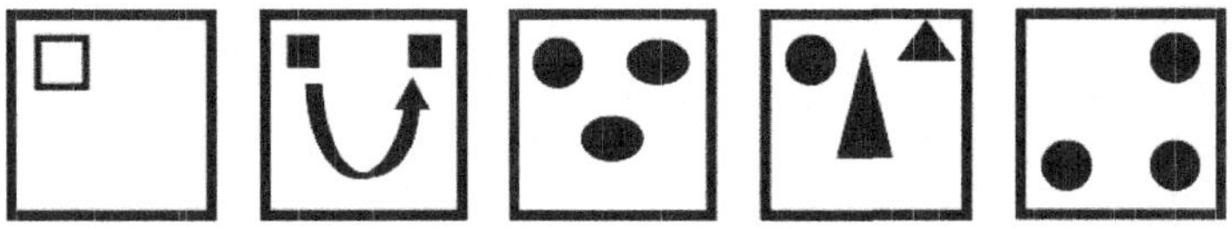

SET 38

Set A **Set B**

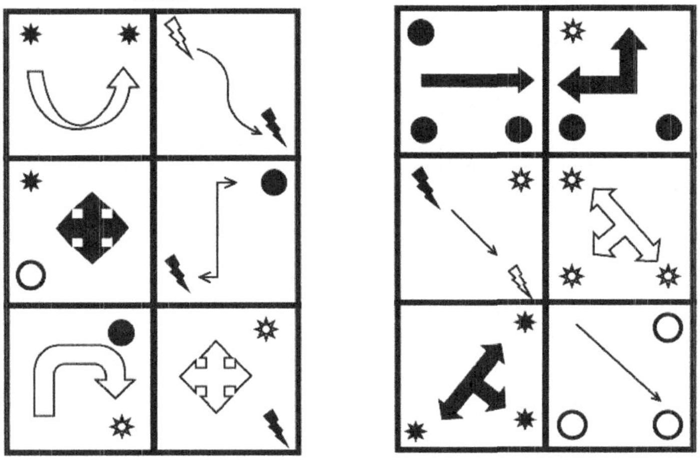

Questions 186-190

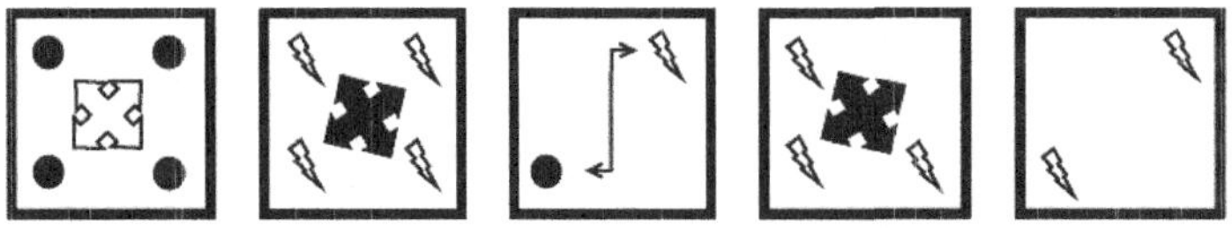

SET 39

Set A

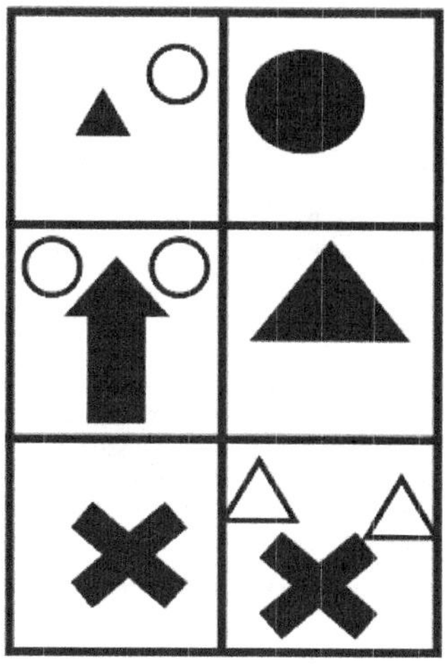

Set B

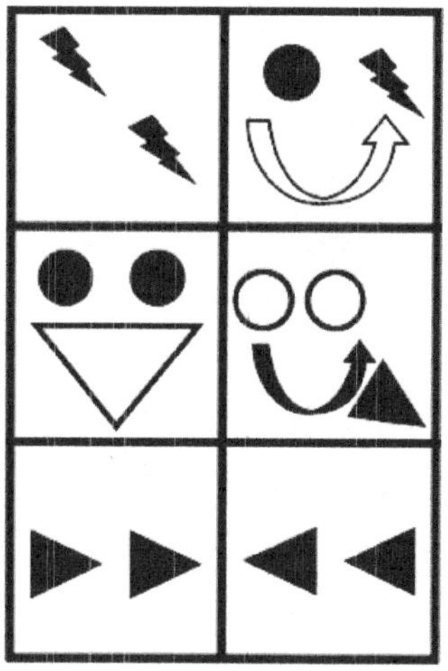

Questions 191-195

SET 40

Set A

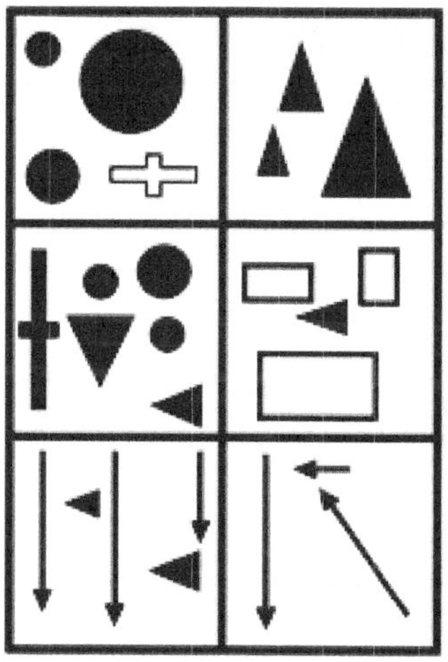

Set B

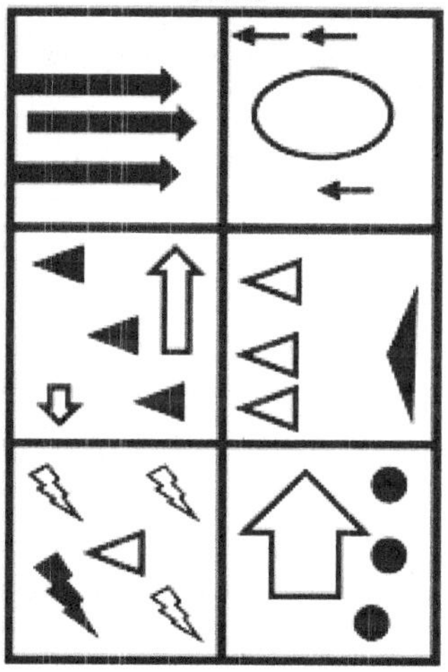

Questions 196-200

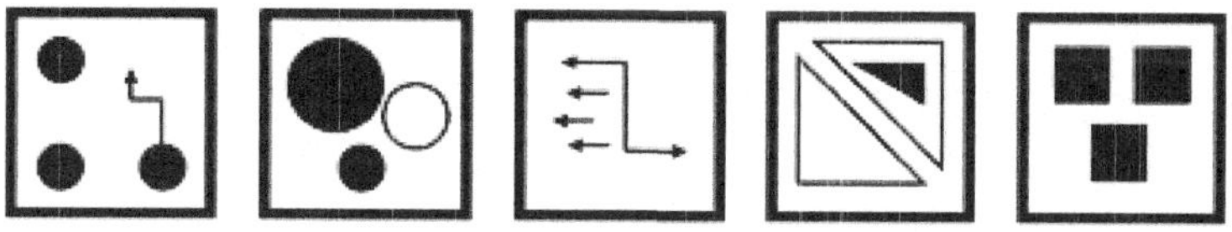

For Questions 201 – 250: Which answer option completes the series?

Q201

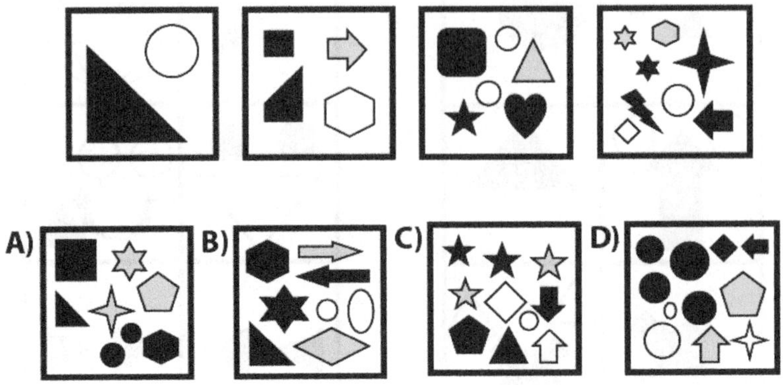

Q202

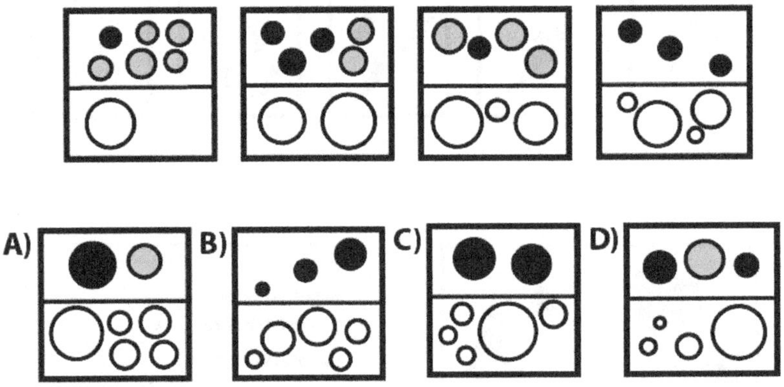

Q203

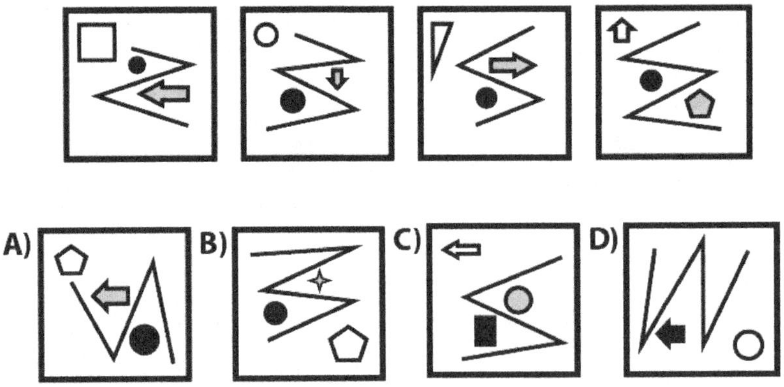

Q204

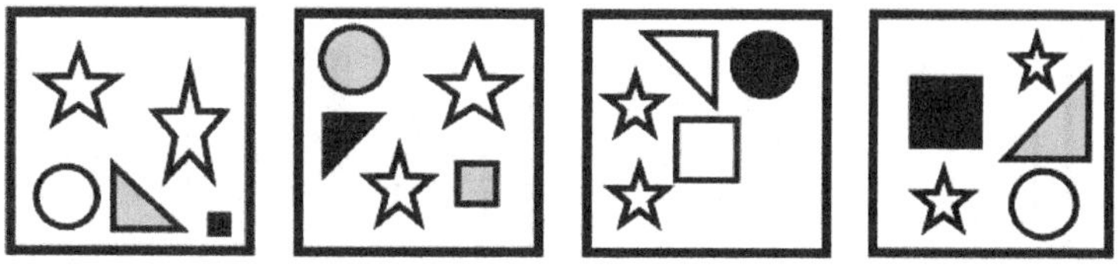

A) 
B) 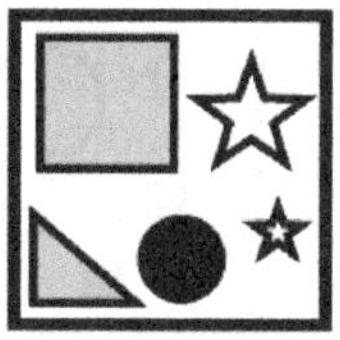
C) 
D) 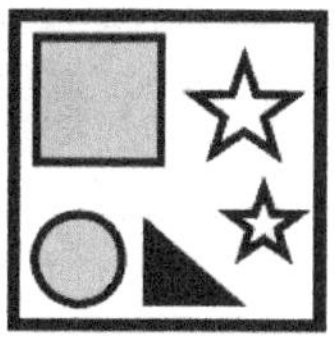

Q205

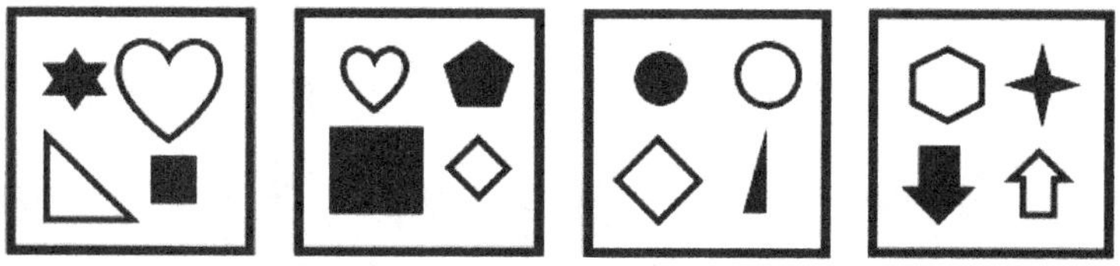

A) 
B) 
C) 
D) 

Q206

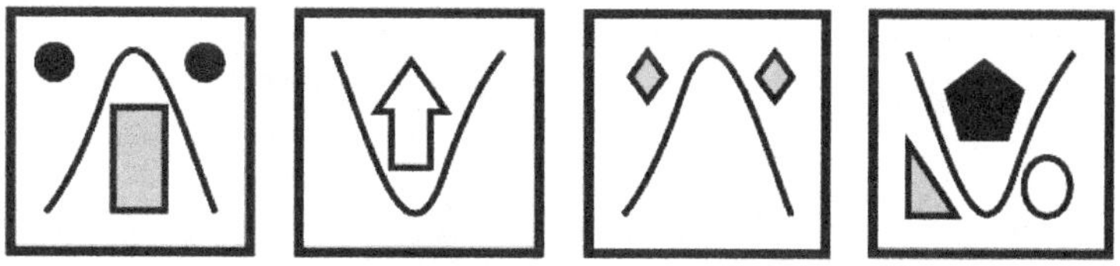

A) 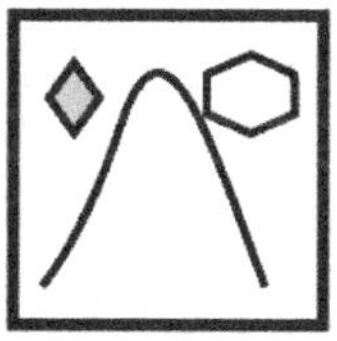
B) 
C) 
D) 

Q207

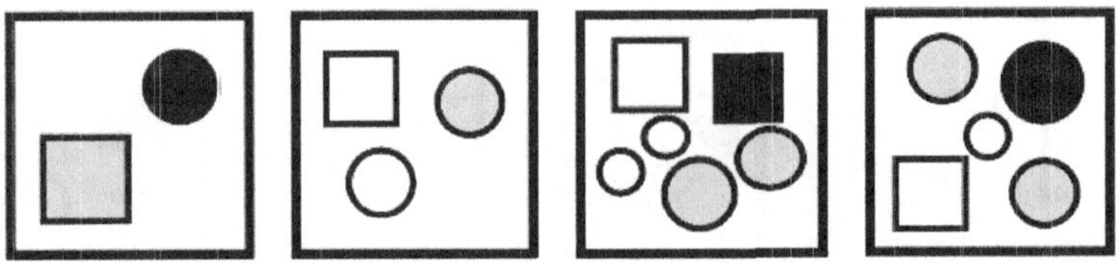

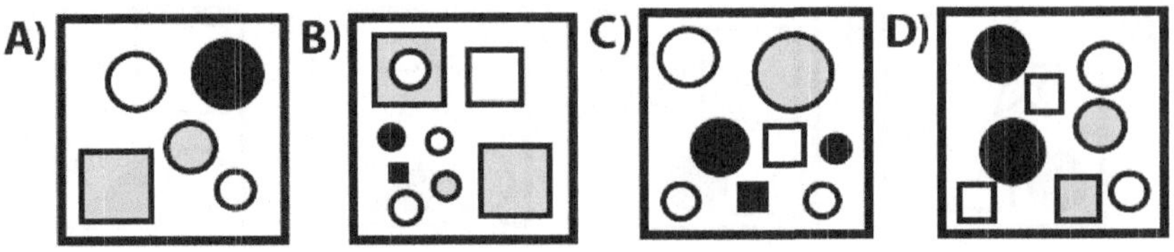

Q208

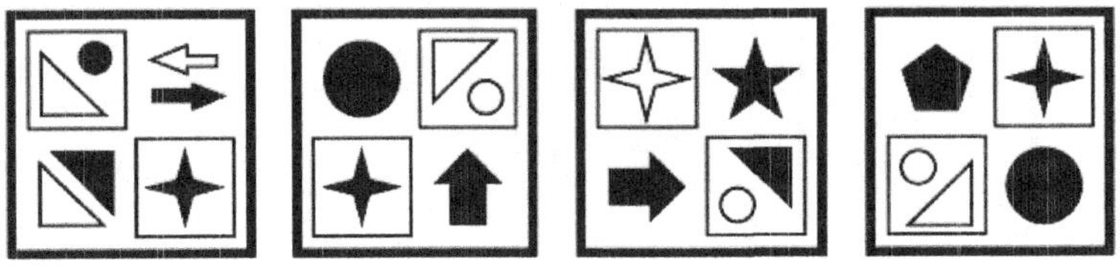

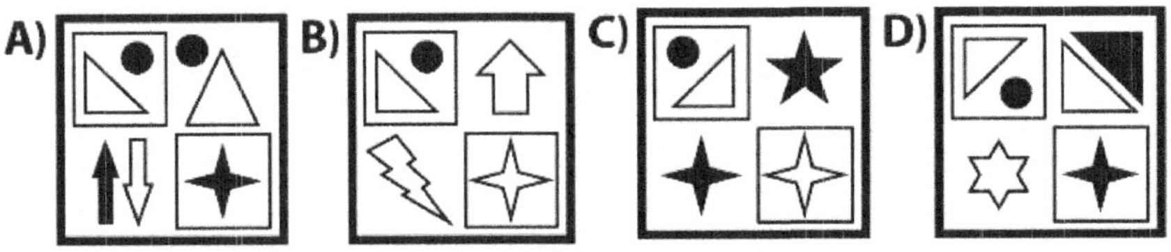

Q209

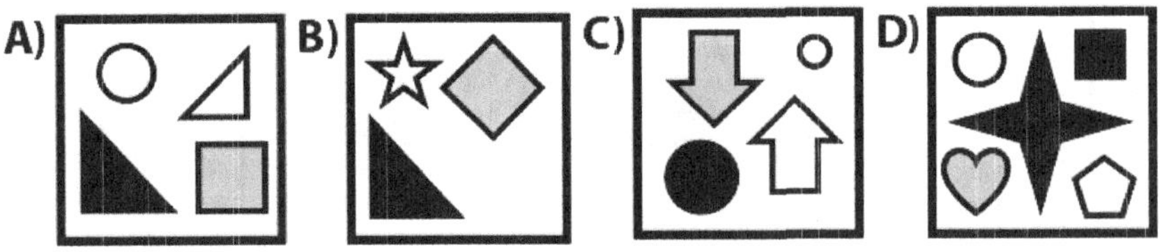

Q210

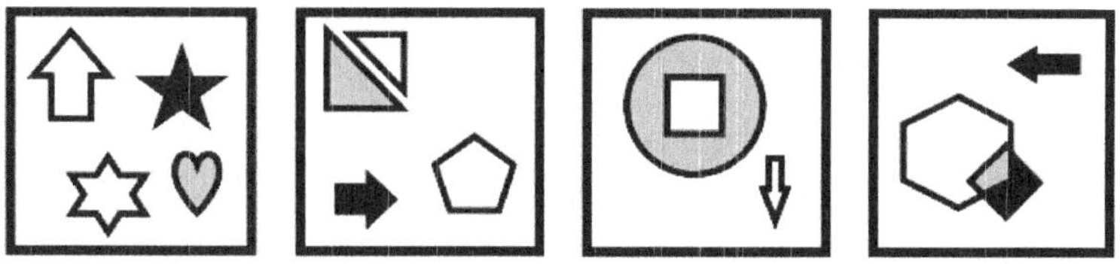

A) 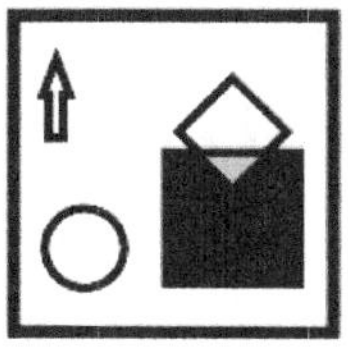 B)  C) 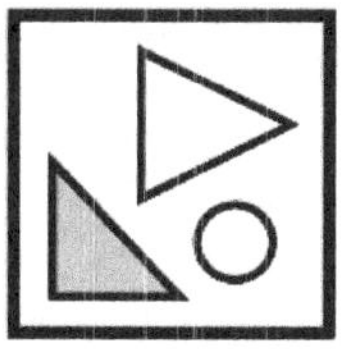 D) 

Q211

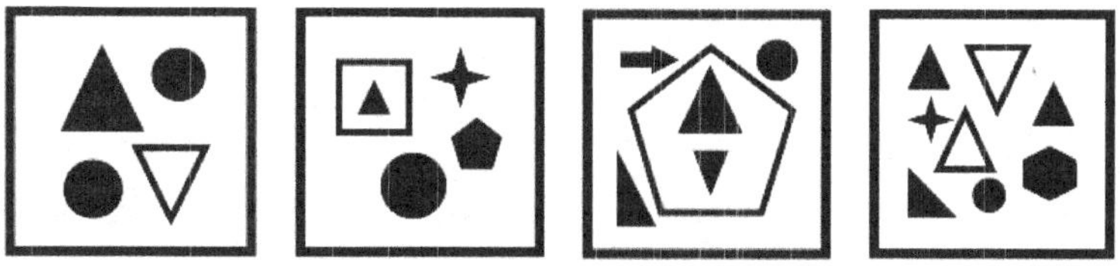

A)  B)  C) 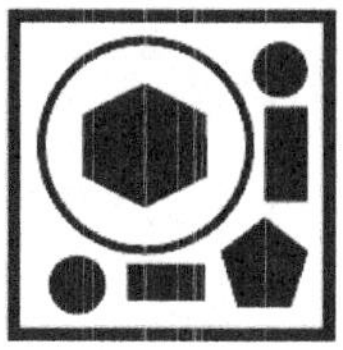 D) 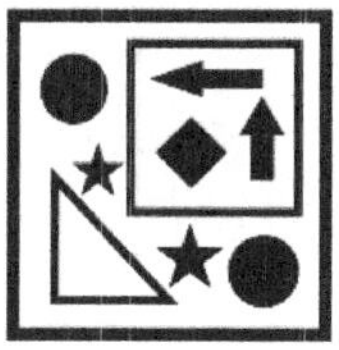

Q212

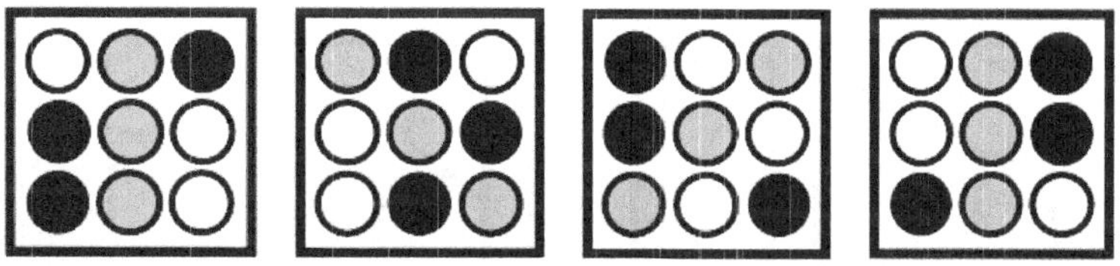

A) 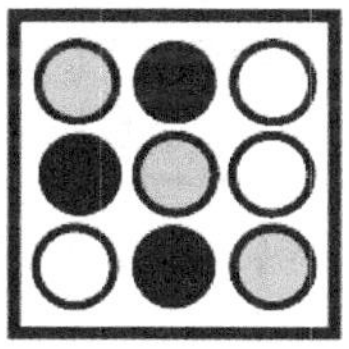 B) 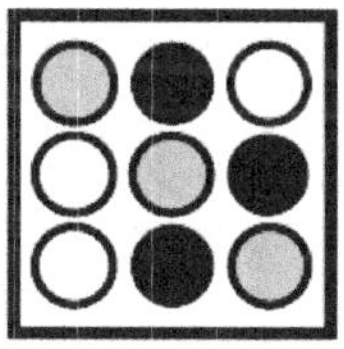 C) 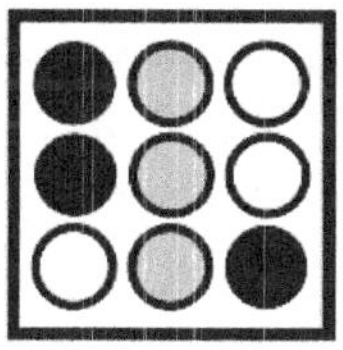 D) 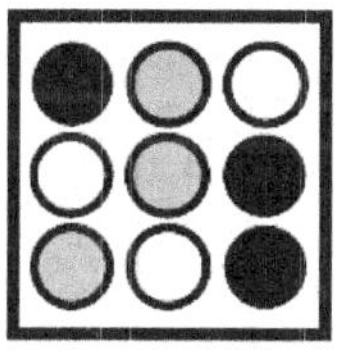

Q213

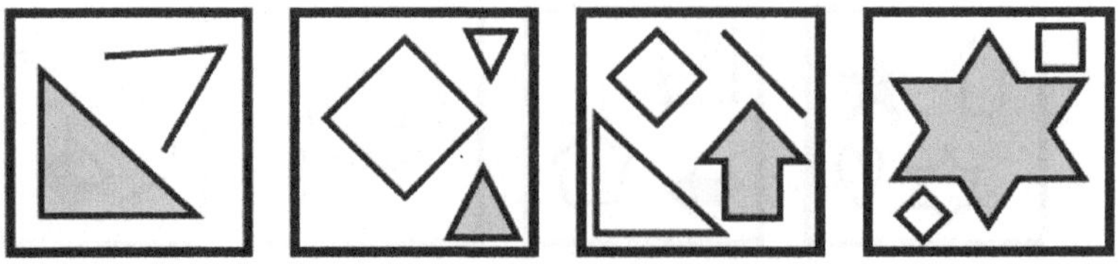

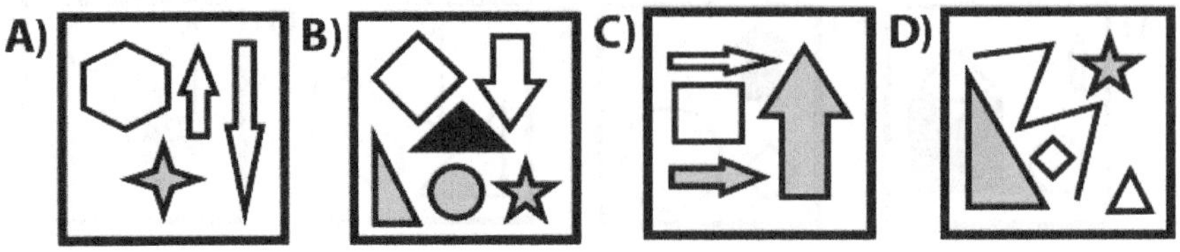

Q214

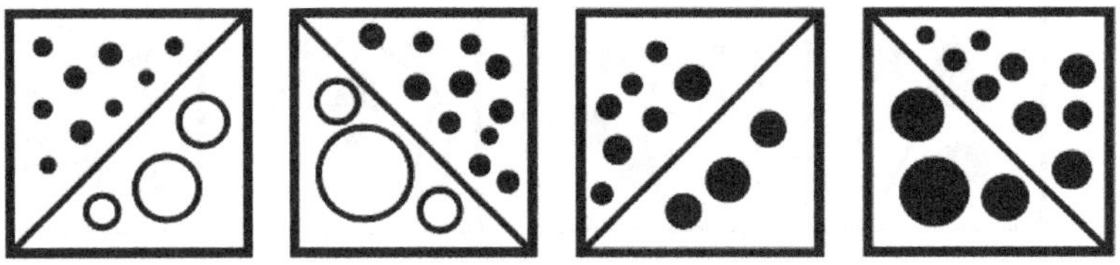

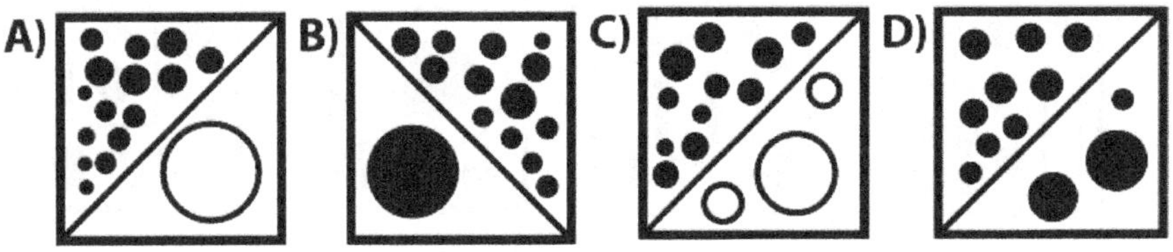

Q215

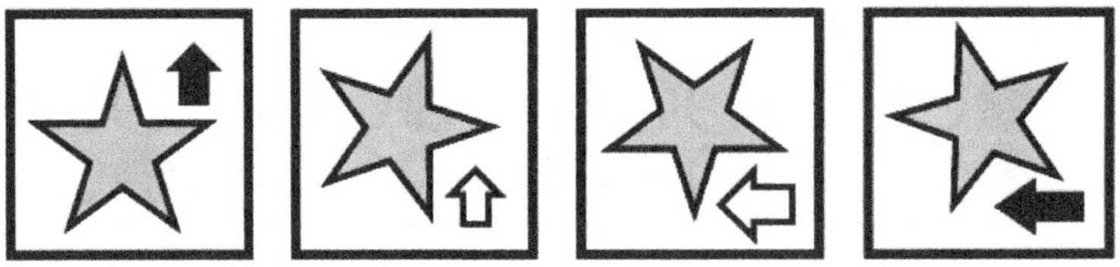

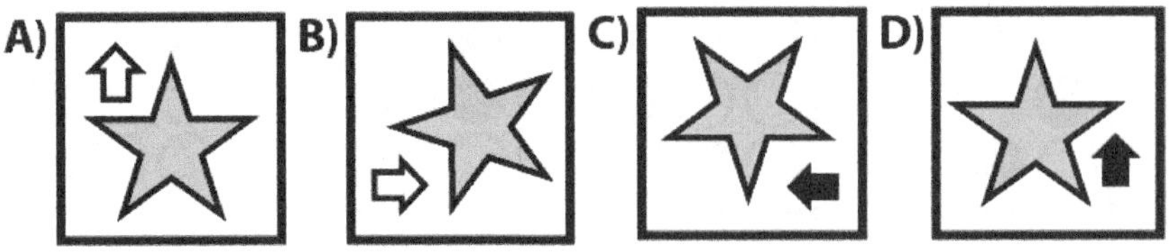

Q216

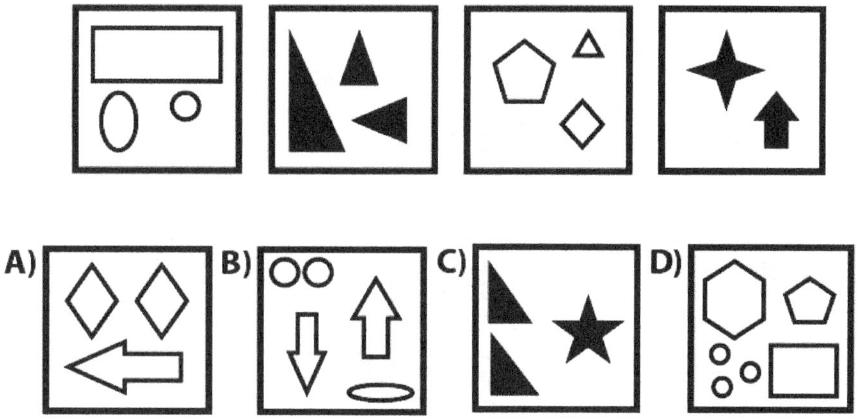

Q217

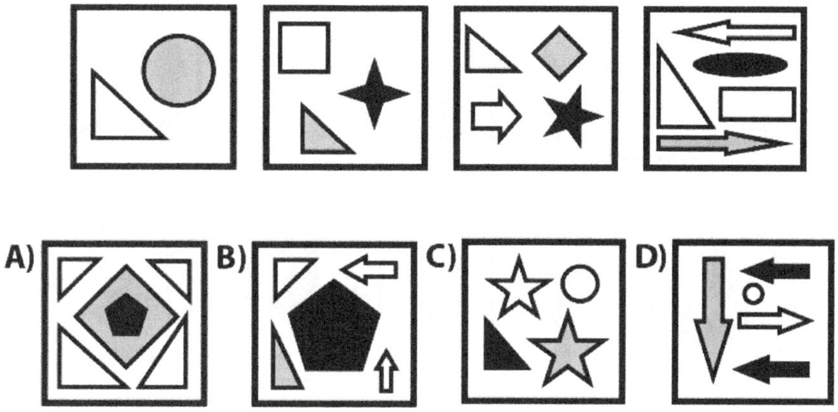

Q218

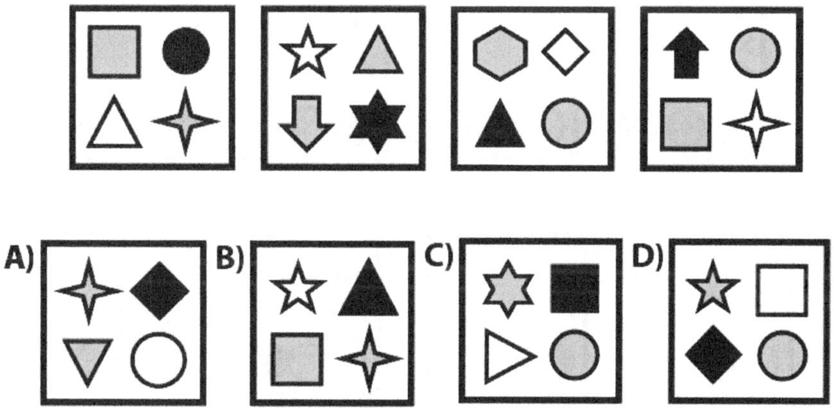

Q219

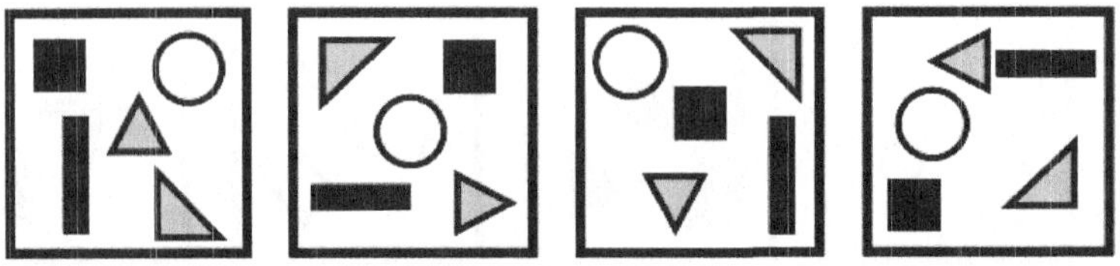

A) 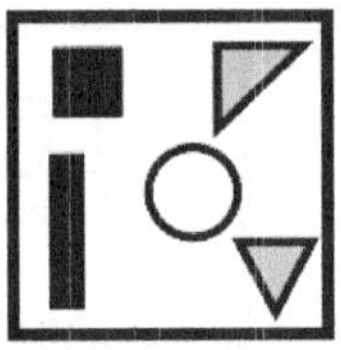 B) 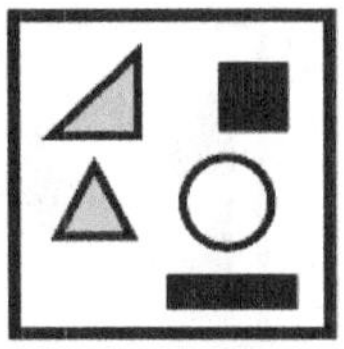 C) 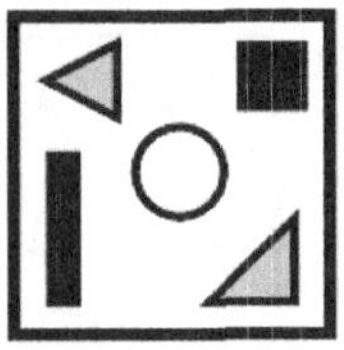 D) 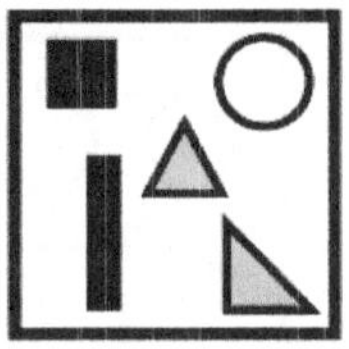

Q220

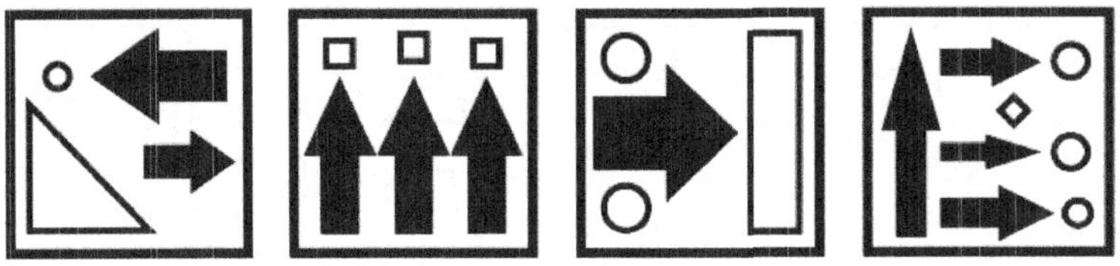

A)  B)  C)  D) 

Q221

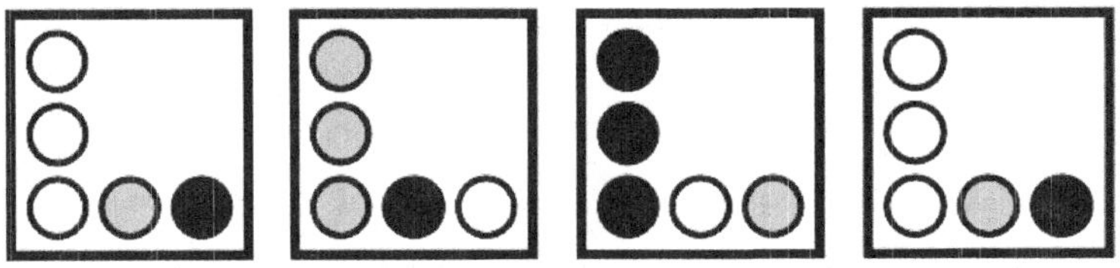

A) 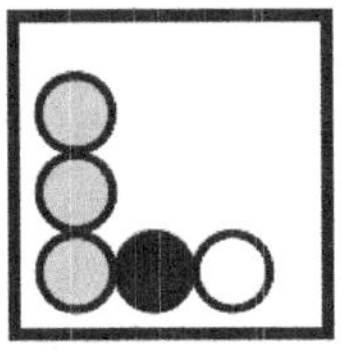 B) 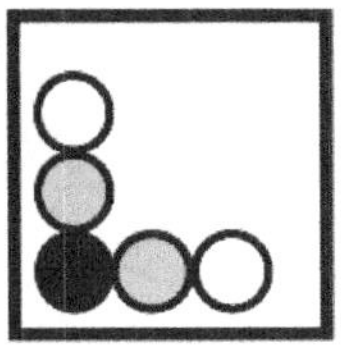 C) 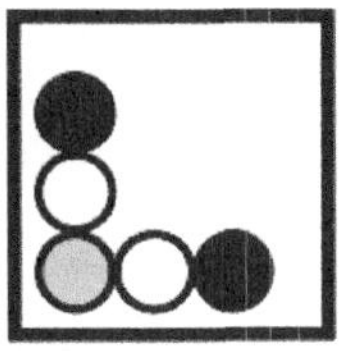 D) 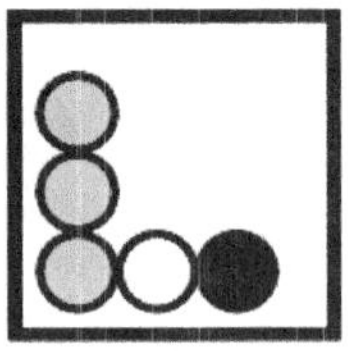

Q222

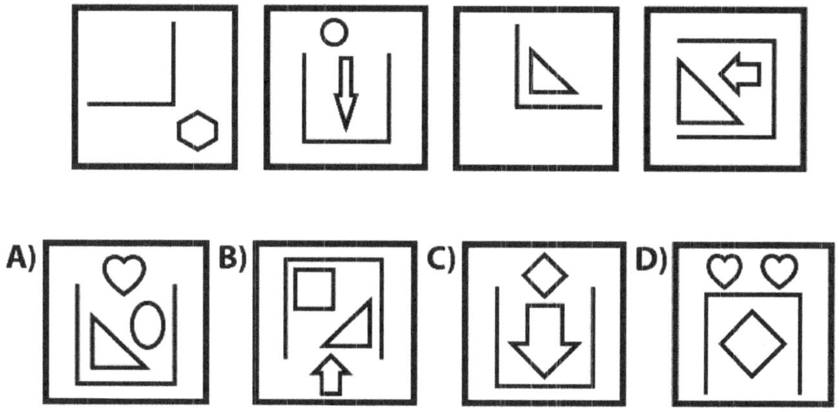

Q223

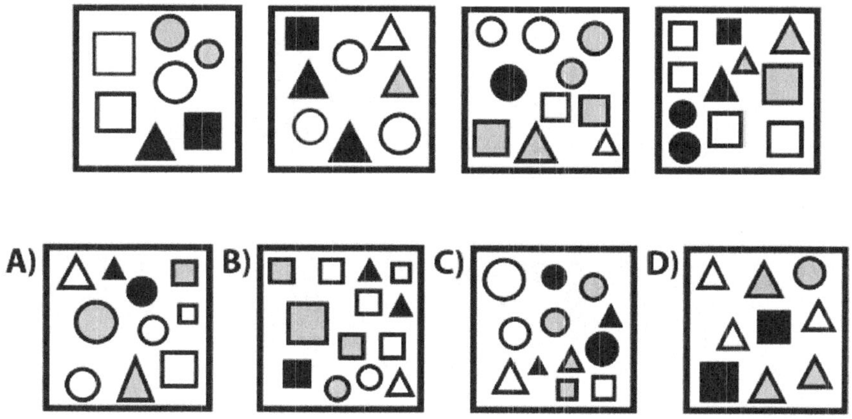

Q224

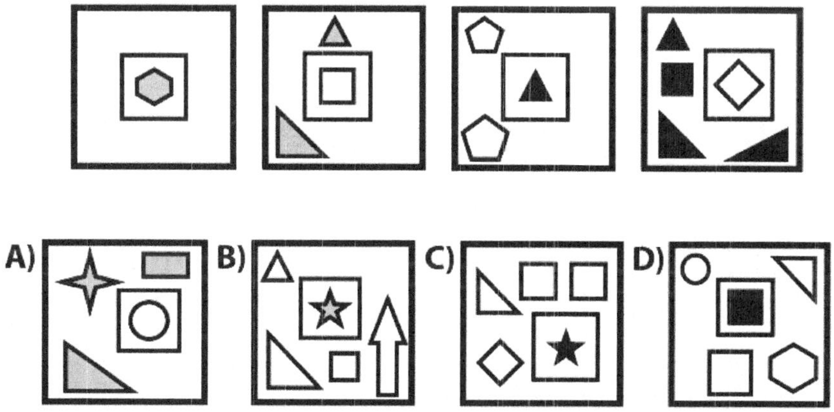

Q225

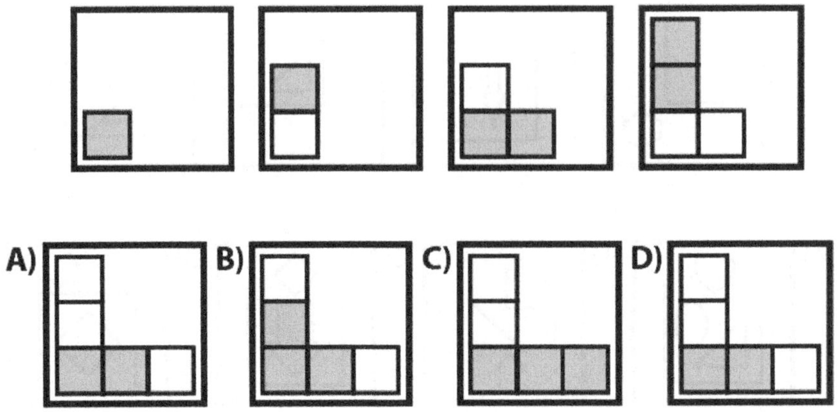

Q226

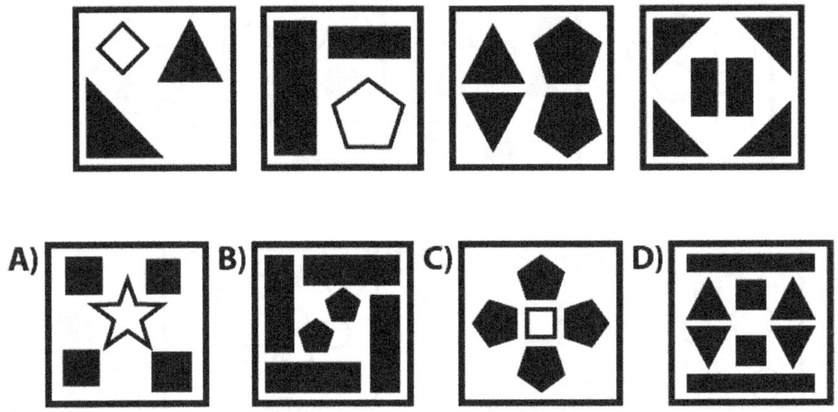

Q227

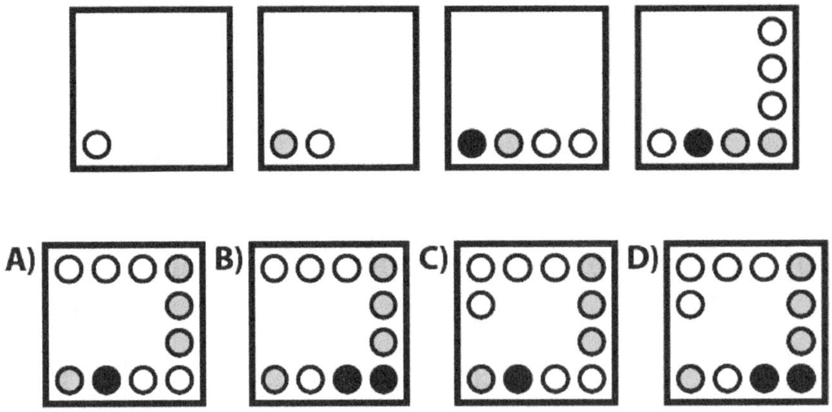

Q228

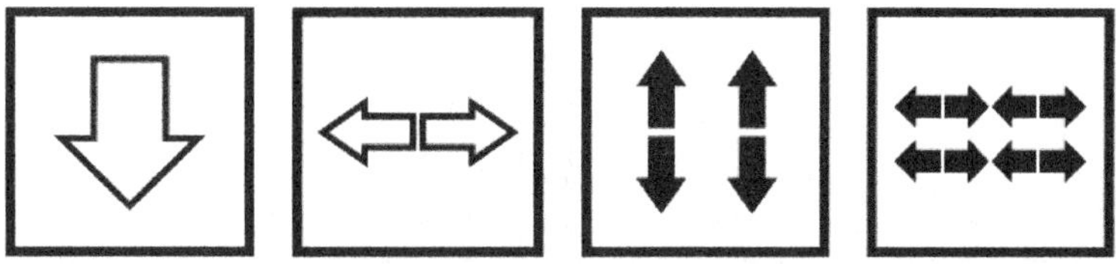

A) 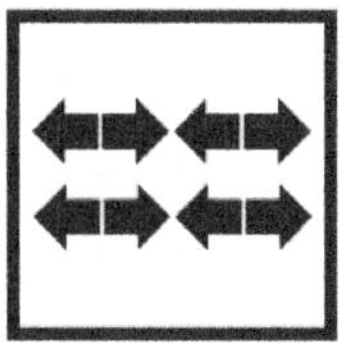
B) 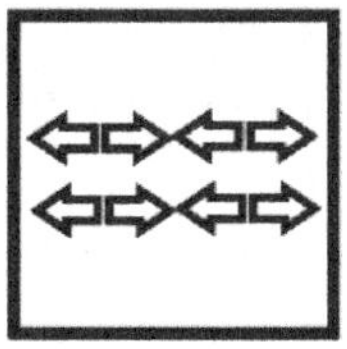
C) 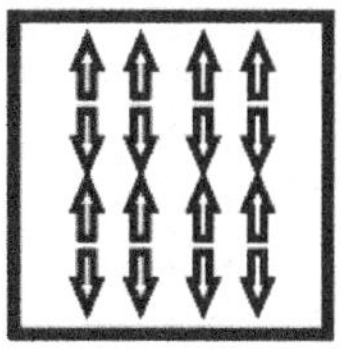
D) 

Q229

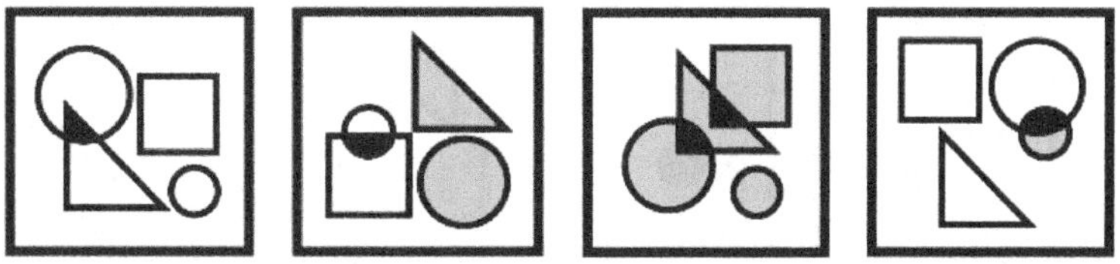

A) 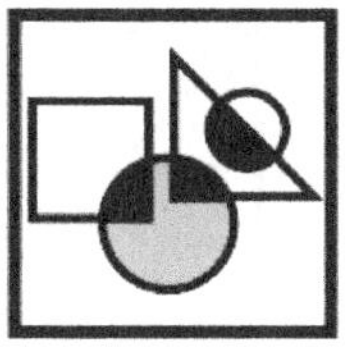
B) 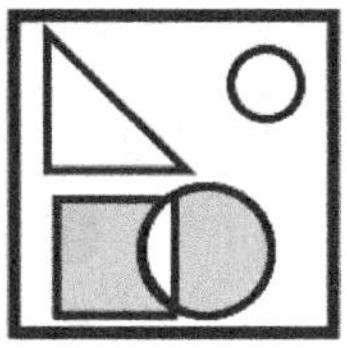
C) 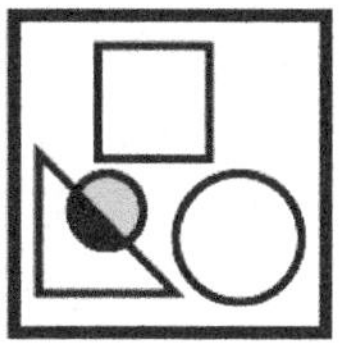
D) 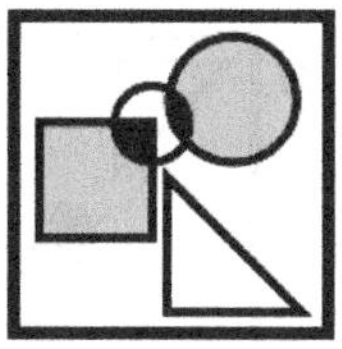

Q230

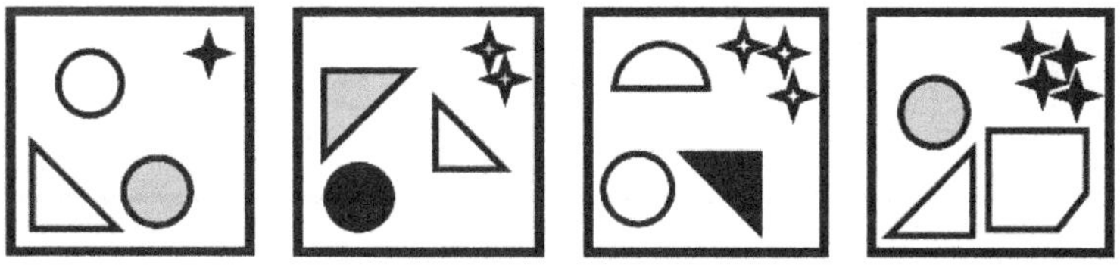

A) 
B) 
C) 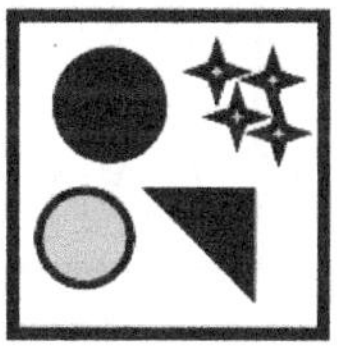
D) 

Q231

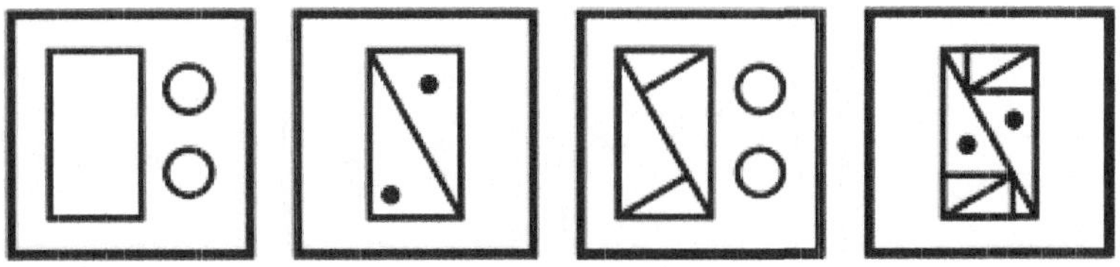

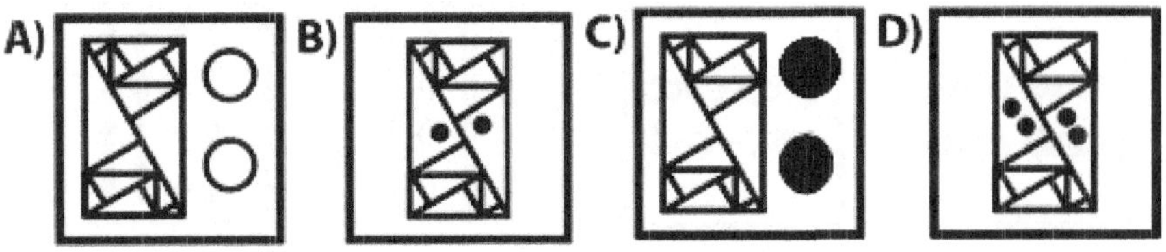

Q232

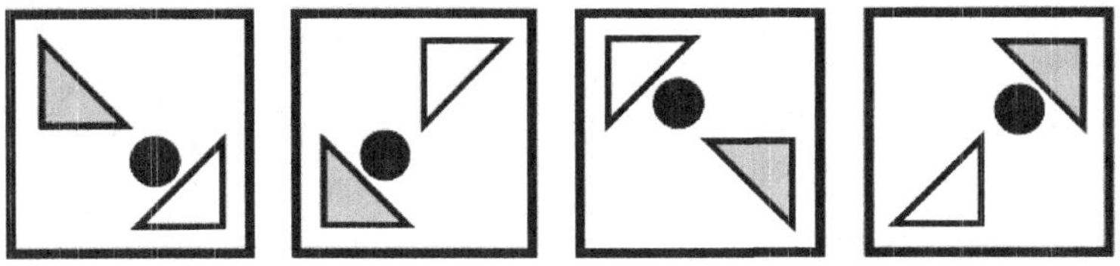

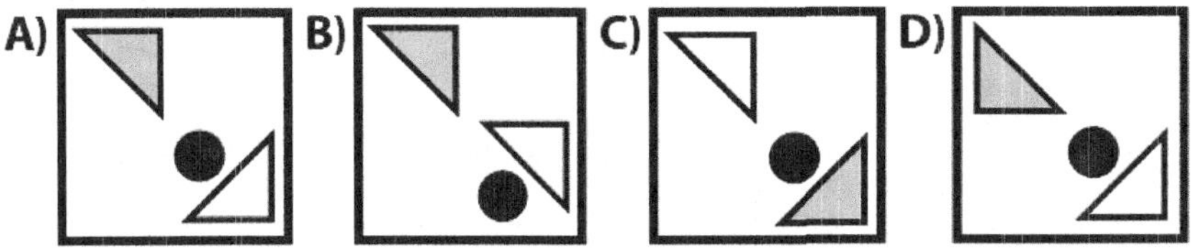

Q233

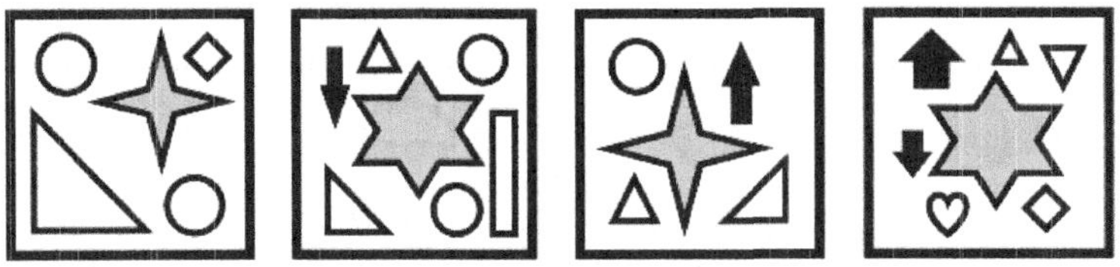

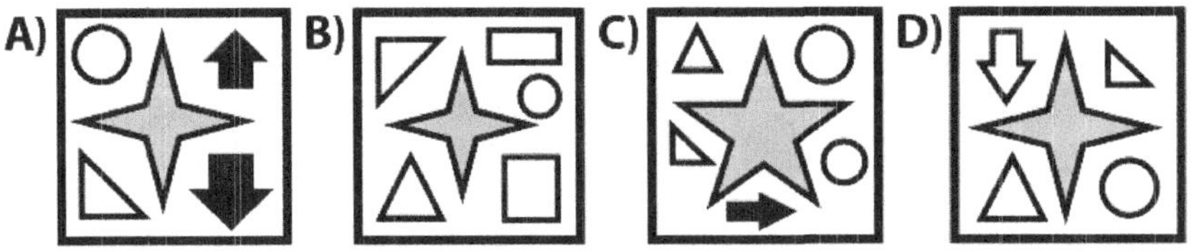

Q234

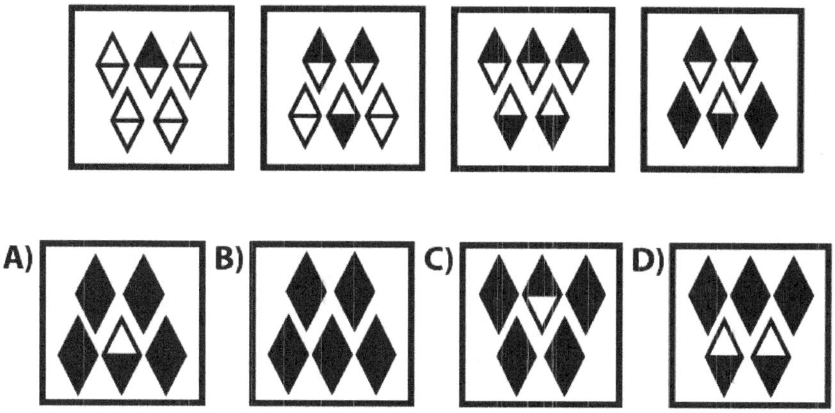

Q235

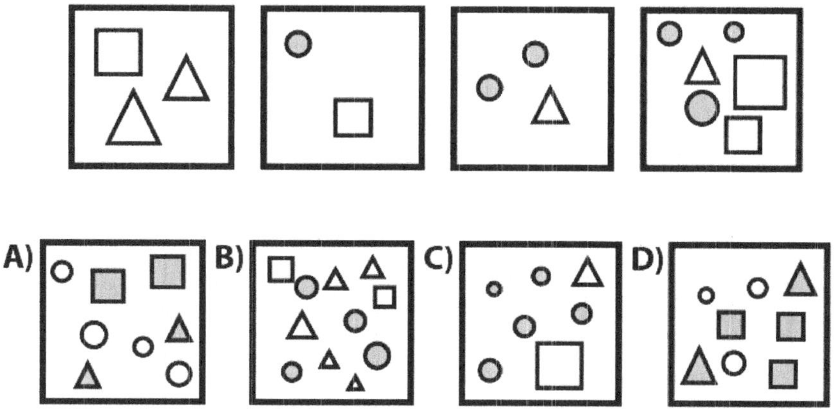

Q236

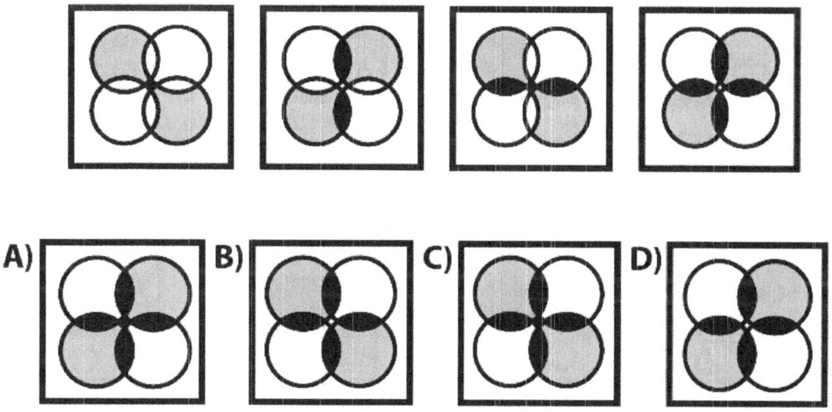

Q237

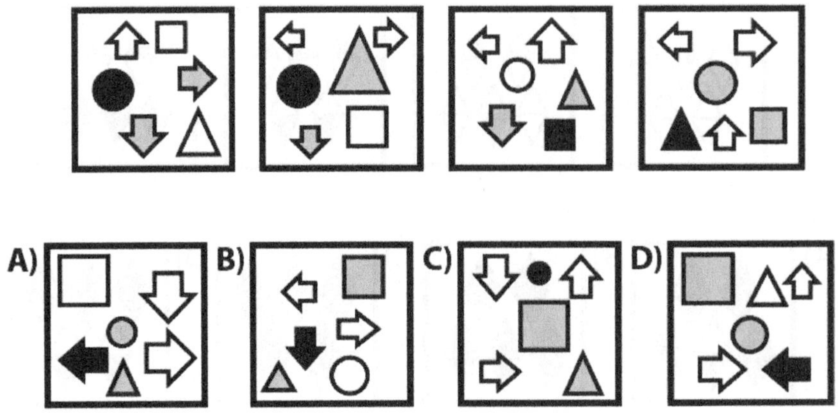

Q238

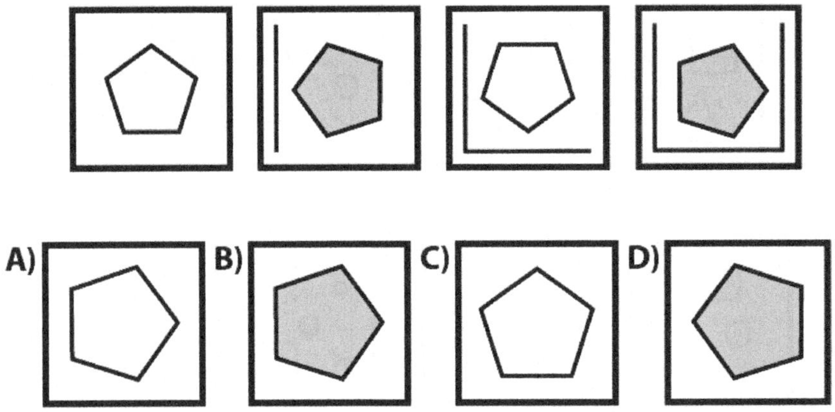

Q239

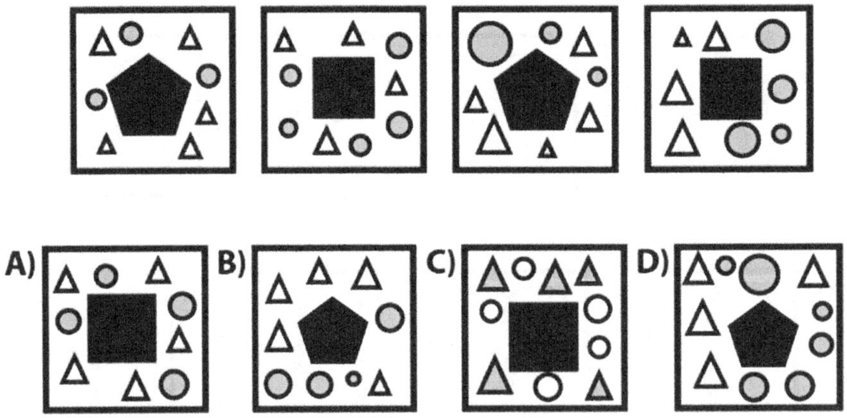

Q240

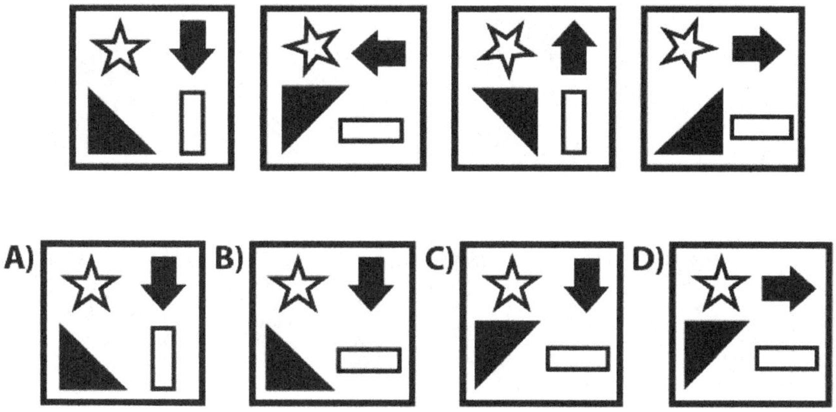

Q241

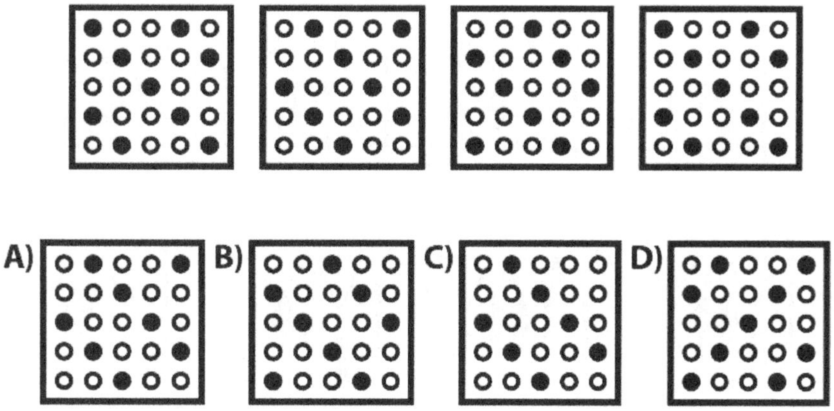

Q242

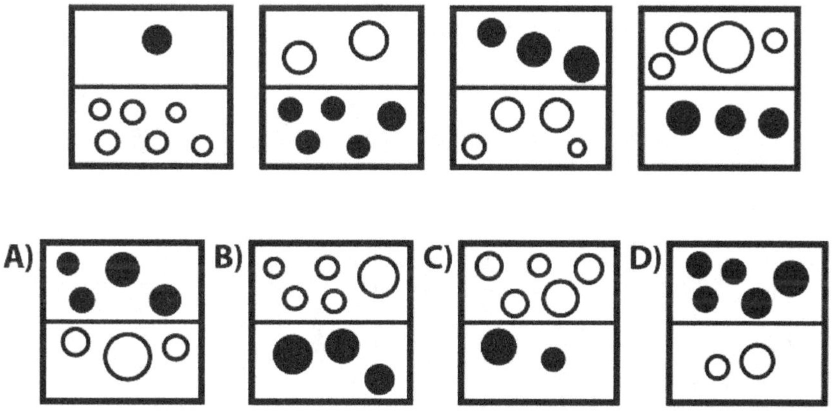

Q243

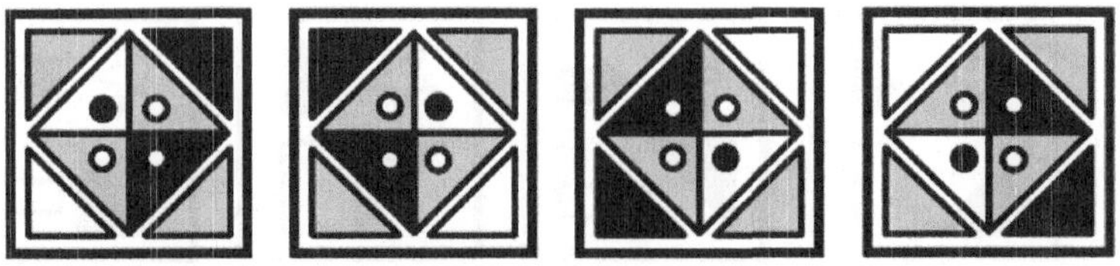

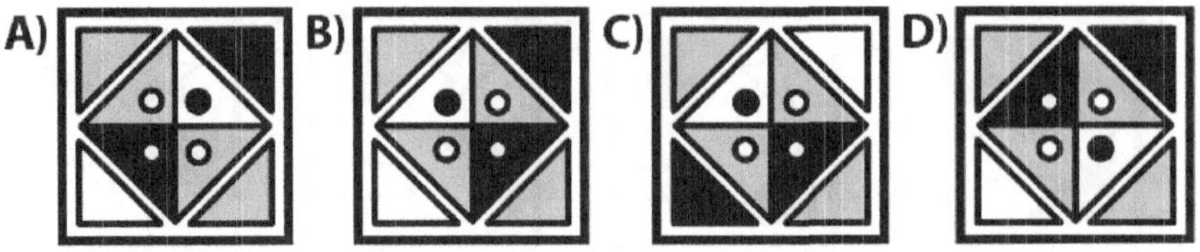

Q244

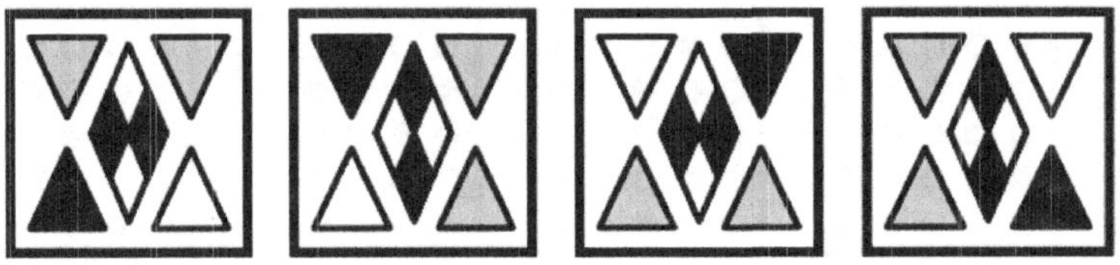

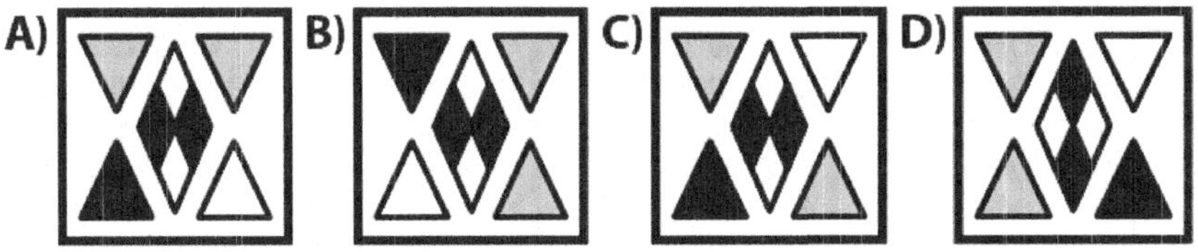

Q245

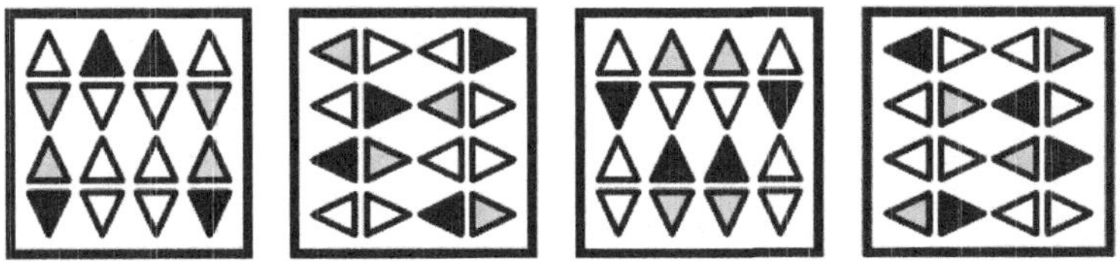

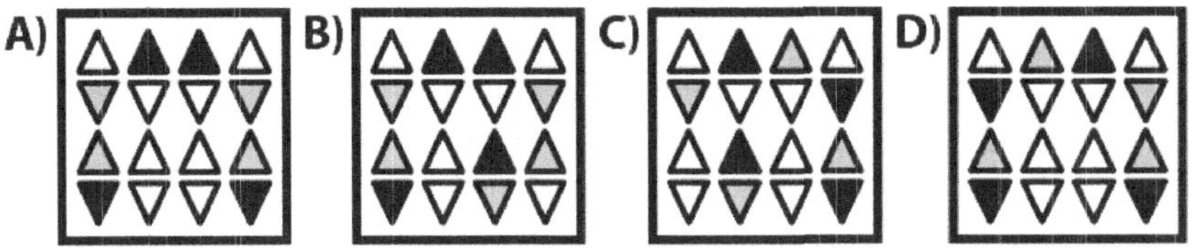

Q246

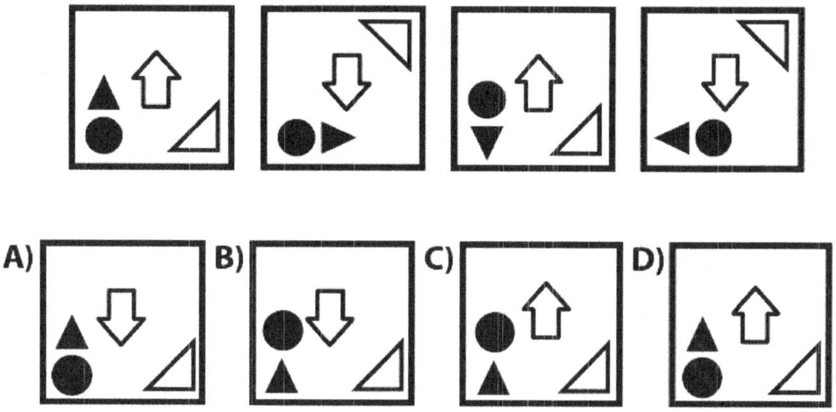

Q247

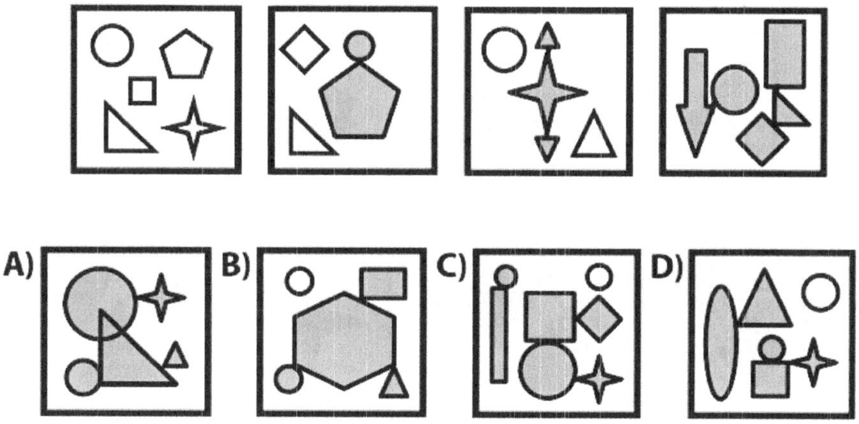

Q248

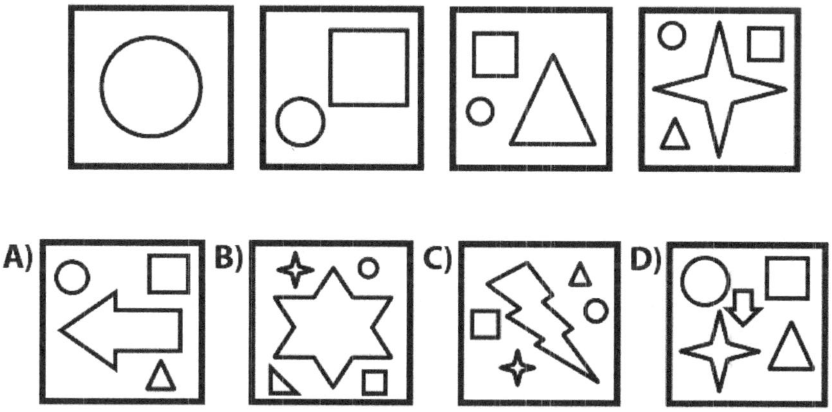

Q249

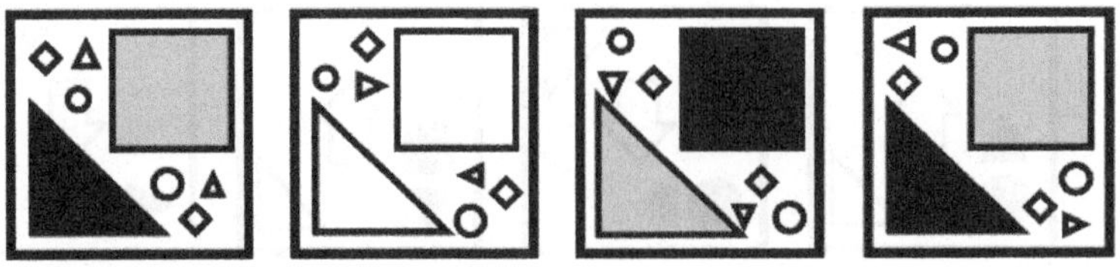

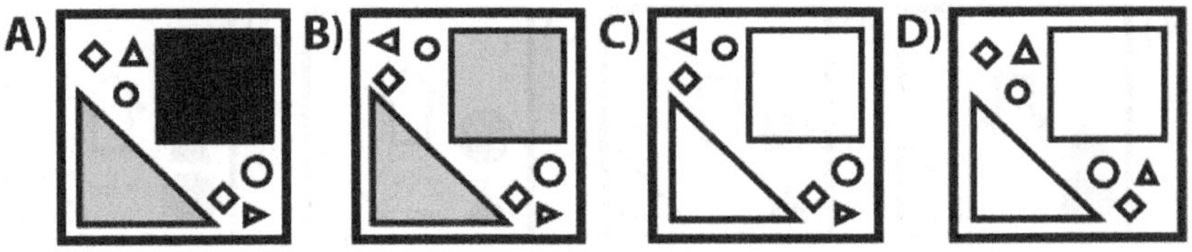

Q250

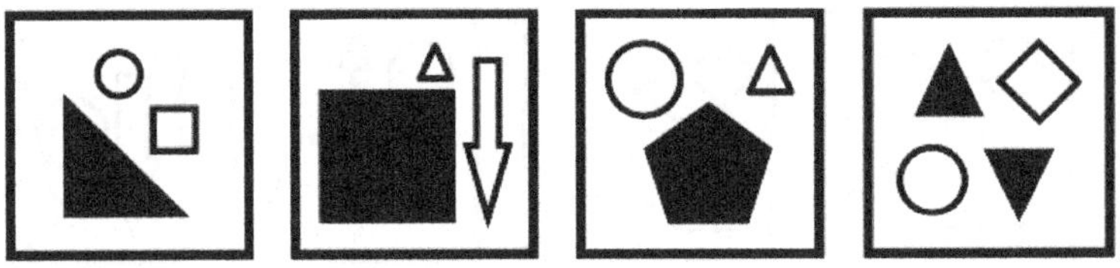

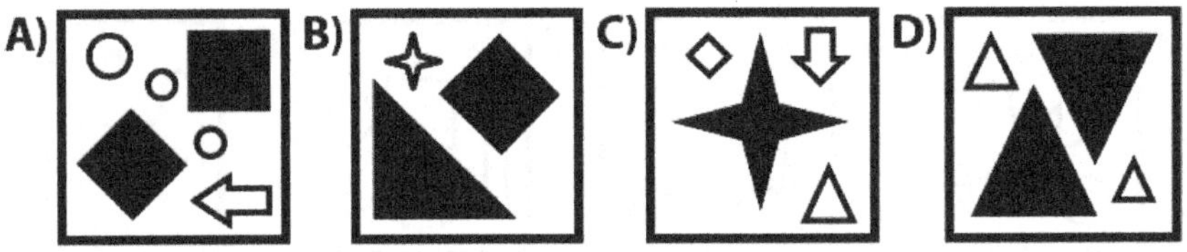

For Questions 251 – 300, which answer option completes the statement?

Q251

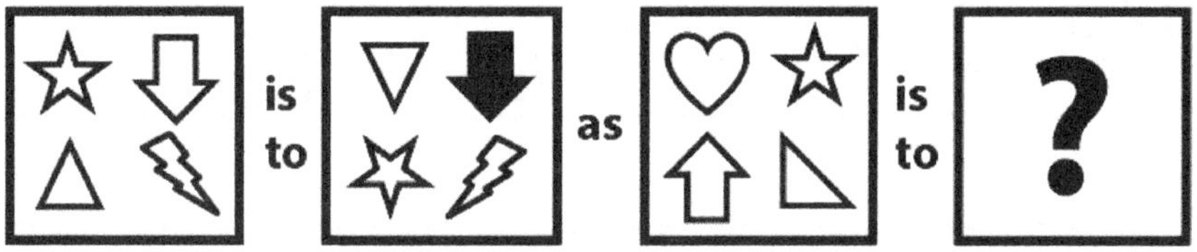

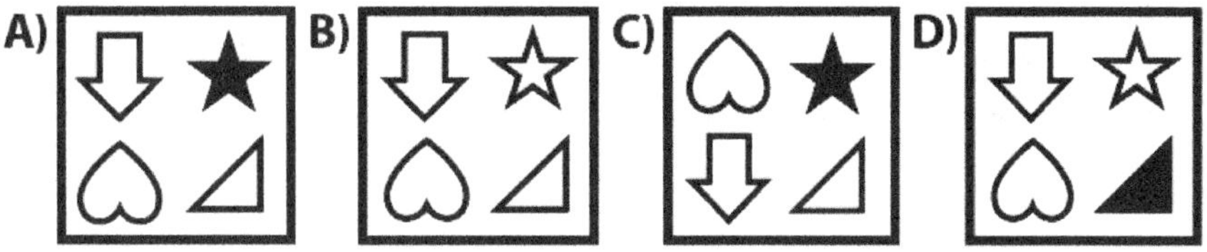

Q252

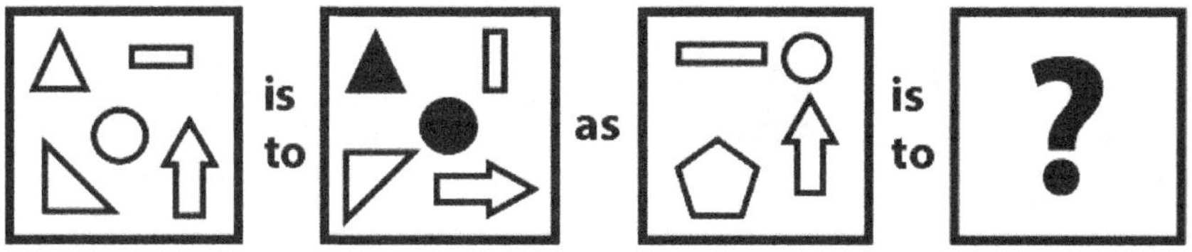

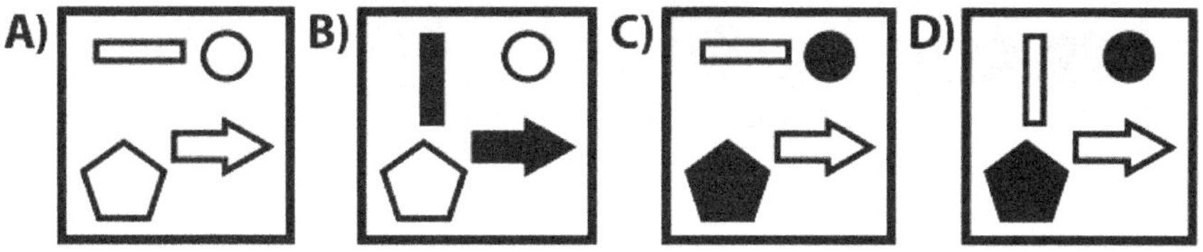

Q253

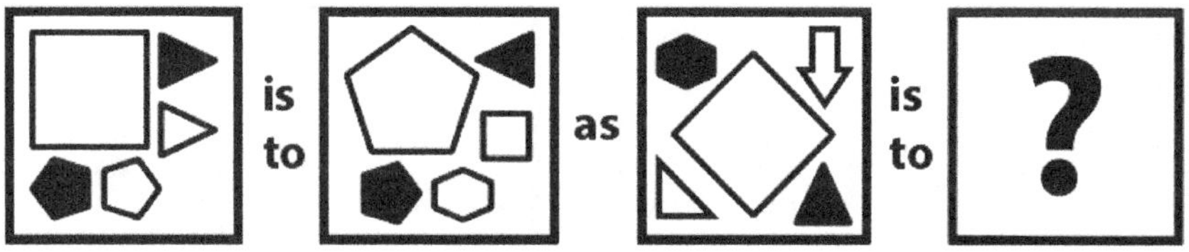

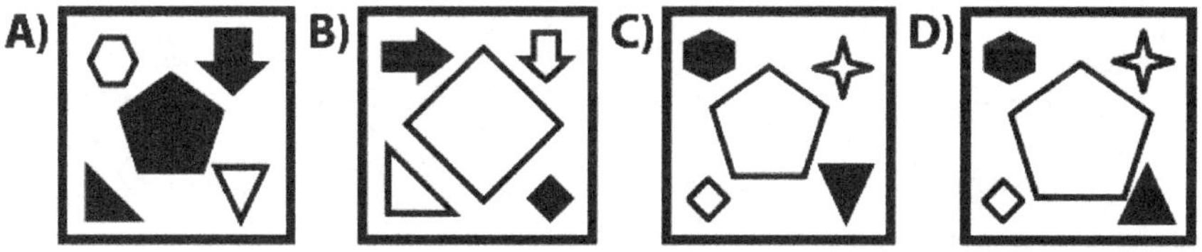

Q254

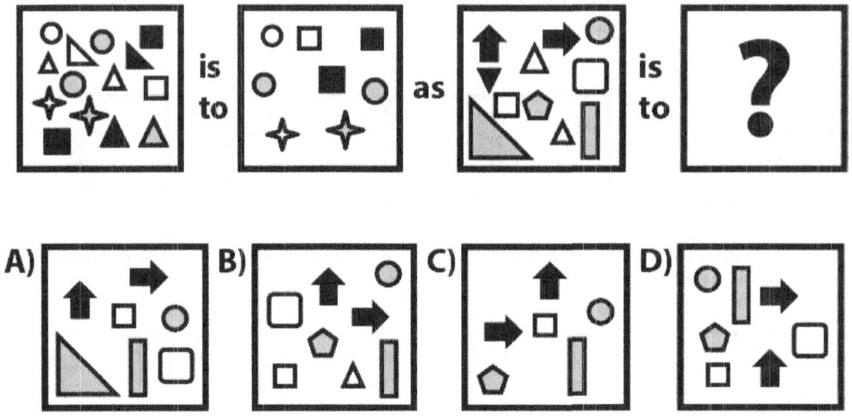

Q255

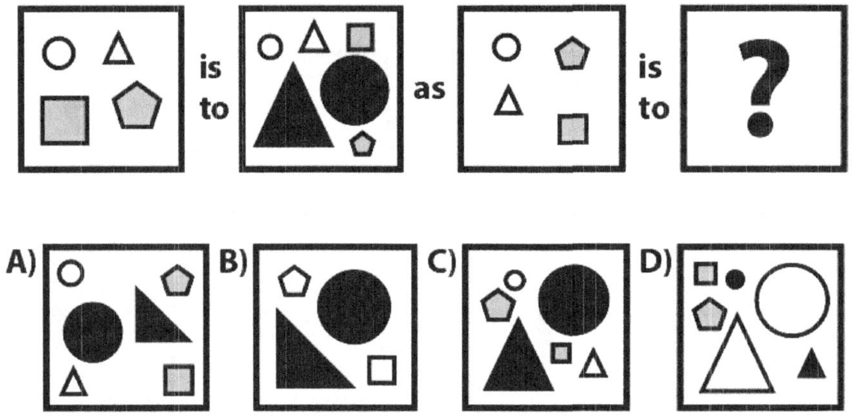

Q256

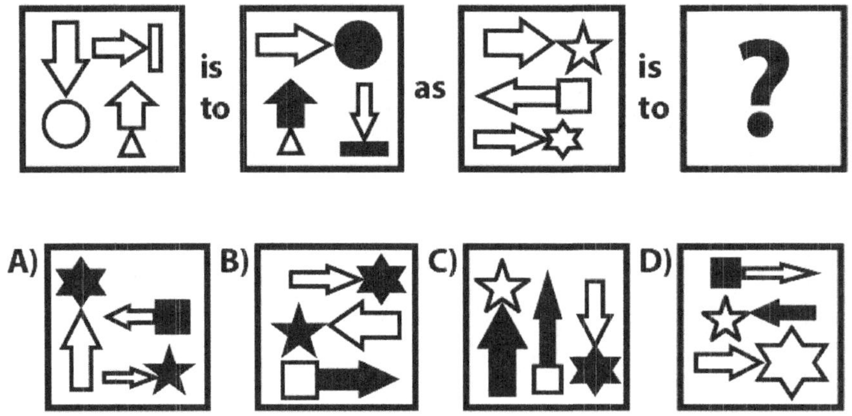

Q257

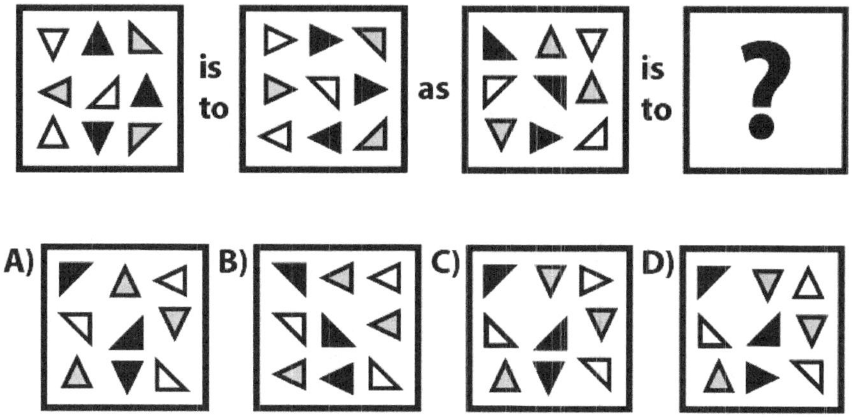

Q258

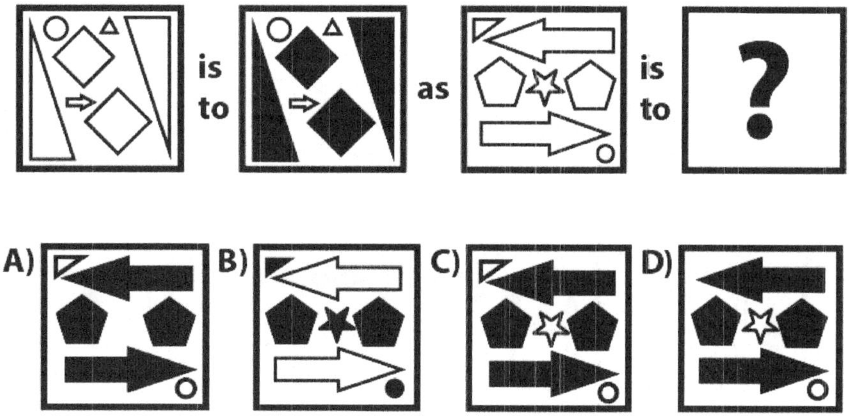

Q259

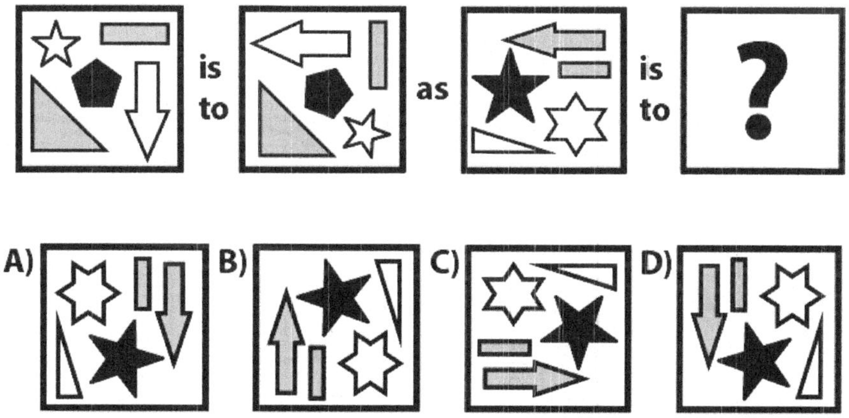

Q260

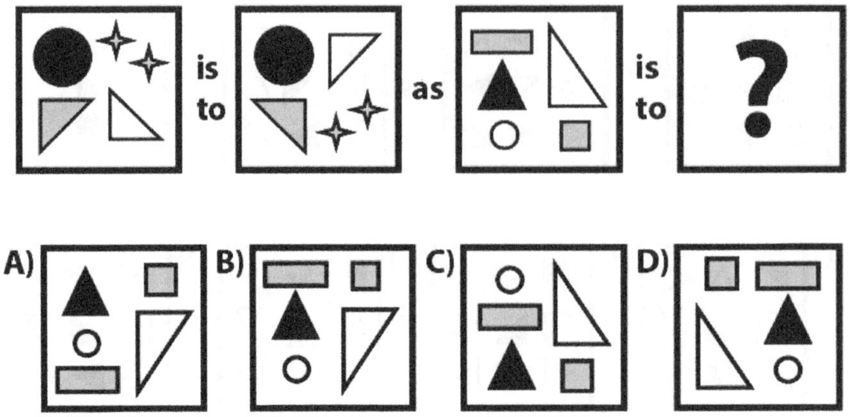

Q261

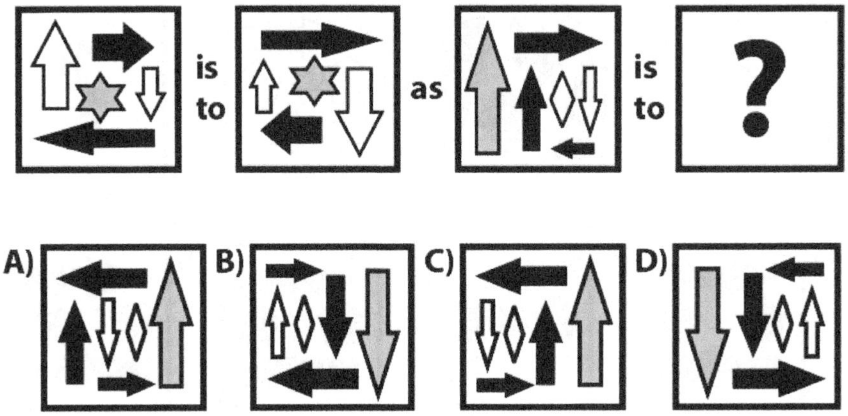

Q262

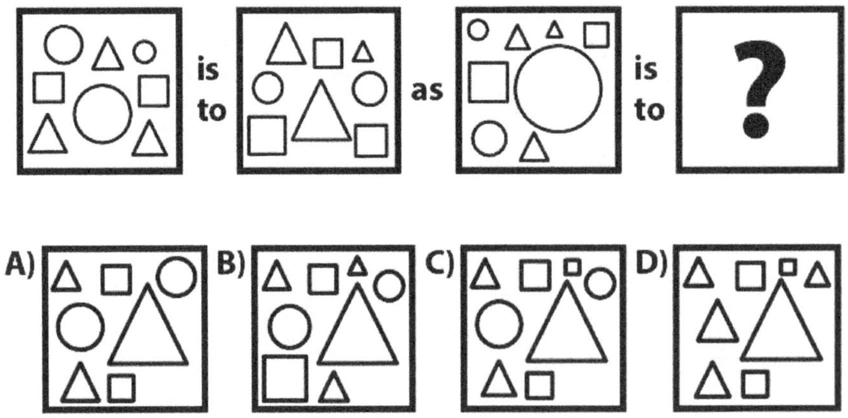

Q263

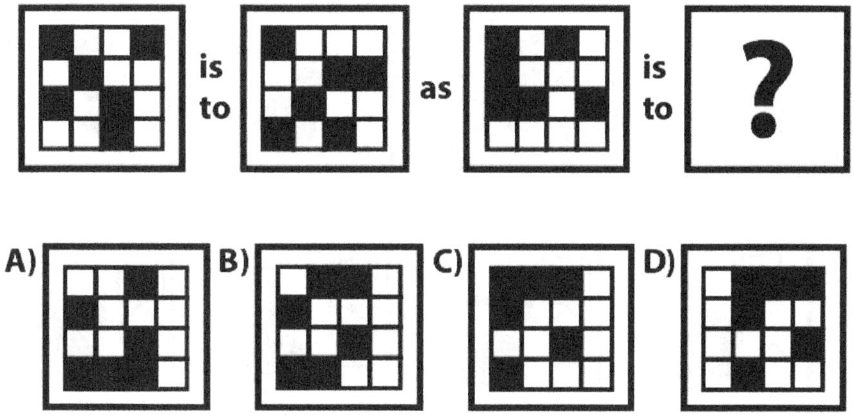

Q264

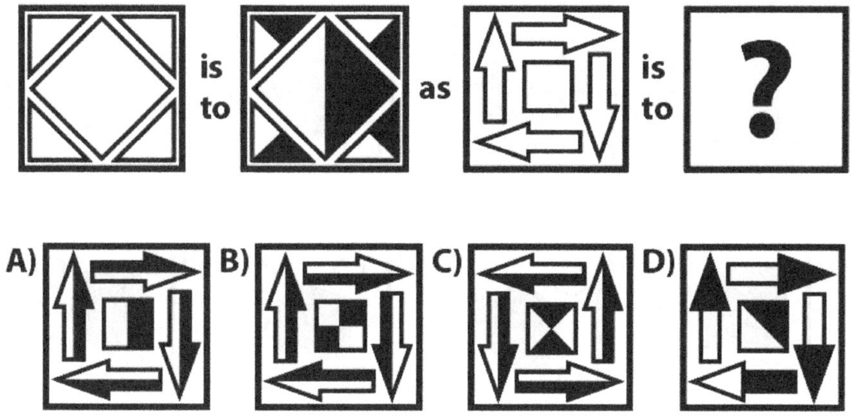

Q265

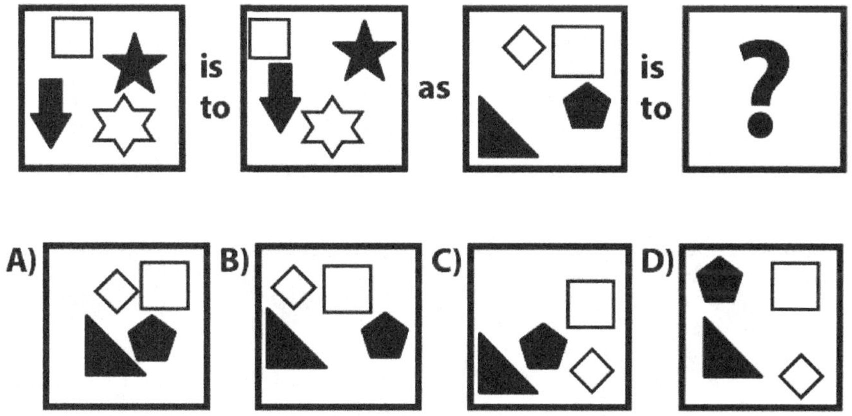

Q266

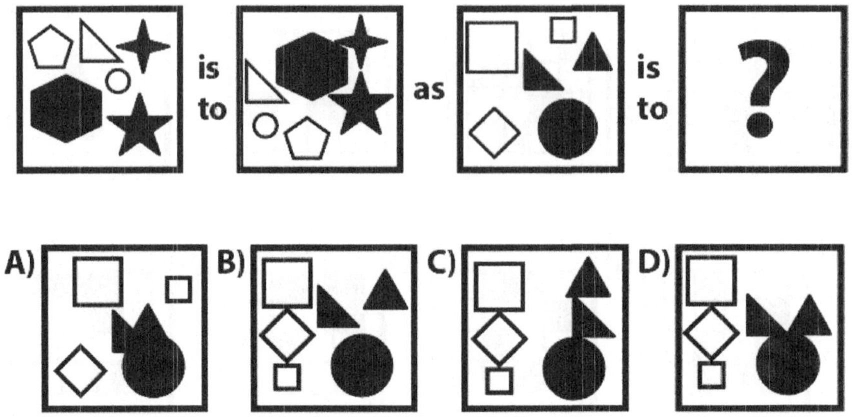

Q267

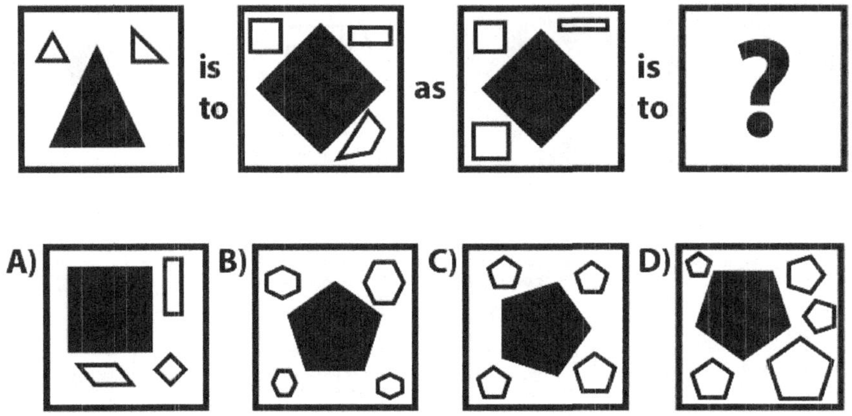

Q268

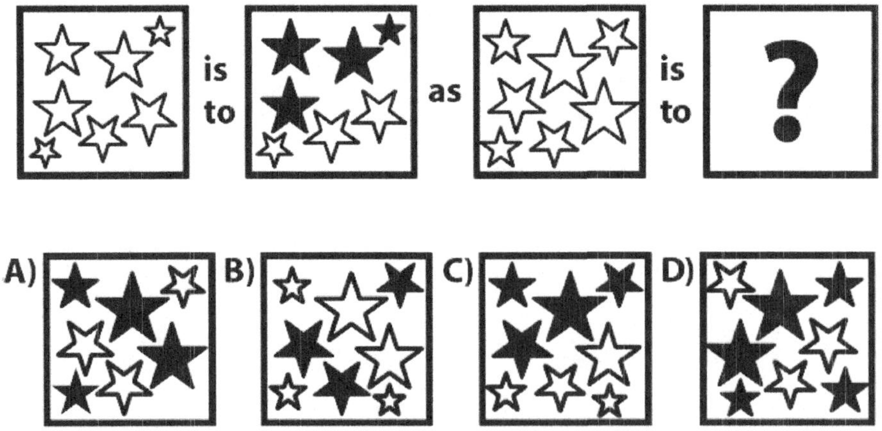

Q269

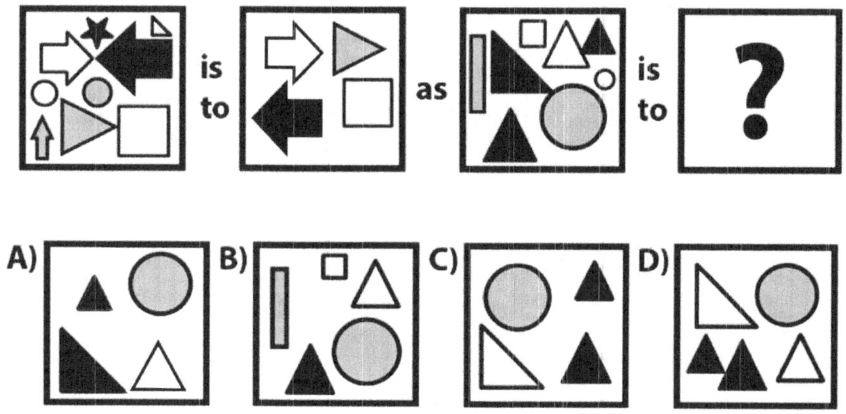

Q270

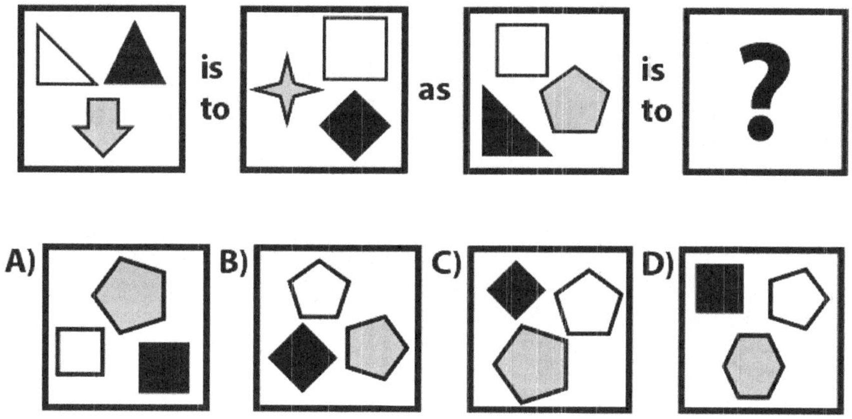

Q271

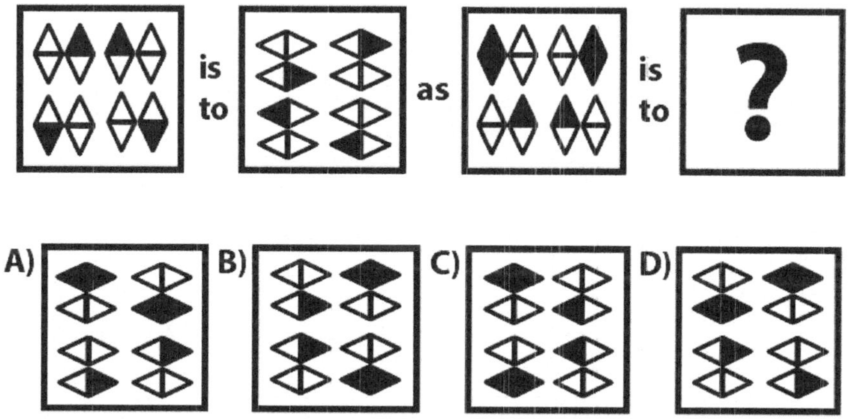

Q272

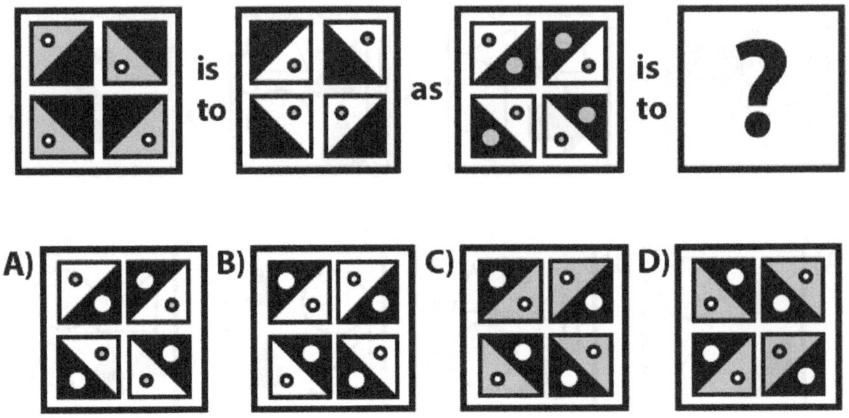

Q273

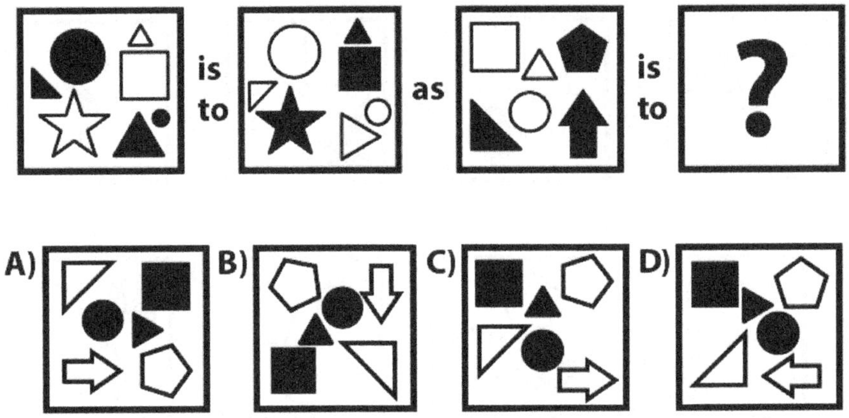

Q274

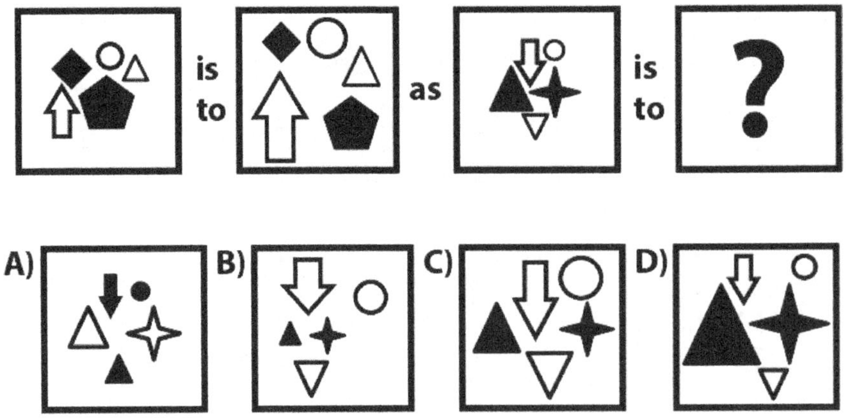

Q275

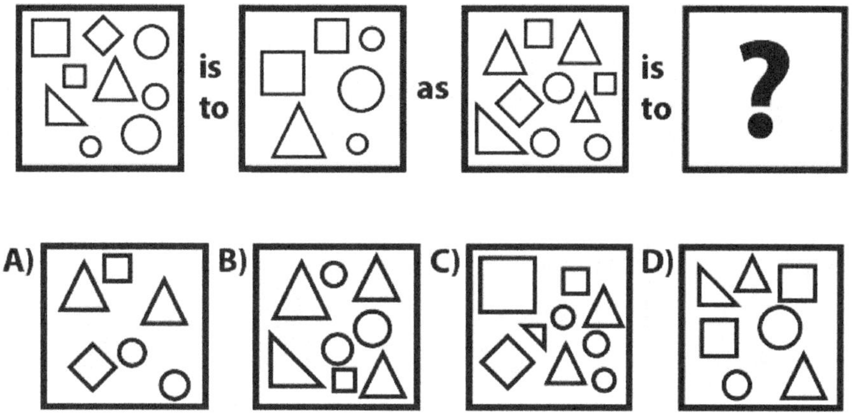

Q276

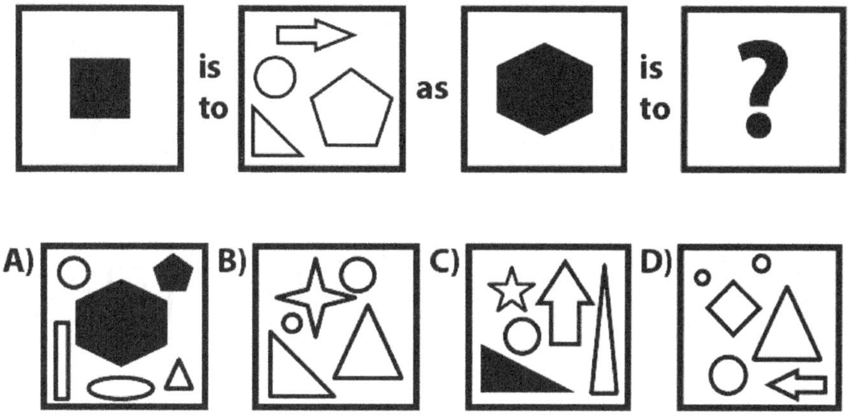

Q277

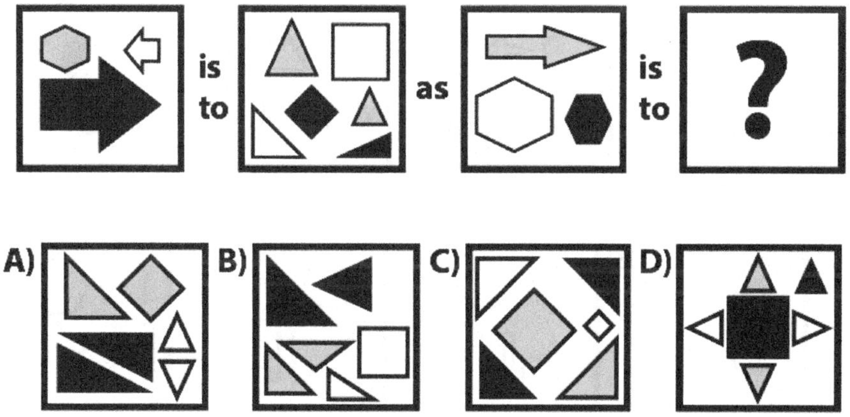

Q278

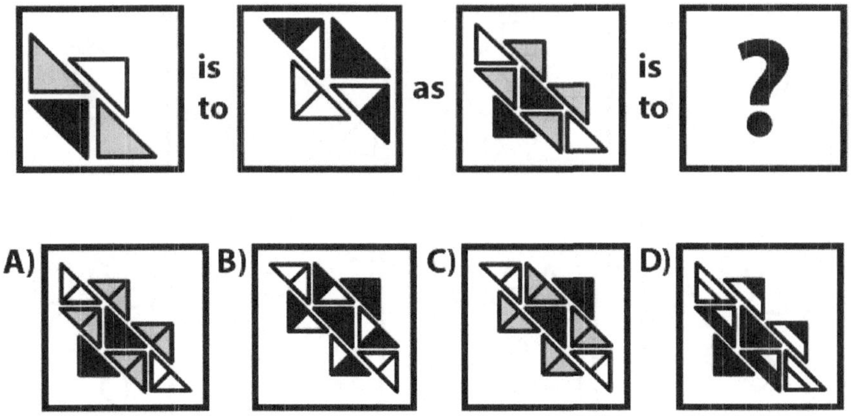

Q279

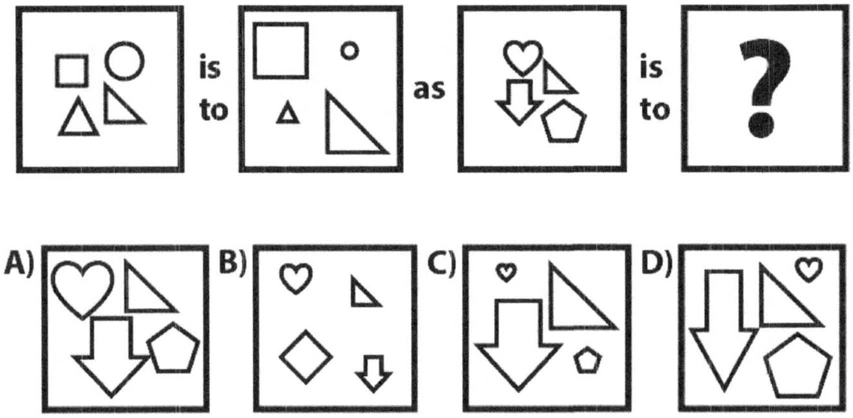

Q280

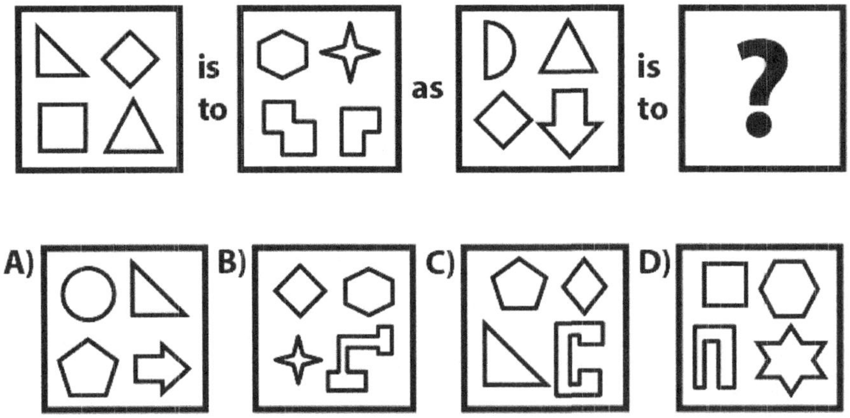

Q281

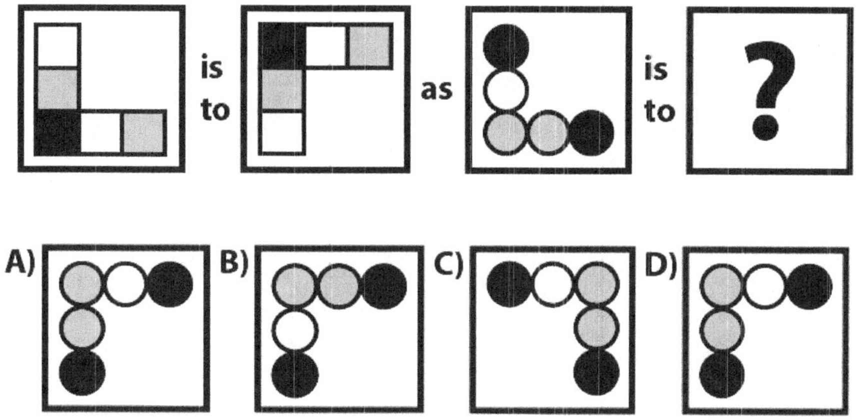

Q282

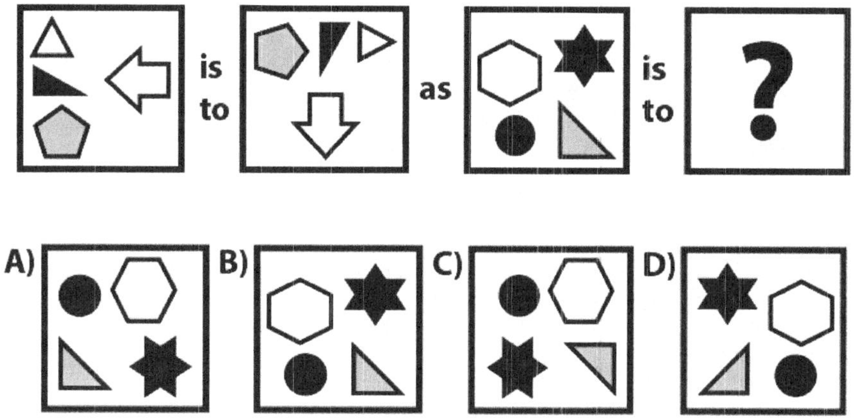

Q283

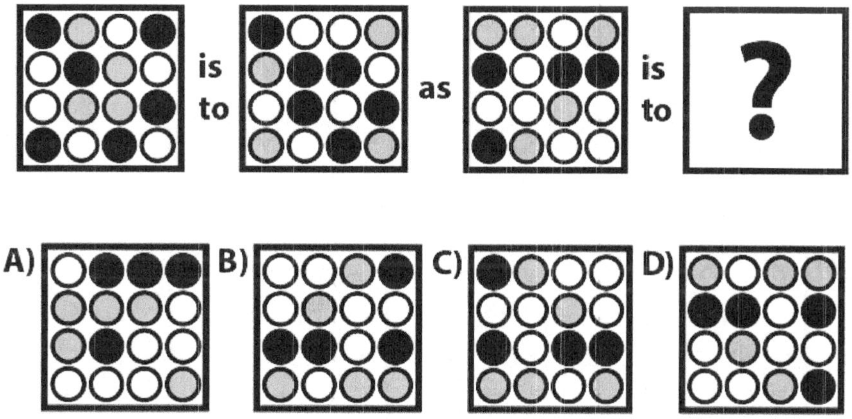

Q284

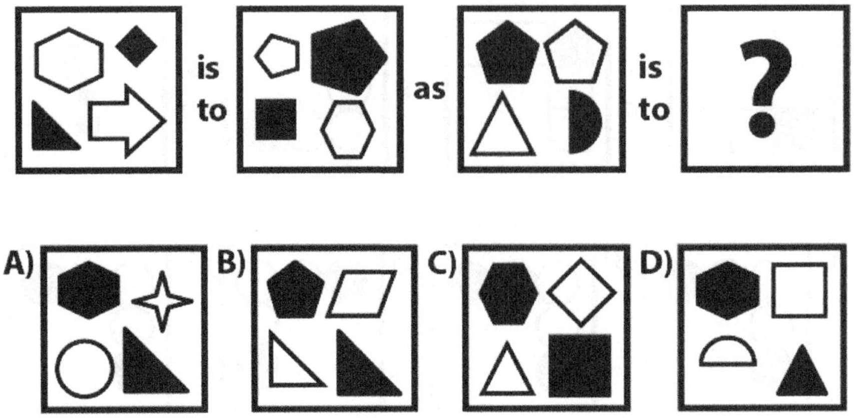

Q285

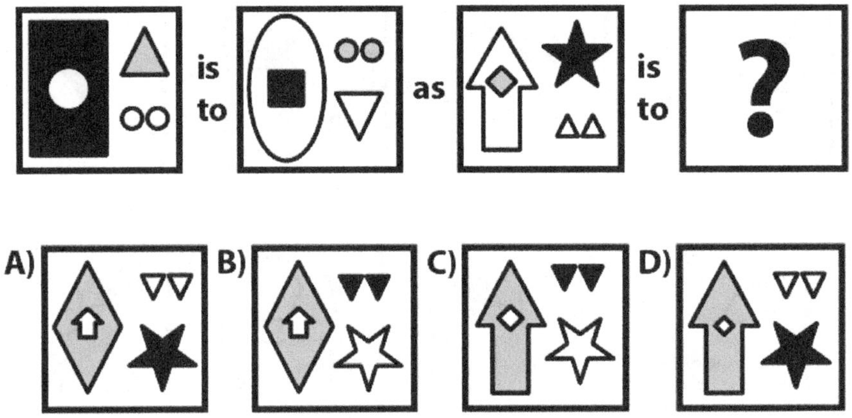

Q286

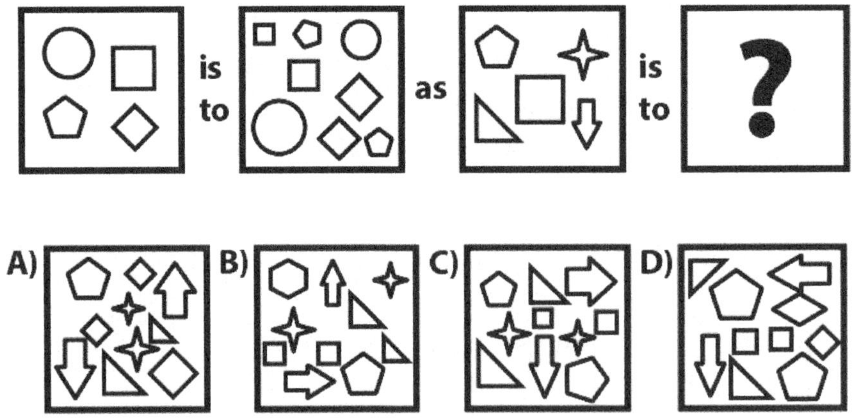

Q287

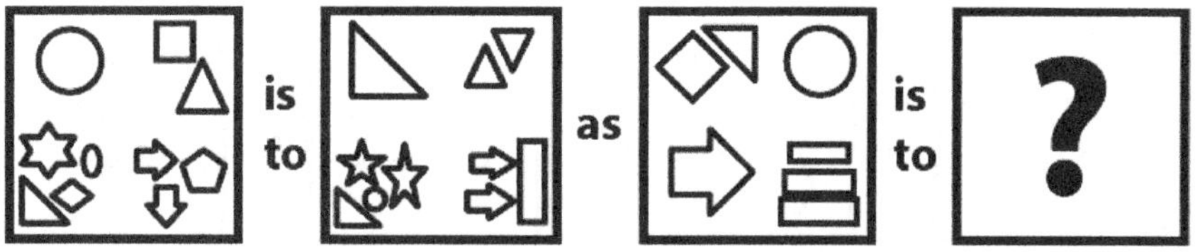

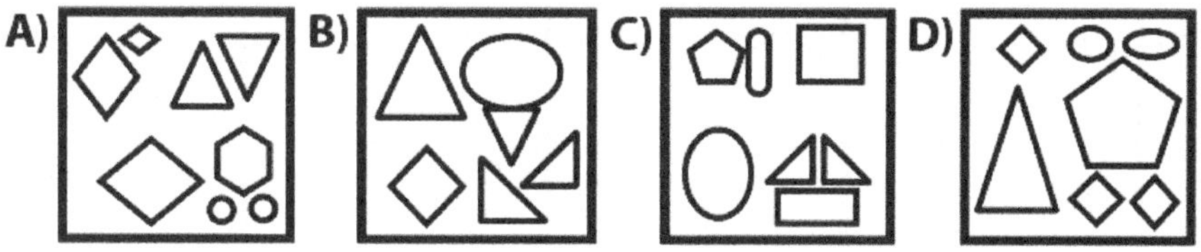

Q288

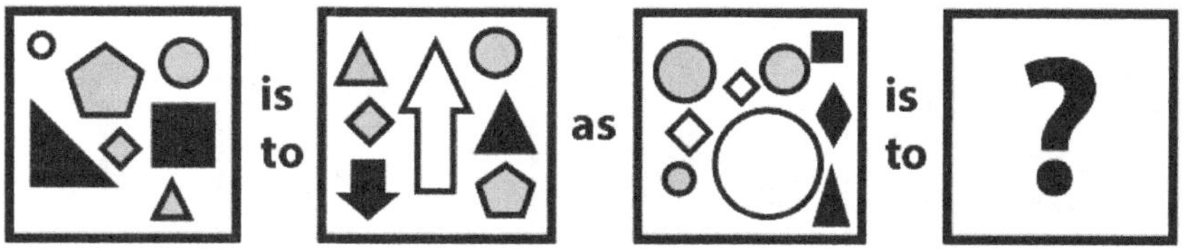

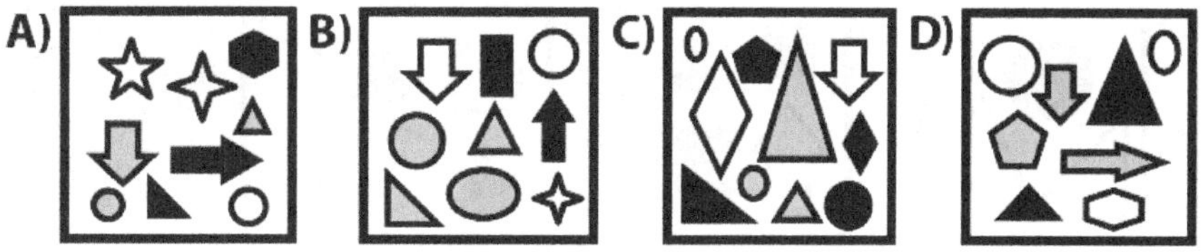

Q289

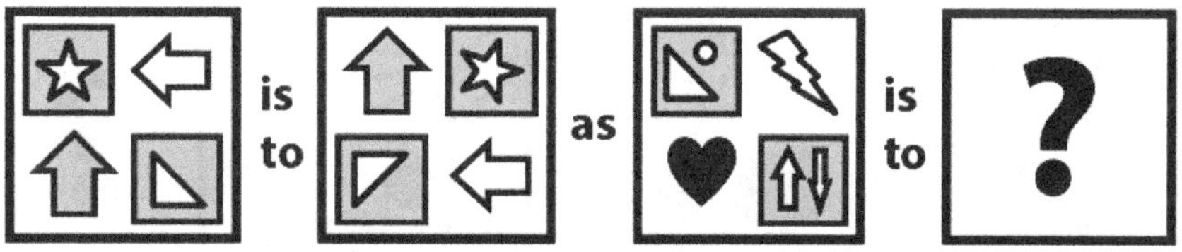

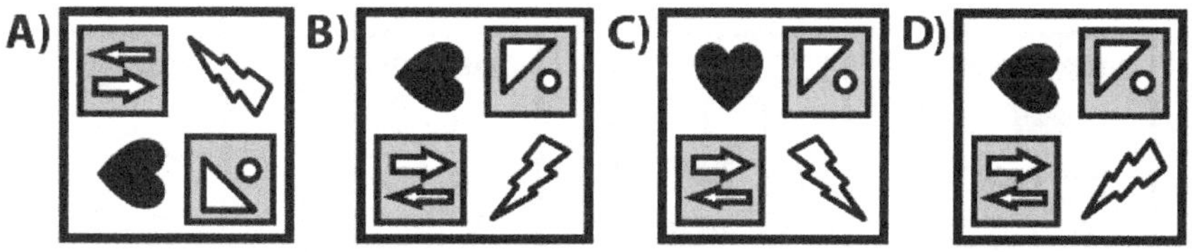

Q290

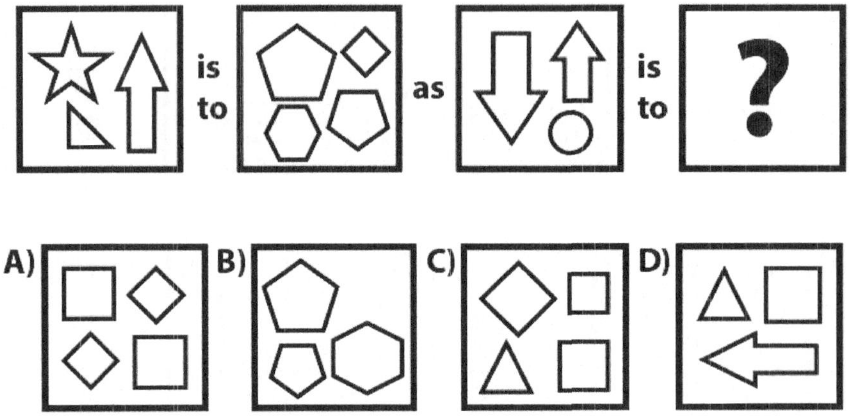

Q291

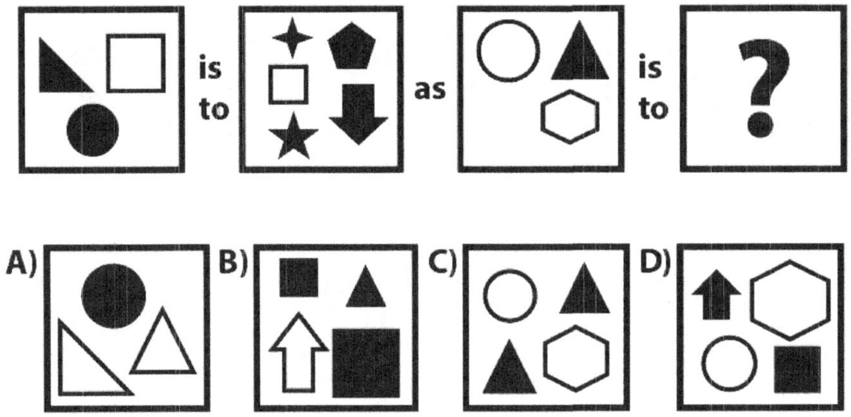

Q292

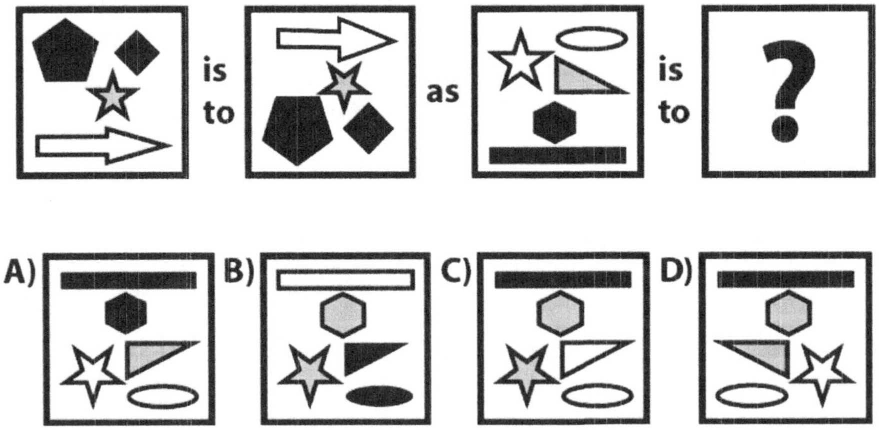

Q293

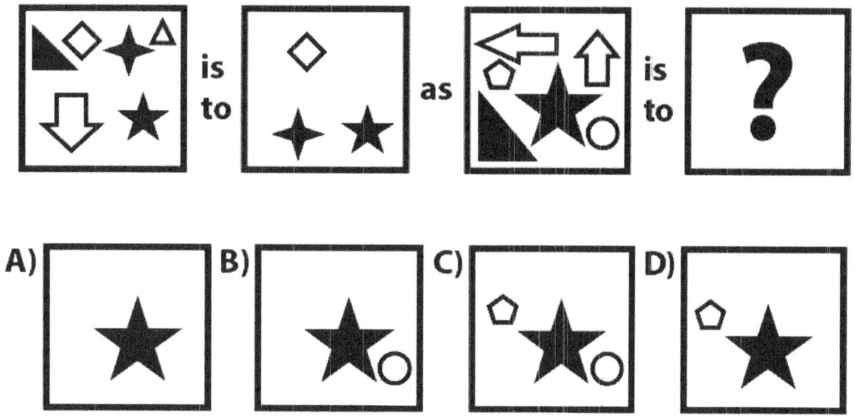

Q294

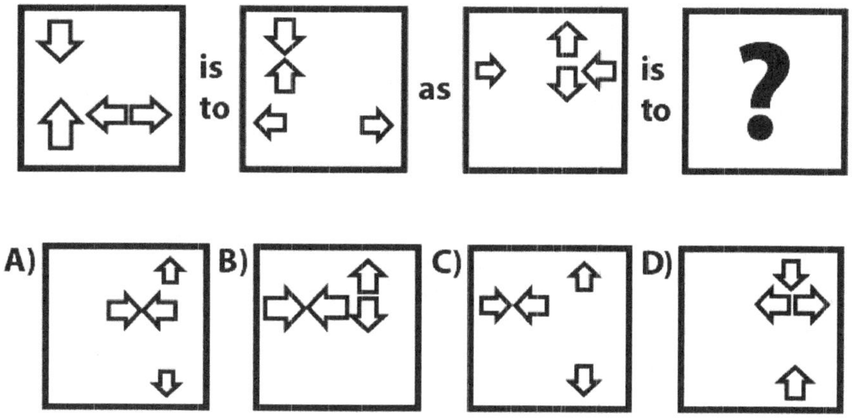

Q295

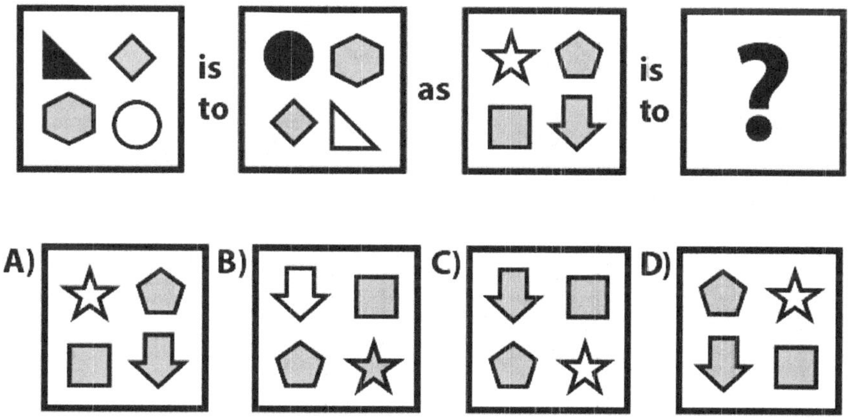

Q296

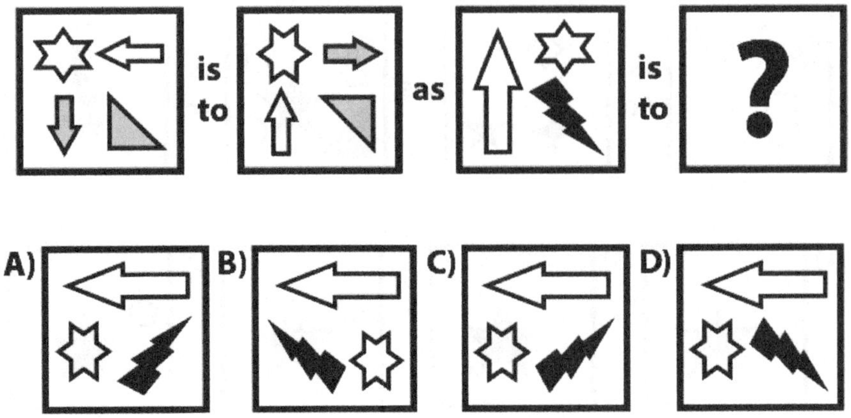

Q297

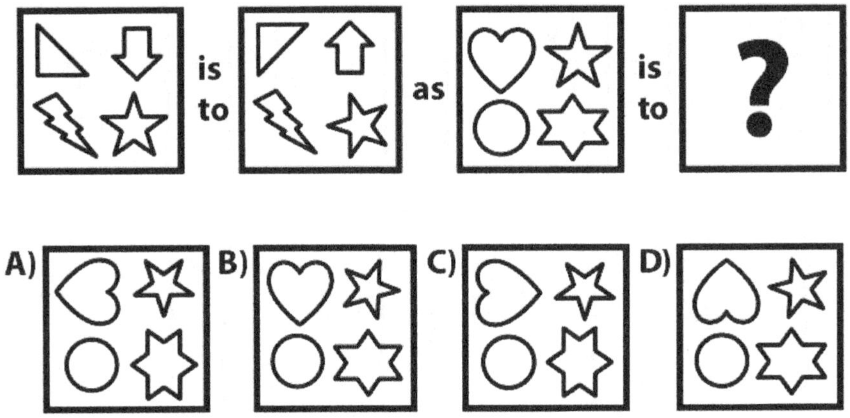

Q298

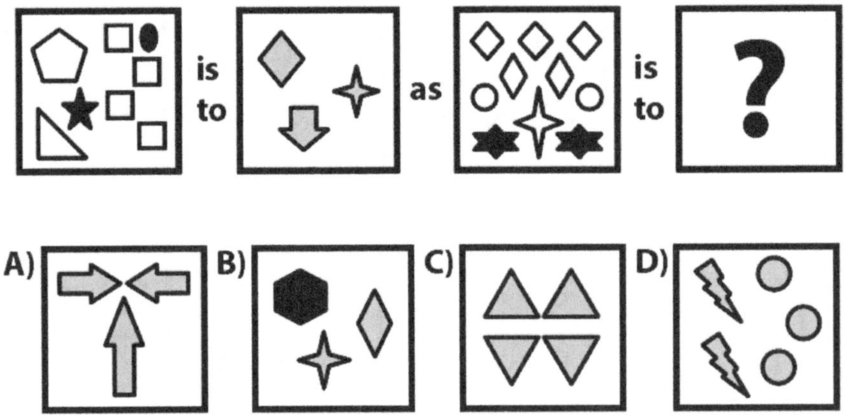

Q299

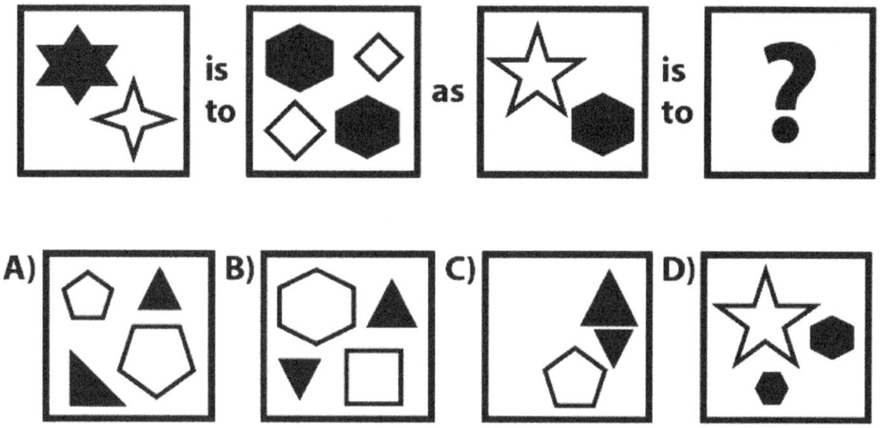

Q300

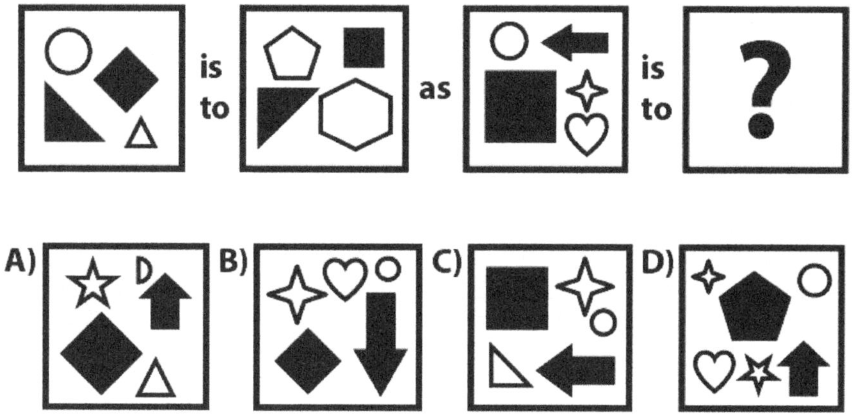

SECTION 1 MATHEMATICAL THINKING QUESTIONS

1. Robert has a box of building blocks. The box contains 8 yellow blocks and 12 red blocks. He picks three blocks from the box and stacks them up high. Calculate the probability that he stacks two red building blocks and one yellow building block, in **any** order.

A. $\frac{8}{20}$ B. $\frac{44}{95}$ C. $\frac{11}{18}$ D. $\frac{8}{19}$ E. $\frac{12}{20}$ F. $\frac{35}{60}$

2. Solve $\frac{3x+5}{5} + \frac{2x-2}{3} = 18$

A. 12.11 B. 13.49 C. 13.95 D. 14.2 E. 19 F. 265

3. Solve $3x^2 + 11x - 20 = 0$

A. $\frac{3}{4}$ and $-\frac{4}{3}$ B. $-\frac{3}{4}$ and $\frac{4}{3}$ C. -5 and $\frac{4}{3}$ D. 5 and $\frac{4}{3}$ E. 12 only F. -12 only

4. Express $\frac{5}{x+2} + \frac{3}{x-4}$ as a single fraction.

A. $\frac{15x-120}{(x+2)(x-4)}$

B. $\frac{8x-26}{(x+2)(x-4)}$

C. $\frac{8x-14}{(x+2)(x-4)}$

D. $\frac{15}{8x}$

E. 24

F. $\frac{8x-14}{x^2-8}$

5. The value of p is directly proportional to the cube root of q. When $p = 12$, $q = 27$. Find q when $p = 24$.

A. 32 B. 64 C. 124 D. 128 E. 216 F. 1728

6. Write 72^2 as a product of its prime factors.

A. $2^6 \times 3^4$ B. $2^6 \times 3^5$ C. $2^4 \times 3^4$ D. 2×3^3 E. $2^6 \times 3$ F. $2^3 \times 3^2$

7. Calculate: $\frac{2.302 \times 10^5 + 2.302 \times 10^2}{1.151 \times 10^{10}}$

A. 0.0000202

B. 0.00020002

C. 0.00002002

D. 0.00000002

E. 0.000002002

F. 0.000002002

8. Given that $y^2 + ay + b = (y+2)^2 - 5$, find the values of a and b.

A. $a = -1, b = 4$
B. $a = 1, b = 9$
C. $a = -1, b = -9$
D. $a = -9, b = 1$
E. $a = 4, b = -1$
F. $a = 4, b = 1$

9. Express $\frac{4}{5} + \frac{m-2n}{m+4n}$ as a single fraction in its simplest form:

A. $\frac{6m+6n}{5(m+4n)}$
B. $\frac{9m+26n}{5(m+4n)}$
C. $\frac{20m+6n}{5(m+4n)}$
D. $\frac{3m+9n}{5(m+4n)}$
E. $\frac{3(3m+2n)}{5(m+4n)}$

10. A is inversely proportional to the square root of B. When A = 4, B = 25. Calculate the value of A when B = 16.

A. 0.8
B. 4
C. 5
D. 6
E. 10
F. 20

11. S, T, U and V are points on the circumference of a circle, and O is the centre of the circle. Given that angle SVU = 89°, calculate the size of the smaller angle SOU.

A. 89°
B. 91°
C. 102°
D. 178°
E. 182°
F. 212°

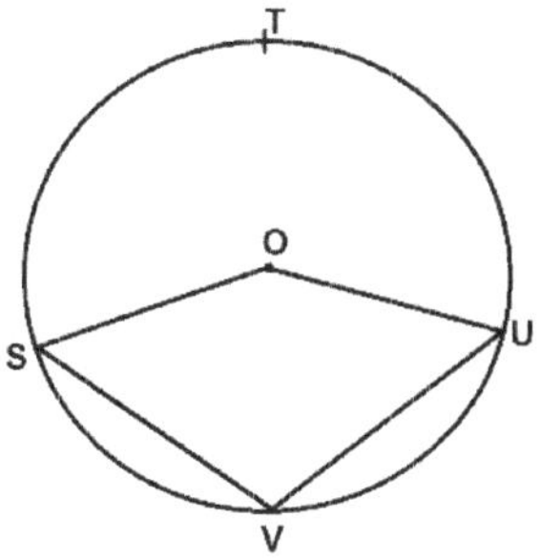

12. Open cylinder A has a surface area of 8π cm² and a volume of 2π cm³. Open cylinder B is an enlargement of A and has a surface area of 32π cm². Calculate the volume of cylinder B.

A. 2π cm³
B. 8π cm³
C. 10π cm³
D. 14π cm³
E. 16π cm³
F. 32π cm³

13. Express $\frac{8}{x(3-x)} - \frac{6}{x}$ in its simplest form.

A. $\frac{3x-10}{x(3-x)}$
B. $\frac{3x+10}{x(3-x)}$
C. $\frac{6x-10}{x(3-2x)}$
D. $\frac{6x-10}{x(3+2x)}$
E. $\frac{6x-10}{x(3-x)}$
F. $\frac{6x+10}{x(3-x)}$

14. A bag contains 10 balls. 9 of those are white and 1 is black. What is the probability that the black ball is drawn in the tenth and final draw if the drawn balls are not replaced?

A. 0 B. $\frac{1}{10}$ C. $\frac{1}{100}$ D. $\frac{1}{10^{10}}$ E. $\frac{1}{362,880}$

15. Gambit has an ordinary deck of 52 cards. What is the probability of Gambit drawing 2 Kings (without replacement)?

A. 0 B. $\frac{1}{169}$ C. $\frac{1}{221}$ D. $\frac{4}{663}$ E. None of the above

16. I have two identical unfair dice. The probability that the dice get a 6 is twice as high as the probability of any other outcome, which are all equally likely. What is the probability that when I roll both dice the total will be 12?

A. 0 B. $\frac{4}{49}$ C. $\frac{1}{9}$ D. $\frac{2}{7}$ E. None of the above

17. A roulette wheel consists of 36 numbered spots and 1 zero spot (i.e., 37 spots in total). What is the probability that the ball will stop in a spot either divisible by 3 or 2?

A. 0 B. $\frac{25}{37}$ C. $\frac{25}{36}$ D. $\frac{18}{37}$ E. $\frac{24}{37}$

18. I have a fair coin that I flip 4 times. What is the probability I get 2 heads and 2 tails?

A. $\frac{1}{16}$ B. $\frac{3}{16}$ C. $\frac{3}{8}$ D. None of the above E. $\frac{9}{16}$

19. Shivun rolls two fair dice. What is the probability that he gets a total of 5, 6 or 7?

A. $\frac{9}{36}$ B. $\frac{7}{12}$ C. $\frac{1}{6}$ D. $\frac{5}{12}$ E. None of the above

20. Dr Savary has a bag that contains x red balls, y blue balls and z green balls (and no others). He pulls out a ball, replaces it, and then pulls out another. What is the probability that he picks one red ball and one green ball?

A. $\frac{2(x+y)}{x+y+z}$

B. $\frac{xz}{(x+y+z)^2}$

C. $\frac{2xz}{(x+y+z)^2}$

D. $\frac{(x+z)}{(x+y+z)^2}$

E. $\frac{4xz}{(x+y+z)^4}$

F. More information needed

21. Mr Kilbane has a bag that contains x red balls, y blue balls and z green balls (and no others). He pulls out a ball, does **NOT** replace it, and then pulls out another. What is the probability that he picks one red ball and one blue ball?

A. $\frac{2xy}{(x+y+z)^2}$

B. $\frac{2xy}{(x+y+z)(x+y+z-1)}$

C. $\frac{2xy}{(x+y+z)^2}$

D. $\frac{xy}{(x+y+z)(x+y+z-1)}$

E. $\frac{4xy}{(x+y+z-1)^2}$

F. More information needed

22. There are two tennis players. The first player wins the point with probability p, and the second player wins the point with probability $1-p$. The rules of tennis say that the first player to score four points wins the game, unless the score is 4 to 3. At this point the first player to get two points ahead wins. What is the probability that the first player wins in exactly 5 rounds?

A. $4p^4(1-p)$

B. $p^4(1-p)$

C. $4p(1-p)$

D. $4p(1-p)^4$

E. $4p^5(1-p)$

F. More information needed

23. Solve the equation $\frac{4x+7}{2} + 9x + 10 = 7$.

A. $\frac{22}{13}$

B. $-\frac{22}{13}$

C. $\frac{10}{13}$

D. $-\frac{10}{13}$

E. $\frac{13}{22}$

F. $-\frac{13}{22}$

24. The volume of a sphere is $V = \frac{4}{3}\pi r^3$, and the surface area of a sphere is $S = 4\pi r^2$. Express S in terms of V.

A. $S = (4\pi)^{\frac{2}{3}}(3V)^{\frac{2}{3}}$

B. $S = (8\pi)^{\frac{1}{3}}(3V)^{\frac{2}{3}}$

C. $S = (4\pi)^{\frac{1}{3}}(9V)^{\frac{2}{3}}$

D. $S = (4\pi)^{\frac{1}{3}}(3V)^{\frac{2}{3}}$

E. $S = (16\pi)^{\frac{1}{3}}(9V)^{\frac{2}{3}}$

25. Express the volume of a cube, V, in terms of its surface area, S.

A. $V = (\frac{S}{6})^{\frac{3}{2}}$

B. $V = S^{\frac{3}{2}}$

C. $V = (\frac{6}{S})^{\frac{3}{2}}$

D. $V = (\frac{S}{6})^{\frac{1}{2}}$

E. $V = (\frac{S}{36})^{\frac{1}{2}}$

F. $V = (\frac{S}{36})^{\frac{3}{2}}$

26. Solve the equations $4x + 3y = 7$ and $2x + 8y = 12$.

A. $(x, y) = \left(\frac{17}{13}, \frac{10}{13}\right)$

B. $(x, y) = \left(\frac{10}{13}, \frac{17}{13}\right)$

C. $(x, y) = (1, 2)$

D. $(x, y) = (2, 1)$

E. $(x, y) = (6, 3)$

F. $(x, y) = (3, 6)$

G. No solutions possible.

27. Rearrange $\frac{(7x+10)}{(9x+5)} = 3y^2 + 2$, to make x the subject.

A. $\frac{15\,y^2}{7-9(3y^2+2)}$
B. $\frac{15\,y^2}{7+9(3y^2+2)}$
C. $-\frac{15\,y^2}{7-9(3y^2+2)}$
D. $-\frac{15\,y^2}{7+9(3y^2+2)}$
E. $-\frac{5\,y^2}{7+9(3y^2+2)}$
F. $\frac{5\,y^2}{7+9(3y^2+2)}$

28. Simplify $3x\left(\frac{3x^7}{x^{\frac{1}{3}}}\right)^3$

A. $9x^{20}$ B. $27x^{20}$ C. $87x^{20}$ D. $9x^{21}$ E. $27x^{21}$ F. $81x^{21}$

29. Simplify $2x[(2x)^7]^{\frac{1}{14}}$

A. $2x\sqrt{2\,x^4}$
B. $2x\sqrt{2x^3}$
C. $2\sqrt{2\,x^4}$
D. $2\sqrt{2x^3}$
E. $8x^3$
F. $8x$

30. What is the circumference of a circle with an area of 10π?

A. $2\pi\sqrt{10}$
B. $\pi\sqrt{10}$
C. 10π
D. 20π
E. $\sqrt{10}$
F. More information needed

31. If $a.b = (ab) + (a + b)$, then calculate the value of $(3.4).5$

A. 19 B. 54 C. 100 D. 119 E. 132

32. If $a.b = \frac{a^b}{a}$, calculate $(2.3).2$

A. $\frac{16}{3}$ B. 1 C. 2 D. 4 E. 8

33. Solve $x^2 + 3x - 5 = 0$

A. $x = -\frac{3}{2} \pm \frac{\sqrt{11}}{2}$
B. $x = \frac{3}{2} \pm \frac{\sqrt{11}}{2}$
C. $x = -\frac{3}{2} \pm \frac{\sqrt{11}}{4}$
D. $x = \frac{3}{2} \pm \frac{\sqrt{11}}{4}$
E. $x = \frac{3}{2} \pm \frac{\sqrt{29}}{2}$
F. $x = -\frac{3}{2} \pm \frac{\sqrt{29}}{2}$

34. How many times do the curves $y = x^3$ and $y = x^2 + 4x + 14$ intersect?

A. 0 B. 1 C. 2 D. 3 E. 4

35. Which of the following graphs **do not** intersect?

I. $y = x$ II. $y = x^2$ III. $y = 1 - x^2$ IV. $y = 2$

A. I and II
B. II and III
C. III and IV
D. I and III
E. I and IV
F. II and IV

36. Calculate the product of $897{,}653$ and 0.009764.

A. 87646.8
B. 8764.68
C. 876.468
D. 87.6468
E. 8.76468
F. 0.876468

37. Solve for x: $\frac{7x+3}{10} + \frac{3x+1}{7} = 14$

A. $\frac{929}{51}$ B. $\frac{949}{47}$ C. $\frac{949}{79}$ D. $\frac{980}{79}$

38. What is the area of an equilateral triangle with side length x

A. $\frac{x^2\sqrt{3}}{4}$ B. $\frac{x\sqrt{3}}{4}$ C. $\frac{x^2}{2}$ D. $\frac{x}{2}$ E. x^2 F. x

39. Simplify $3 - \frac{7x(25x^2-1)}{49x^2(5x+1)}$

A. $3 - \frac{5x-1}{7x}$
B. $3 - \frac{5x+1}{7x}$
C. $3 + \frac{5x-1}{7x}$
D. $3 + \frac{5x+1}{7x}$
E. $3 - \frac{5x^2}{49}$
F. $3 + \frac{5x^2}{49}$

40. Solve the equation $x^2 - 10x - 100 = 0$

A. $-5 \pm 5\sqrt{5}$
B. $-5 \pm \sqrt{5}$
C. $5 \pm 5\sqrt{5}$
D. $5 \pm \sqrt{5}$
E. $5 \pm 5\sqrt{125}$
F. $-5 \pm \sqrt{125}$

41. Rearrange $x^2 - 4x + 7 = y^3 + 2$ to make x the subject.

A. $x = 2 \pm \sqrt{y^3 + 1}$
B. $x = 2 \pm \sqrt{y^3 - 1}$
C. $x = -2 \pm \sqrt{y^3 - 1}$
D. $x = -2 \pm \sqrt{y^3 + 1}$
E. x cannot be made the subject for this equation.

42. Rearrange $3x + 2 = \sqrt{7x^2 + 2x + y}$ to make y the subject.

A. $y = 4x^2 + 8x + 2$
B. $y = 4x^2 + 8x + 4$
C. $y = 2x^2 + 10x + 2$
D. $y = 2x^2 + 10x + 4$
E. $y = x^2 + 10x + 2$
F. $y = x^2 + 10x + 4$

43. Rearrange $y^4 - 4y^3 + 6y^2 - 4y + 2 = x^5 + 7$ to make y the subject.

A. $y = 1 + (x^5 + 7)^{\frac{1}{4}}$
B. $y = -1 + (x^5 + 7)^{\frac{1}{4}}$
C. $y = 1 + (x^5 + 6)^{\frac{1}{4}}$
D. $y = -1 + (x^5 + 6)^{\frac{1}{4}}$

44. The aspect ratio of my television screen is 4:3 and the diagonal is 50 inches. What is the area of my television screen?

A. 1,200 inches²
B. 1,000 inches²
C. 120 inches²
D. 100 inches²
E. More information needed.

45. Rearrange the equation $\sqrt{1 + 3x^{-2}} = y^5 + 1$ to make x the subject.

A. $x = \frac{(y^{10} + 2y^5)}{3}$
B. $x = \frac{3}{(y^{10} + 2y^5)}$
C. $x = \sqrt{\frac{3}{y^{10} + 2y^5}}$
D. $x = \sqrt{\frac{y^{10} + 2y^5}{3}}$
E. $x = \sqrt{\frac{y^{10} + 2y^5 + 2}{3}}$
F. $x = \sqrt{\frac{3}{y^{10} + 2y^5 + 2}}$

46. Solve $3x - 5y = 10$ and $2x + 2y = 13$

A. $(x, y) = (\frac{19}{16}, \frac{85}{16})$
B. $(x, y) = (\frac{85}{16}, -\frac{19}{16})$
C. $(x, y) = (\frac{85}{16}, \frac{19}{16})$
D. $(x, y) = (-\frac{85}{16}, -\frac{19}{16})$
E. No solutions possible.

47. The two inequalities $x + y \leq 3$ and $x^3 - y^2 < 3$ define a region on a plane. Which of the following points is inside the region?

A. $(2, 1)$
B. $(2.5, 1)$
C. $(1, 2)$
D. $(3, 5)$
E. $(1, 2.5)$
F. None of the above.

48. How many times do $y = x + 4$ and $y = 4x^2 + 5x + 5$ intersect?

A. 0 B. 1 C. 2 D. 3 E. 4

49. How many times do $y = x^3$ and $y = x$ intersect?

A. 0 B. 1 C. 2 D. 3 E. 4

50. A cube has unit length sides. What is the length of a line joining a vertex to the midpoint of the opposite side?

A. $\sqrt{2}$
B. $\sqrt{\frac{3}{2}}$
C. $\sqrt{3}$
D. $\sqrt{5}$
E. $\frac{\sqrt{5}}{2}$

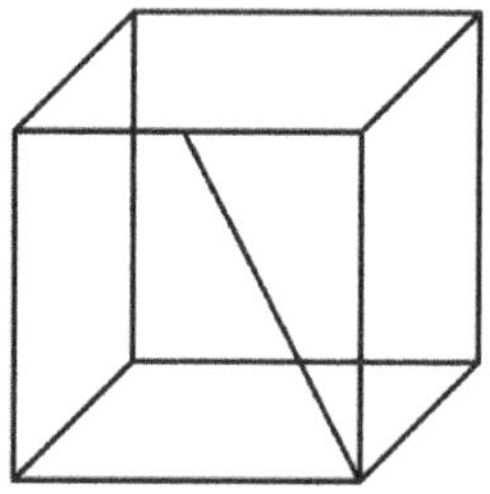

51. Solve for x, y, and z.

$x + y - z = -1$
$2x - 2y + 3z = 8$
$2x - y + 2x = 9$

A. $x = 2, y = -15, z = -14$
B. $x = 15, y = 2, z = 14$
C. $x = 14, y = 15, z = -2$
D. $x = -2, y = 15, z = 14$
E. $x = 2, y = -15, z = 14$
F. No solutions possible

52. Fully factorise: $3a^3 - 30a^2 + 75a$

A. $3a(a - 3)^3$
B. $a(3a - 5)^2$
C. $3a(a^2 - 10a + 25)$
D. $3a(a - 5)^2$
E. $3a(a + 5)^2$

53. Solve for *x* and *y*:

$4x + 3y = 48$
$3x + 2y = 34$

A. $x = 8, y = 6$
B. $x = 6, y = 8$
C. $x = 3, y = 4$
D. $x = 4, y = 3$
E. $x = 30, y = 12$
F. $x = 12, y = 30$
G. No solutions possible

54. Evaluate: $\frac{-(5^2-4\times7)^2}{-6^2+2\times7}$

A. $-\frac{3}{50}$
B. $\frac{11}{22}$
C. $-\frac{3}{22}$
D. $\frac{9}{50}$
E. $\frac{9}{22}$
F. 0

55. All license plates are 6 characters long. The first 3 characters consist of letters and the next 3 characters of numbers. How many unique license plates are possible?

A. 676,000
B. 6,760,000
C. 67,600,000
D. 1,757,600
E. 17,576,000
F. 175,760,000

56. How many solutions are there for $2(2(x^2 - 3x)) = -9$

A. 0
B. 1
C. 2
D. 3
E. Infinite solutions

57. Evaluate: $\left(x^{\frac{1}{2}}y^{-3}\right)^{\frac{1}{2}}$

A. $\frac{x^{\frac{1}{2}}}{y}$

B. $\frac{x}{y^{\frac{3}{2}}}$

C. $\frac{x^{\frac{1}{4}}}{y^{\frac{3}{2}}}$

D. $\frac{y^{\frac{1}{4}}}{x^{\frac{3}{2}}}$

58. Bryan earned a total of £1,240 last week from renting out three flats. From this, he had to pay 10% of the rent from the 1-bedroom flat for repairs, 20% of the rent from the 2-bedroom flat for repairs, and 30% from the 3-bedroom flat for repairs. The rent on the 3-bedroom flat costs twice as much as the 1-bedroom flat. Given that the total repair bill was £276 calculate the rent for each apartment.

	1 Bedroom	2 Bedrooms	3 Bedrooms
A	280	400	560
B	140	200	280
C	420	600	840
D	250	300	500
E	500	600	1,000

59. Evaluate: $5\,[5(6^2 - 5 \times 3) + 400^{\frac{1}{2}}]^{\frac{1}{3}} + 7$

A. 0
B. 25
C. 32
D. 49
E. 56
F. 200

60. What is the area of a regular hexagon with side length 1?

A. $3\sqrt{3}$
B. $\frac{3\sqrt{3}}{2}$
C. $\sqrt{3}$
D. $\frac{\sqrt{3}}{2}$
E. 6
F. More information needed

61. Dexter moves into a new rectangular room that is 19 metres longer than it is wide, and its total area is 780 square metres. What are the room's dimensions?

A. Width = 20m; Length = −39m
B. Width = 20m; Length = 39m
C. Width = 39m; Length = 20m
D. Width = −39m; Length = 20m
E. Width = −20m; Length = 39m

62. Tom uses 34 meters of fencing to enclose his rectangular lot. He measured the diagonals to 13 metres long. What is the length and width of the lot?

A. 3m by 4m
B. 5m by 12m
C. 6m by 12m
D. 8m by 15m
E. 9m by 15m
F. 10m by 10m

63. Solve $\frac{3x-5}{2} + \frac{x+5}{4} = x + 1$

A. 1
B. 1.5
C. 3
D. 3.5
E. 4.5
F. None of the above

64. Calculate: $\frac{5.226\times10^6 + 5.226\times10^5}{1.742\times10^{10}}$

A. 0.033
B. 0.0033
C. 0.00033
D. 0.000033
E. 0.0000033

65. Calculate the area of the triangle shown to the right:

A. $3 + \sqrt{2}$
B. $\frac{2 + 2\sqrt{2}}{2}$
C. $2 + 5\sqrt{2}$
D. $3 - \sqrt{2}$
E. 3
F. 6

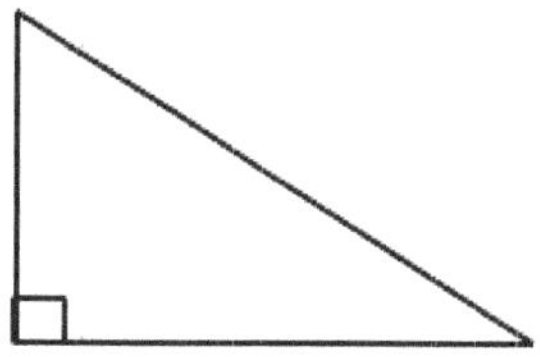

66. Rearrange $\sqrt{\frac{4}{x} + 9} = y - 2$ to make x the subject.

A. $x = \frac{11}{(y-2)^2}$
B. $x = \frac{9}{(y-2)^2}$
C. $x = \frac{4}{(y+1)(y-5)}$
D. $x = \frac{4}{(y-1)(y+5)}$
E. $x = \frac{4}{(y+1)(y+5)}$
F. $x = \frac{4}{(y-1)(y-5)}$

67. When 5 is subtracted from $5x$ the result is half the sum of 2 and $6x$. What is the value of x?

A. 0
B. 1
C. 2
D. 3
E. 4
F. 6

68. Estimate $\frac{54.98 + 2.25^2}{\sqrt{905}}$

A. 0
B. 1
C. 2
D. 3
E. 4
F. 5

69. At a pizza parlour, you can order one of three types of crust: single, double or triple cheese. You also have the option to include ham, olives, pepperoni, bell pepper, meat balls, tomato slices, and pineapples. How many different types of pizza are available at the Pizza Parlour?

A. 10
B. 96
C. 192
D. 384
E. 768
F. None of the above

70. Solve the simultaneous equations $x^2 + y^2 = 1$ and $x + y = \sqrt{2}$ for $x, y > 0$

A. $(x, y) = (\frac{\sqrt{2}}{2}, \frac{\sqrt{2}}{2})$
B. $(x, y) = (\frac{1}{2}, \frac{\sqrt{3}}{2})$
C. $(x, y) = (\sqrt{2} - 1, 1)$
D. $(x, y) = (\sqrt{2}, \frac{1}{2})$

71. How many negative roots does $f(x) = 16x^4 + 32x^3 + 24x^2 + 8x + 1$ have?

A. 0
B. 1
C. 2
D. 3
E. 4
F. 5

72. Solve the inequality $x^2 \geq 6 - x$

A. $x \leq -3$ and $x \leq 2$
B. $x \leq -3$ and $x \geq 2$
C. $x \geq -3$ and $x \leq 2$
D. $x \geq -3$ and $x \geq 2$
E. $x \geq 2$ only
F. $x \geq -3$ only

73. The hypotenuse of an equilateral right-angled triangle is x cm. What is the area of the triangle in terms of x?

A. $\frac{\sqrt{x}}{2}$
B. $\frac{x^2}{4}$
C. $\frac{x}{4}$
D. $\frac{3x^2}{4}$
E. $\frac{x^2}{10}$

74. Mr Heard derives a formula: $Q = \frac{(X+Y)^2 A}{3B}$. He doubles the values of X and Y, halves the value of A and triples the value of B. What happens to value of Q?

A. Decreases by $\frac{1}{3}$
B. Increases by $\frac{1}{3}$
C. Decreases by $\frac{2}{3}$
D. Increases by $\frac{2}{3}$
E. Increases by $\frac{4}{3}$
F. Decreases by $\frac{4}{3}$

75. Consider the graphs $y = x^2 - 2x + 3$, and $y = x^2 - 6x - 10$. Which of the following is true?

A. Both equations intersect the x-axis.
B. Neither equation intersects the x-axis.
C. The first equation does not intersect the x-axis; the second equation intersects the x-axis.
D. The first equation intersects the x-axis; the second equation does not intersect the x-axis.

76. A crocodile's tail weighs 30kg. Its head weighs as much as the tail and one half of the body and legs. The body and legs together weigh as much as the tail and head combined. What is the total weight of the crocodile?

A. 220kg
B. 240kg
C. 260kg
D. 280kg
E. 300kg

77. Evaluate the following: $\frac{4.2\times10^{10} - 4.2\times10^{6}}{2\times10^{3}}$

A. 2.09979×10^{6}
B. 2.09979×10^{7}
C. 2.09979×10^{8}
D. 2.09979×10^{9}
E. 2.09979×10^{10}

78. Calculate $a - b$

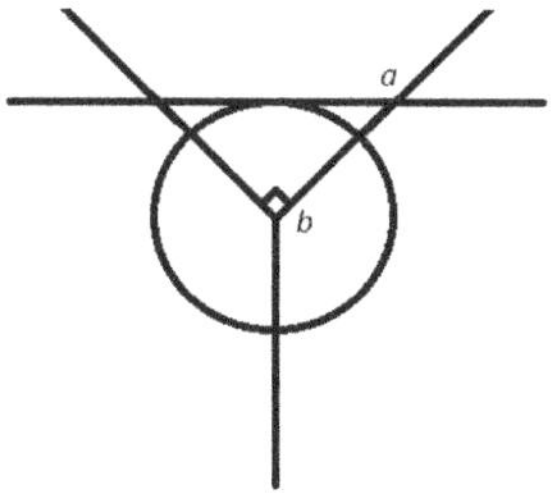

A. $0°$
B. $5°$
C. $10°$
D. $15°$
E. $20°$

79. Jack has a bag with a complete set of snooker balls (15 red, 1 yellow, 1 green, 1 brown, 1 blue, 1 pink and 1 black ball) within it. Blindfolded Jack draws two balls from the bag. What is the probability that he draws a blue and a black ball in any order?

A. $\frac{2}{41}$
B. $\frac{1}{210}$
C. $\frac{2}{210}$
D. $\frac{1}{105}$
E. $\frac{2}{441}$

80. Which is the equivalent function to: $y = 9x^{-\frac{1}{3}}$

A. $y = \frac{1}{x}$
B. $y = \sqrt[3]{9x}$
C. $y = \frac{1}{\sqrt[3]{9x}}$
D. $y = \frac{9}{\sqrt[3]{x}}$
E. $y = \frac{3}{\sqrt[3]{x}}$

81. Make y the subject of the formula: $\frac{y+x}{x} = \frac{x}{a} + \frac{a}{x}$

A. $y = \frac{x^2}{a} + a$
B. $y = \frac{x^2+a^2-ax}{a}$
C. $y = \frac{-ax}{x^2+a^2}$
D. $y = \frac{x^2}{ax} + a - x$
E. $y = a^2 - ax$

82. The graph below shows a circle with radius 5 and centre $(0,0)$.

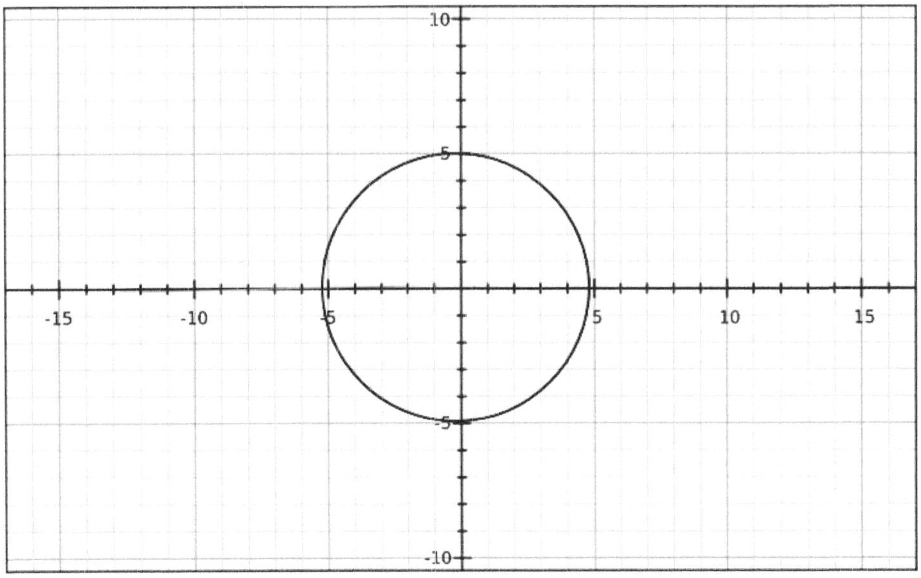

What are the values of x when the line $y = 3x - 5$ meets the circle?

A. $x = 0$ or $x = 3$
B. $x = 0$ or $x = 3.5$
C. $x = 1$ or $x = 3.5$
D. $x = 1.5$ or $x = -3$
E. $x = 1.5$ or $x = -2$

83. There are 1000 international airports in the world. If 4 flights take off every hour from each airport, estimate the annual number of commercial flights worldwide, to the nearest 1 million

A. 20 million
B. 35 million
C. 37 million
D. 40 million
E. 42 million
F. 44 million

84. How many seconds are there in 66 weeks? $[n! = 1 \times 2 \times 3 \times \ldots \times n]$

A. 7!
B. 8!
C. 9!
D. 10!
E. 11!
F. 12!

85. Write $\frac{\sqrt{20}-2}{\sqrt{5}+3}$ in the form: $p\sqrt{5} + q$

A. $2\sqrt{5} - 4$
B. $3\sqrt{5} - 4$
C. $3\sqrt{5} - 5$
D. $4\sqrt{5} - 6$
E. $5\sqrt{5} + 4$

86. Consider the triangle below where BE = 4cm, EC = 2cm and AC = 9cm. What is the length of side DE?

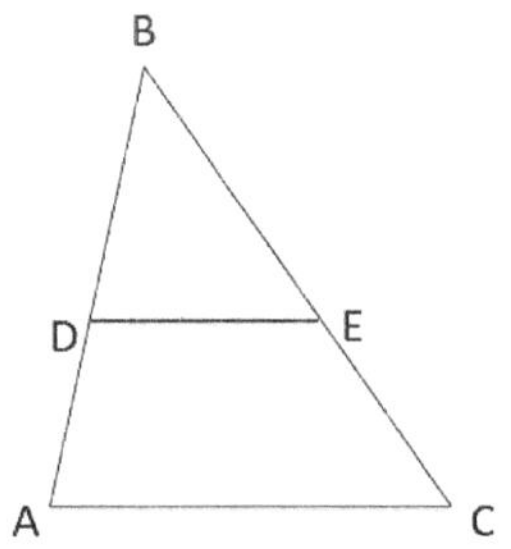

A. 4cm
B. 5.5cm
C. 6cm
D. 7.5cm
E. 8cm

87. An investment of £500 is made in a compound interest account that compounds annually. At the end of 3 years the balance reads £1687.50. What is the interest rate?

A. 20% B. 35% C. 50% D. 65% E. 80%

88. Rupert plays one game of tennis and one game of squash. The probability that he will win the tennis game is $\frac{3}{4}$. The probability that he will win the squash game is $\frac{1}{3}$. What is the probability that he will win one game only?

A. $\frac{3}{12}$ B. $\frac{7}{12}$ C. $\frac{4}{5}$ D. $\frac{13}{12}$ E. $\frac{7}{6}$

89. Calculate the perimeter of a regular polygon each interior angle is 150° and each side is 15 cm.

A. 75 cm
B. 150 cm
C. 180 cm
D. 225 cm
E. 1,500 cm
F. More information is needed.

90. Calculate $\frac{1.25\times10^{10}+1.25\times10^{9}}{2.5\times10^{8}}$

A. 0
B. 1
C. 55
D. 110
E. 1.25×10^8
F. 5.5×10^7
G. 5.5×10^8

91. Solve $y = 2x - 1$ and $y = x^2 - 1$ for x and y

A. $(0,-1)$ and $(2,3)$
B. $(1,-1)$ and $(2,2)$
C. $(1,4)$ and $(3,2)$
D. $(2,-3)$ and $(4,5)$
E. $(3,-1)$ and $(3,1)$
F. $(4,-2)$ and $(-2,4)$

92. Simplify fully: $\frac{(3x^{\frac{1}{2}})^3}{3x^2}$

A. $\frac{3x}{\sqrt{x}}$
B. $\frac{9}{x}$
C. $3x^{\frac{1}{2}}$
D. $3x\sqrt{x}$
E. $\frac{9}{\sqrt{x}}$

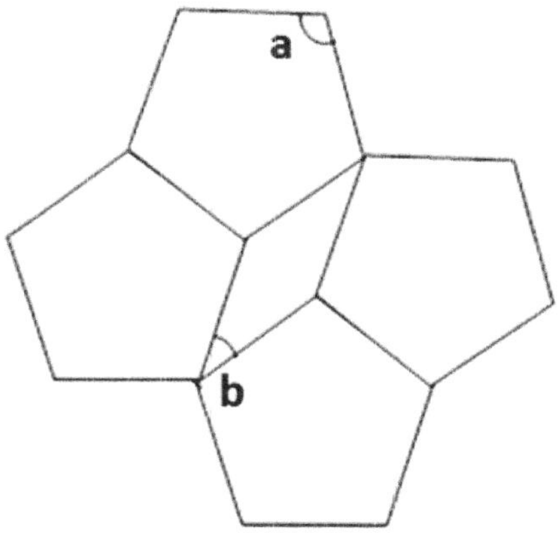

93. Study the diagram, comprising regular pentagons. What is the product of a and b?

A. 580°
B. 1,111°
C. 3,888°
D. 7,420°
E. 9,255°
F. 15,552°

94. Tim stands at the waterfront and holds a 30 cm ruler horizontally at eye level one metre in front of him. It lines up so it appears to be exactly the same length as a cruise ship 1 km out to sea. How long is the cruise ship?

A. 299.7 m
B. 300.0 m
C. 333.3 m
D. 29,970 m
E. 30,000 m

95. Bob is twice as old as Kerry, and Kerry is three times as old as Bob's son. Their ages combined make 50 years. How old was Bob when his son was born?

A. 15
B. 20
C. 25
D. 30
E. 35

96. The mean of a set of 11 numbers is 6. Two numbers are removed, and the mean is now 5. Which of the following is not a possible combination of removed numbers?

A. 1 and 20
B. 6 and 9
C. 10 and 11
D. 15 and 6
E. 19 and 2

97. Evaluate: $\frac{3.4\times10^{11} + 3.4\times10^{10}}{6.8\times10^{12}}$

A. 5.5×10^{-12}
B. 5.5×10^{-2}
C. 5.5×10^{1}
D. 5.5×10^{2}
E. 5.5×10^{10}
F. 5.5×10^{12}

98. A circle has a radius of 3 m. A line passes through the circle's centre and intersects with a tangent 4 m from its tangent point. How far is this point of intersection from the centre of the circle?

A. 1 m
B. 3 m
C. 5 m
D. 7 m
E. 9 m

99. Consider A: $y = 3x$ and B: $y = \frac{6}{x} - 7$. At what values of x do the two equations intersect

A. $x = 2$ and $x = 9$
B. $x = 3$ and $x = -6$
C. $x = \frac{2}{3}$ and $x = -3$
D. $x = 6$
E. $x = -\frac{2}{3}$

100. Calculate the radius of a sphere which has a surface area three times as great as its volume.

A. 0.5
B. 1
C. 1.5
D. 2
E. 2.5
F. More information is needed

101. The diagram shows a series of identical rectangular sports fields, calculate the shortest distance between points A and B.

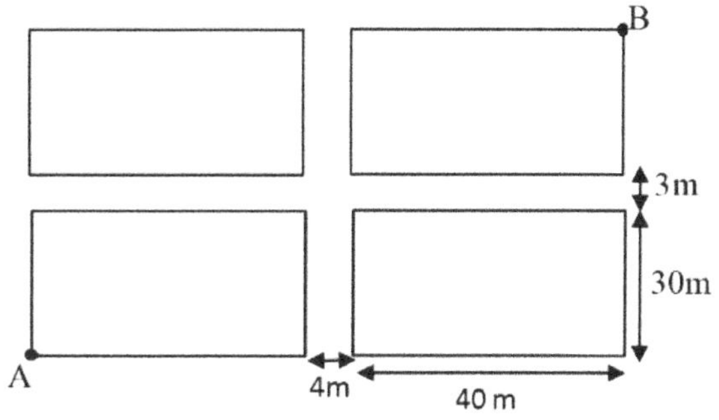

A. 100 m
B. 105 m
C. 146 m
D. 148 m
E. 154 m
F. None of the above.

102. Simplify fully: $1 + (3\sqrt{2} - 1)^2 + (3 + \sqrt{2})^2$

A. $30 + 6\sqrt{2} - 2\sqrt{18}$
B. $30 + 6\sqrt{2} + 2\sqrt{18}$
C. $3\,[2\,(\sqrt{2} - 1) + 2]$
D. 24
E. 29
F. 31

103. Each vertex of a square lies directly on the edge of a circle with a radius of 1cm. Calculate the area of the circle that is not occupied by the square. Use $\pi = 3$.

A. 0.25 cm² B. 0.5 cm² C. 0.75 cm² D. 1.0 cm² E. 1.25 cm² F. 1.5 cm²

104. If $(3p + 5)^2 = 24p + 49$, calculate p

A. −5 or −9 B. −3 or −6 C. −4 or 6 D. −6 or 4 E. 4 or −2

105. Find the values of angles b and c.

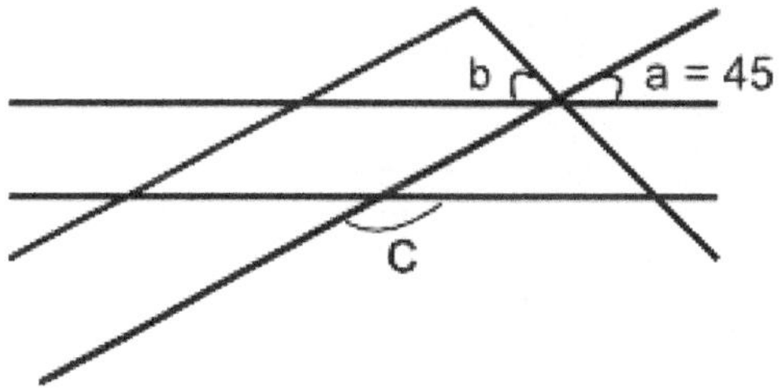

A. 45° and 135°
B. 45° and 130°
C. 50° and 135°
D. 55° and 130°
E. More information needed.

106. If the lines $y_1 = (n + 1)x + 10$ and $y_2 = (n + 3)x + 2$ are perpendicular, then n must equal which of the following?

A. 2 B. −2 C. 3 D. −3 E. 0 F. 1

107. A formula: $\frac{z(x+y)(l-m+n)}{3}$ is given. If each variable in the equation was measured in metres, what would you expect this formula to calculate?

A. A length
B. An area
C. A volume
D. A volume of rotation
E. A geometric average

108. What is the equation of the line of best fit for the scatter graph below?

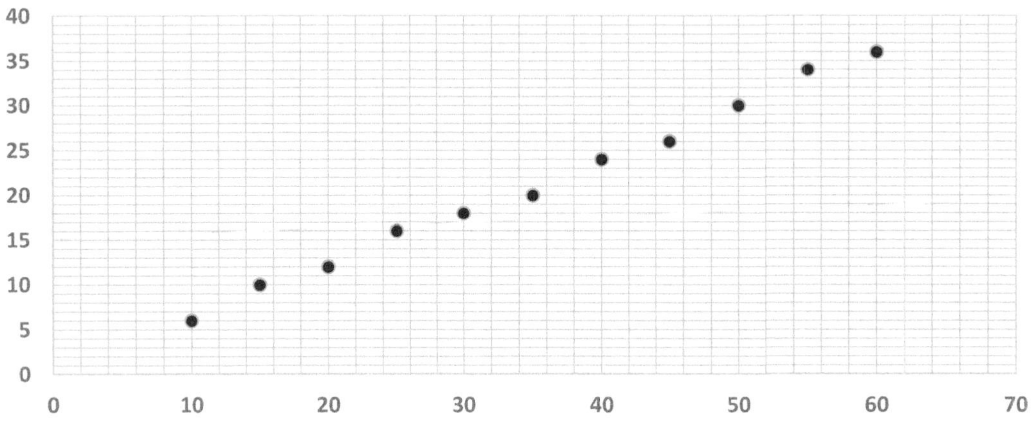

A. $y = 0.2x + 0.35$
B. $y = 0.2x - 0.35$
C. $y = 0.4x + 0.35$
D. $y = 0.4x - 0.35$
E. $y = 0.6x + 0.35$

109. What is the median of the following numbers: $\frac{7}{36}$; $0.\dot{3}$; $\frac{11}{18}$; 0.25; 0.75; $\frac{62}{72}$; $\frac{7}{7}$

A. $\frac{7}{36}$
B. $0.\dot{3}$
C. $\frac{11}{18}$
D. $\frac{62}{72}$
E. 0.75

110. The table below shows the results of a study investigating antibiotic resistance in staphylococcus populations.

Antibiotic	Number of Bacteria tested	Number of Resistant Bacteria
Benzyl-penicillin	10^{11}	98
Chloramphenicol	10^{9}	1200
Metronidazole	10^{8}	256
Erythromycin	10^{5}	2

A single staphylococcus bacterium is chosen at random from a similar population. Resistance to any one antibiotic is independent of resistance to others. Calculate the probability that the bacterium selected will be resistant to all four drugs.

A. 1 in 10^{12}
B. 1 in 10^{6}
C. 1 in 10^{20}
D. 1 in 10^{25}
E. 1 in 10^{30}
F. 1 in 10^{35}

111. Solve $y = x^2 - 3x + 4$ and $y - x = 1$ as (x, y).

A. $(-1,2)$ and $(3,4)$
B. $(1,2)$ and $(3,4)$
C. $(7,-2)$ and $(6,5)$
D. $(2,-3)$ and $(4,-1)$
E. $(1,-1)$ and $(-7,-1)$

112. Evaluate the following: $((\frac{6}{8} \times \frac{7}{3}) \div (\frac{7}{5} \times \frac{2}{6})) \times 0.40 \times 15\% \times 5\% \times \pi \times (\sqrt{e^2}) \times 0.20 \times (e\pi)^{-1}$

A. $\frac{4}{55}$ B. $\frac{8}{770}$ C. $\frac{9}{4{,}000}$ D. $\frac{8}{54{,}321}$ E. $\frac{9}{67{,}800}$

113. Bill wants to lay down laminate flooring in his living room, which has an in-built circular fish tank that he will have to lay the flooring around. He has decided to buy planks that he can cut to fit the dimensions of his room. He must, however, buy whole planks and cut them down himself. The room's dimensions are given below, as are those of one plank. Calculate the number of planks needed to cover the whole floor. Take $\pi = 3$.

A. 30
B. 417
C. 600
D. 589
E. 43

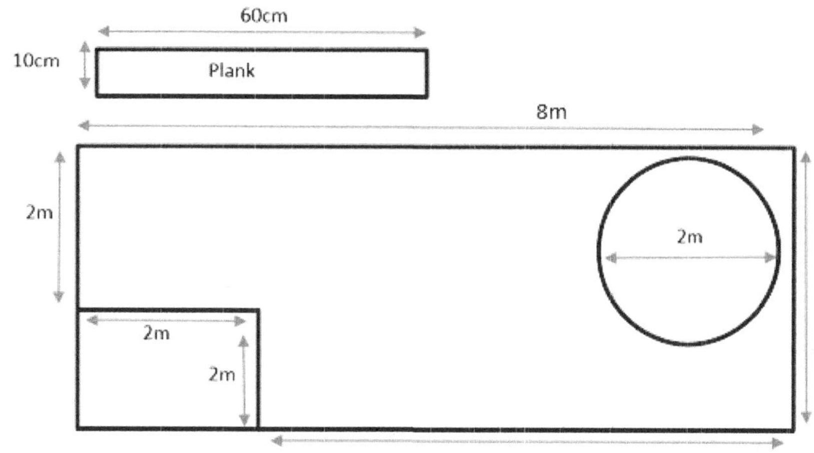

114. Rearrange $\frac{(16x+11)}{(4x+5)} = 4y^2 + 2$ to make x the subject

A. $x = \frac{20y^2-1}{[16-4\,(4y^2+2)]}$
B. $x = \frac{20y^2-8}{[16-6\,(4y^2+2)]}$
C. $x = \frac{6y^2-1}{[16-4\,(4y^2+2)]}$
D. $x = \frac{21y^2-1}{[16-4\,(2y^2+2)]}$
E. $x = \frac{7y^2-1}{[6-14\,(6+7)]}$

115. Four unbiased coins are tossed. What is the probability of getting at most two heads?

A. $\frac{3}{4}$ B. $\frac{7}{8}$ C. $\frac{11}{16}$ D. $\frac{1}{2}$ E. $\frac{5}{8}$

116. What is the probability of rolling the same number exactly three times with five six-sided dice?

A. $\frac{10}{36}$ B. $\frac{17}{32}$ C. $\frac{125}{648}$ D. $\frac{108}{124}$ E. $\frac{133}{648}$

117. What is the digit in the $10{,}000$s place in the number 301^5?

A. 0
B. 9
C. 3
D. 5
E. 1
F. 2
G. 7

118. Calculate the value of $\sqrt{20 - 20\sqrt{5} + 25} + \sqrt{5 - 8\sqrt{5} + 16}$.

A. $9 - 3\sqrt{5}$
B. $1 - \sqrt{5}$
C. $\sqrt{5} - 1$
D. $3\sqrt{5} - 9$
E. $\sqrt{66 - 28\sqrt{5}}$
F. 13
G. -3

119. A hospital has two wards, one for critically ill patients called Ward A and one for general patients, called Ward B. The probability a patient in Ward A survives is $\frac{1}{9}$, and the probability a patient in Ward B survives is $\frac{3}{5}$. (Every patient is in one of the two wards). Given that there are p people in Ward A, and the overall survival rate of the hospital is $\frac{1}{4}$, what is q, the number of people in Ward B, in terms of p?

A. $\frac{3p}{45}$
B. $\frac{45p}{3}$
C. $\frac{25p}{63}$
D. $\frac{63p}{25}$
E. 50
F. $\frac{45p}{12p-45}$
G. $\frac{12p-45}{45p}$

120. A man tosses a fair coin 7 times. What is P(he gets more than 4 heads and two of the last 3 tosses are heads)?

A. $\frac{3}{16}$
B. $\frac{7}{8}$
C. $\frac{33}{128}$
D. $\frac{3}{8}$
E. $\frac{33}{64}$
F. $\frac{279}{512}$

121. I have 2 blue balls and 3 red balls which I will throw into 5 indistinguishable boxes. Assuming I don't miss, how many distinct situations could I be in after all the balls are thrown?

A. 14
B. 5^5
C. 32
D. 16
E. 8
F. 4
G. $5^3 + 5^2$

122. What angle is swept by the minute hand on a clock between $08{:}34$ and $11{:}12$?

A. $1260°$
B. $948°$
C. $924°$
D. $720°$
E. $724°$

123. An inflated spherical football is packaged in the smallest possible box that it will fit inside of. What is the ratio of volume taken up by the football to the volume of the box?

A. $\frac{\pi}{12} : 1$
B. $\frac{12}{\pi} : 1$
C. $\frac{6}{\pi} : 1$
D. $\frac{\pi}{6} : 1$
E. $\frac{8}{\pi} : 1$

124. The diagram below shows a scalene triangle with a line crossing through it parallel to the base. What is the length of the base, which is marked x?

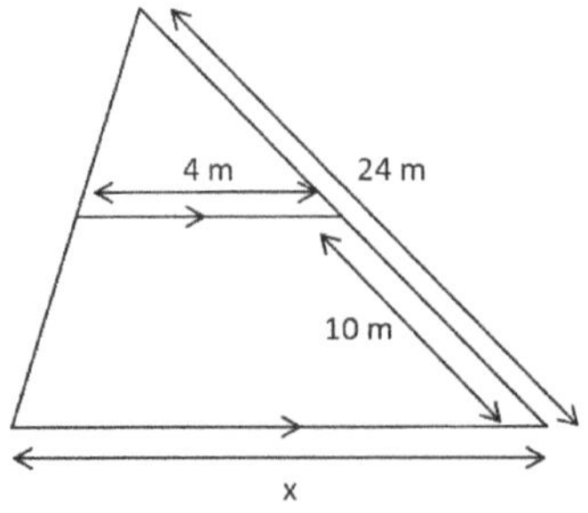

A. $6\frac{1}{7}$ m
B. $7\frac{5}{8}$ m
C. $6\frac{3}{8}$ m
D. $6\frac{6}{7}$ m
E. $7\frac{1}{6}$ m

125. There are five rides in a theme park which are arranged on the corners of a regular pentagon, as shown in the diagram below. If someone wants to walk from ride 2 to ride 4, what bearing should they walk on?

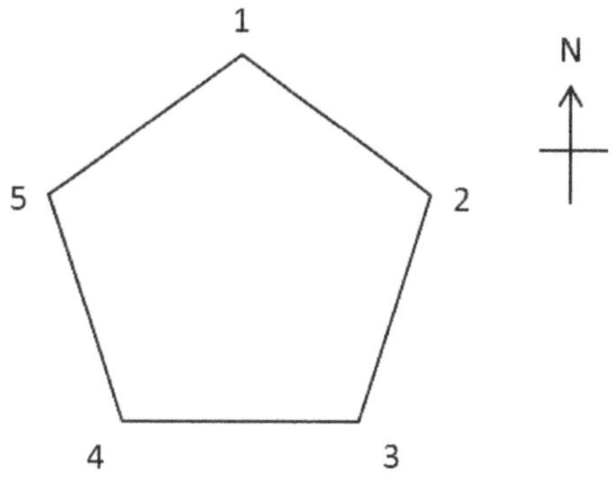

A. 45°
B. 54°
C. 112°
D. 234°
E. 245°

126. What is the area of the grey section in the diagram below?

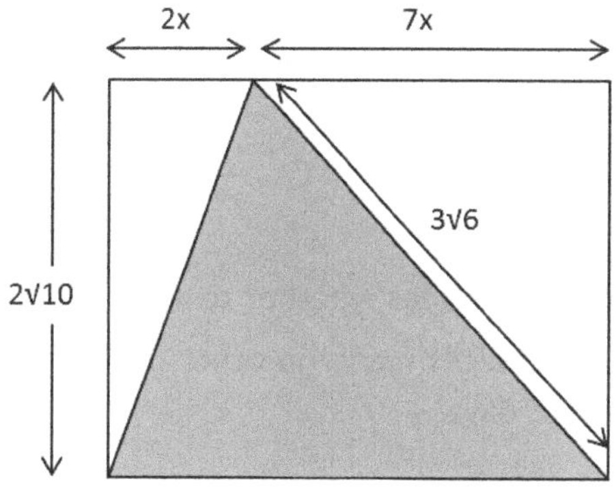

A. $12\sqrt{15}$
B. $18\sqrt{10}$
C. $\frac{18}{7}\sqrt{35}$
D. $\frac{6}{5}\sqrt{15}$
E. $\frac{43}{9}\sqrt{35}$

127. The diagram shows a garden, the grey area is to be covered with grass. The grass comes in rolls that are 1 m by 10 m. How many rolls are needed to cover the garden?

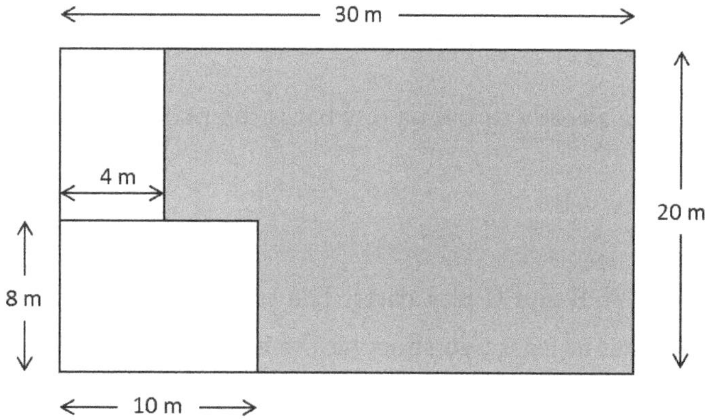

A. 47
B. 48
C. 49
D. 50
E. 51

128. In a household there are 2 people with size 6 feet and 3 people with size 11 feet. Each person owns 4 pairs of shoes. All of the shoes are randomly mixed up in a large bag. If someone pulls out a left size 11 shoe, what is the probability that the next shoe that they pull out is a right size 11 shoe?

A. $\frac{1}{2}$ B. $\frac{12}{39}$ C. $\frac{3}{10}$ D. $\frac{11}{39}$ E. $\frac{16}{39}$

129. What is the surface area to volume ratio of a solid cylinder with radius 'r' and length '$3r$'?

A. $3:r$
B. $4\frac{1}{3}:r$
C. $8:3r$
D. $1:6r$
E. $4:1r$

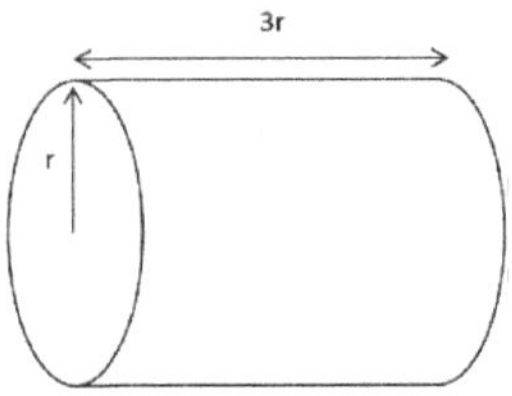

130. The volume of a cylinder is between 2 and 3 times the value of its overall surface area. If its height is 8, what values can r take? (Assuming r is non-zero)

A. $1 \leq r \leq 3$
B. $r \leq 8$
C. $8 \leq r \leq 24$
D. $r \geq 16$
E. $\frac{3}{2} \leq r \leq \frac{7}{4}$
F. $2 \leq r \leq 3$

131. On Mondays Professor X takes class A or B. The probability he picks class A is $\frac{2}{7}$. On Tuesdays, he takes class A if he took class B the day before, otherwise he picks in the same way he did on Monday. Prof. X took class A on Tuesday; what is the probability he took class A on Monday?

A. $\frac{2}{7}$
B. $\frac{5}{7}$
C. $\frac{10}{49}$
D. $\frac{10}{39}$
E. $\frac{4}{39}$
F. $\frac{7}{39}$
G. $\frac{31}{49}$

132. Every day, a man decides whether to walk his dog with probability $\frac{1}{3}$ that he does take it for a walk, independently of choices made on other days. After 4 days, what is the probability that he walked his dog at least once every 2 days?

A. $\frac{1}{27}$
B. $\frac{7}{27}$
C. $\frac{8}{27}$
D. $\frac{11}{27}$
E. $\frac{1}{9}$
F. $\frac{1}{3}$

133. There is a box that is 3m by 4m by 5m. What is the maximum length of stick that can fit in this box?

A. 6 m
B. $5\sqrt{2}$ m
C. $\sqrt{77}$ m
D. $2\sqrt{3}$ m
E. $\sqrt{39}$ m

134. Given you have already thrown a 6, what is the probability of throwing three consecutive 6s using a fair die?

A. $\frac{1}{216}$
B. $\frac{1}{36}$
C. $\frac{1}{6}$
D. $\frac{1}{2}$
E. 1

135. Three people, A, B and C play darts. The probability that they hit a bullseye are respectively $\frac{1}{5}, \frac{1}{4}, \frac{1}{3}$. What is the probability that at least two shots hit the bullseye?

A. $\frac{1}{60}$
B. $\frac{1}{30}$
C. $\frac{1}{12}$
D. $\frac{1}{6}$
E. $\frac{3}{20}$

136. If probability of having blonde hair is 1 in 4, the probability of having brown eyes is 1 in 2 and the probability of having both is 1 in 8, what is the probability of having neither blonde hair nor brown eyes?

A. $\frac{1}{2}$
B. $\frac{3}{4}$
C. $\frac{3}{8}$
D. $\frac{5}{8}$
E. $\frac{7}{8}$

SECTION 2 ACADEMIC LITERACY QUESTIONS

Note: Many of these practice questions have a slightly shorter passage length than you will find in this year's HUMAT. However, the techniques and questions used are *identical* in form, and should mean that when you face the practice papers, you feel fully prepared.

SET 1

The Kyoto Protocol is an international agreement written by the United Nations in order to reduce the effects of climate change. This agreement sets targets for countries in order for them to reduce their greenhouse gas emissions. These gases are believed to be responsible for causing global warming as a result of recent industrialisation.

The Protocol was written in 1997 and each country that signed the protocol agreed to reduce their emissions to their own specific target. This agreement could only become legally binding when two conditions had been fulfilled: When 55 countries agreed to be legally bound by the agreement and when 55% of emissions from industrialised countries had been accounted for.

The first condition was met in 2002, however countries such as Australia and the United States refused to be bound by the agreement so the minimum of 55% of emissions from industrialised countries was not met. It was only after Russia joined in 2004 that allowed the protocol to come into force in 2005.

Some climate scientists have argued that the target combined reduction of 5.2% emissions from industrialised nations would not be enough to avoid the worst consequences of global warming. In order to have a significant impact, we would need to aim at reducing emissions by 60% and to get larger countries such as the US to support the agreement.

1. The Kyoto Protocol is legally binding in all industrialised countries.
2. The greenhouse gas emissions from Australia and the United States represent 45% of emissions from industrialised countries.
3. Each country chose the amount by which they would reduce their own emissions.
4. The global emission of greenhouse gases has reduced since 2005.
5. The harmful effects of climate change would be avoided if all countries reduced their emissions by 60%.

SET 2

The space race was a competition between the Soviet Union and the United States to show off their technological superiority and economic power. It took place during the Cold War when there was a tense relationship between these nations. As the technology used in space exploration could also have military applications, both nations had many scientists and technicians involved.

In 1957, the USSR launched the first artificial satellite into the Earth's orbit, named Sputnik. The launch of this satellite was one of the first steps towards space exploration. The Americans were worried that the Soviets could use similar technology to launch nuclear warheads. This prompted urgency within the Americans, leading President Eisenhower to found NASA, and so began the space race.

The Soviets took another step forward in April 1961 when they sent the first person into space, a cosmonaut named Yuri Gagarin. This prompted President John F. Kennedy to make the unexpected claim that the US would beat the Soviets to land a man on the moon and that they would do so before the end of the decade. This led to the foundation of Project Apollo, a programme designed to do this.

In 1969, Neil Armstrong and Buzz Aldrin set off for the moon on the Apollo 11 space mission and became the first astronauts to walk on the moon. Neil Armstrong famously said, "one small step for man, one giant leap for mankind." This lunar landing led the US to win the space race that started with Sputnik's launch in 1957.

6. The Soviet Union were mainly concerned with launching satellites into space for a military advantage over the United States.
7. Project Apollo was founded in order for the United States to defeat the Soviet Union in the Cold War.
8. Yuri Gagarin did not become the first man on the moon because the Soviet technology could not handle the conditions on the moon.
9. The United States began their attempts at space exploration when the Soviets launched Sputnik.
10. The United States were losing the space race when John F. Kennedy said they would land a man on the moon.

SET 3

A marathon is a long-distance running event that is 26.2 miles long. This race was named after the famous Battle of Marathon. The first Persian invasion of Greece took place in 490 BC. The Greek soldiers did not expect to defeat the Persian army, which had greater numbers and superior cavalry. The Greek commander utilised a tactical flank to defeat the Persians forcing them to retreat back to Asia. According to legend, the fastest Greek runner, Pheidippides, was ordered to run from Marathon to Athens to announce the Greek victory over the Persians, but then collapsed and died of exhaustion. This legendary 25 mile journey from Marathon to Athens is the basis for modern marathons.

The initial organisers of the Olympic Games in 1896 wanted an event that would celebrate the glory of Ancient Greece. They therefore chose to use the same course that Pheidippides ran. In subsequent Olympic Games, the exact length of the route depended on the location but was roughly similar to the 25 mile distance. The current standardised distance of 26.2 miles has been chosen by the IAAF and used since 1921, and has been taken from the distance used at the 1908 Olympics in London. Nowadays, more than 500 marathons are organised each year.

11. Pheidippides was chosen as he was the only Greek runner determined enough to make the journey to Athens.
12. Marathon distances have been standardised since the 1908 Olympics.
13. The Persian commander believed he would defeat the Greeks in the Battle of Marathon.
14. The original route from Marathon to Athens is used for IAAF marathons today.
15. The Persian soldiers were trained better than the Greek soldiers.

SET 4

Many species of bird migrate northwards in the spring to take advantage of the abundance of nesting locations and insects to eat. As the availability of food resources decreases during the winter to the point where the birds cannot survive, the birds migrate south again. Some species are capable of flying all the way around the earth.

The act of migration itself can be risky for birds due to the amount of energy required to sustain flight over these long distances. Many juvenile birds can die from exhaustion during their first migration. Due to this inherent risk of migration, many species of birds have acquired different adaptations to increase the efficiency of flight. Flying with other birds in certain formations can allow their flight patterns to be more energy efficient.

The Northern bald ibis migrates from Austria to Italy. The behaviour of these birds is such that they migrate together within a flock and each individual bird continuously changes its position within the flock. Each individual bird benefits by spending some time flying in the updraft produced by the leading birds and a proportional amount of time leading the formation. Although it would theoretically be possible for an individual bird to take advantage of this energy-efficient flight without leading the formation itself, no Northern bald ibis has been shown to do this.

16. As migration is risky and dangerous, it would be better for birds not to migrate.
17. All migrating birds do so in flocks to increase their efficiency.
18. All the birds within a flock of Northern bald ibis benefit from flocking behaviour.
19. A bird within a Northern bald ibis flock that does not lead will be forbidden from flying with the rest of the flock.
20. The migration timing depends on different seasons.

SET 5

The dramatic decline of the bee population in the UK has been attributed to a number of causes such as the loss of wildflowers in the countryside. Bees require these wildflowers for food, and it has been estimated that 97% of the flower-rich grassland has been lost since the 1930s. Other causes include climate change and pesticides that are toxic to bees. This is particularly problematic in the UK, which has had a 50% reduction in the honey bee population between 1985 and 2005 whilst the rest of Europe has only averaged a 20% reduction during the same time period.

This loss of flowers from the British countryside has been caused by agricultural pressures. In order to increase food production, traditional farming methods have been abandoned in favour of techniques that increase productivity. These techniques, however, involve the reduction of wildflowers.

Bumblebees are required to pollinate wildflowers and commercial crops. A reduction of wildflower pollination will result in their decline, which will ultimately affect other wildlife as they can be involved in a complex food chain. The commercial crops will need to be pollinated artificially using expensive methods that will ultimately drive up the price of fruits and vegetables. The global economic value of pollination from bees has been estimated at €265 billion annually.

21. The bee population in the UK has decreased by 97% since the 1930s.
22. The UK is the country with the largest decline in bee population.
23. Reverting back to traditional farming methods will decrease the overall production of food.
24. Artificial pollination will be capable of replacing bees if it becomes cheap enough.
25. Increasing pesticide-free fruit and vegetable growth will slow the decline in bee population.

SET 6

Driving in snowy and icy conditions can be dangerous as it increases stopping distances. The stopping distance represents how far a car will travel before slowing down to a halt. It is made up of the thinking distance, which is how long it takes for a driver to react, and the braking distance, which represents the time taken for the brakes to fully stop the car.

It is advised to fit winter tyres during the winter season as these have much better grip on snow and ice. These tyres are made out of a softer material than regular tyres, allowing them to have more traction at colder temperatures. This ultimately reduces the braking distance.

As the brakes are not very effective at stopping a vehicle on icy roads, it is recommended to steer out of trouble if possible rather than applying the brakes. It is therefore important to be travelling at slower speeds to avoid the need to suddenly brake.

If the car is stuck and cannot move, the driver can stay warm by running the engine to generate heat. However, if the exhaust pipe becomes blocked by snow and the fumes cannot escape then the engine must be turned off. This is because the engine produces carbon monoxide, which is extremely toxic and odourless.

26. Driving whilst tired increases the braking distance.
27. Regular tyres are more dangerous than winter tyres in cold conditions as they are harder.
28. It is always safe to run the engine for heat in cold conditions.
29. It is dangerous to use winter tyres in hot summer conditions.
30. To avoid a collision on icy surfaces, it is important to gently apply the brakes.

SET 7

The Socratic method is a form of philosophical questioning named after the Greek philosopher Socrates. It takes place as a dialogue between Socrates and another individual, and attempts to investigate difficult concepts such as justice and ethics. In this dialogue, Socrates' partner puts forward an opinion or a thesis. Socrates then proposes extra premises that will attempt to disprove the original thesis. If there is an opposition, this shows that the original thesis is false and that the opposite is true.

In this dialogue, Socrates often showed other philosophers and thinkers how their reasoning was wrong. Some respected him for doing so as he was aware of the fact that his knowledge was limited and that he was merely questioning everything critically. However, many people were angered by him asking questions without providing any answers to these difficult questions himself. This led to him making a number of enemies in Greece.

In 399 BC, Socrates was accused of heresy and corruption of the youth by three of his enemies. He was then trialled and found guilty by the jury and so sentenced to death by drinking the poison hemlock. One of his friends, Crito, bribed the guards to allow Socrates to escape; however, he chose not to flee away. Many have referred to him as a martyr as he chose to die standing for knowledge and wisdom.

31. Socrates was the first person to use this method of questioning.
32. The Socratic method questions the wisdom of the person forming the opinions.
33. As described in the passage, the Socratic method involved corrupting the youth and heresy.
34. Socrates chose not to escape from prison because he was afraid his enemies would find him again.
35. Socrates was able to define concepts such as justice and ethics himself.

SET 8

The Anglo-Saxons were the group of people who lived in England between the 5th Century and the Norman conquest in 1066 AD. When the Germanic tribes of the Saxons, Angles and Jutes came to Britain in 449 AD, they pushed the Celtic Britons who were there before them up into Wales. The combination of the Germanic dialects of these different tribes became Anglo-Saxon or Old English.

Old English is very different from Modern English and uses more Germanic words and its grammar is closer to Old German. If English speakers were to read a passage of Old English, they would struggle to understand any more than a few words. It is thought that this Old English is most similar to the Dutch dialect spoken in Friesland, a province in the north of the Netherlands. One of the famous literary works written in Old English was the poem Beowulf. It is not known who wrote this poem and only one original manuscript of the poem still exists today. The story involves the hero Beowulf, who fights and kills the giant Grendel. All the people celebrate the death of Grendel; however, Grendel's mother comes to the town and attempts to kill as many people for revenge. Beowulf then fights Grendel's mother and kills her as well.

36. The Jute tribe did not contribute to the Anglo-Saxon language.
37. German speakers would be able to read Beowulf in its original language.
38. Beowulf was the strongest warrior at that time.
39. A dialect of Old English is currently spoken in the Netherlands.
40. The Celts lived in England in 449 AD.

SET 9

A constellation is a group of stars that are often visible, forming a pattern in the sky. The constellation's visibility depends on a number of factors. The biggest factor is your position on the Earth, for example the constellation Cassiopeia is only visible in the northern hemisphere. As the Earth orbits the Sun, another significant factor affecting constellation visibility is the season on Earth.

As the Earth rotates on its own axis, certain stars and constellations can appear to rise and fall in the night sky. Constellations that do not move in this manner are called circumpolar. This factor can allow people to navigate on the Earth using the positioning of the stars. This is especially useful during marine navigation, as there are no visible landmarks. The most commonly used star for navigation is the North Star Polaris, as its position is constant within the night sky.

There are 12 constellations that take the form of animals or humans known as the zodiac signs. This is the basis for the origin of star signs in astrology, which suggests that human behaviour is influenced by the celestial phenomena. The star sign of a person represents the position of the sun at the moment of their birth. The zodiac sign which shares the same position as the sun in the sky becomes their star sign.

41. Certain stars are not visible from the southern hemisphere.
42. The constellation Cassiopeia is circumpolar.
43. Star signs are chosen by the constellations visible at birth.
44. Polaris is used for navigation as it is the brightest star in the sky.
45. Different constellations are visible from London and Sydney.

SET 10

Maple syrup is a sweet syrup made from maple trees. The sap from the trees is harvested during March. It is then boiled to evaporate water, making it denser and sweeter. It takes roughly 40 litres of maple sap to produce 1 litre of maple syrup. This current process is very similar to that used by the Native Americans, except it uses more advanced equipment.

According to American Indian legend, the maple trees originally made life free from hardship. They produced a thick syrup all year round which the people would drink. A mythological creature named Glooskap saw that the people of a village were strangely silent. The men were not getting ready to hunt and the women were not minding the fires. He found the villagers sitting near the maple trees letting its syrup drip into their mouth.

Glooskap was angered by their laziness and used his powers to fill the trees with water so that they would only produce a dilute, watery sap. This meant that the people had to boil the sap to produce the sweet syrup. Although it wasn't very difficult to do this, it meant that they had to look after their fires and gather firewood. Furthermore, it meant that the trees were not able to produce enough sap to sustain the people all year so they would be forced to hunt and forage during the spring and summer.

46. Sweet syrup can be made from the sap from other trees.
47. Glooskap was angered because there was no syrup left for him to drink.
48. The technique for making maple syrup is similar to that used in the time of the American Indian legends.
49. Sap is only harvested from maple trees for one month a year.
50. Hunting animals was more difficult than drinking maple syrup.

SET 11

Stockholm syndrome is an interesting phenomenon that sometimes happens to people who have been kidnapped or held hostage. They may feel some loyalty or attraction towards the person that has kidnapped them.

This phenomenon was named after a bank robbery in Stockholm, Sweden in 1973. Four bank workers were kept hostage by two criminals who wanted to rob the bank. After being held against their will for six days, they showed that they had formed a positive relationship with their captors. The hostages were seen to be hugging and kissing the men who had kidnapped them.

It can be hard to explain why this might be the case, as it involves the captor putting the hostage in a terrifying situation. In the mind of the hostage, it is this person who can ultimately decide if the hostage is going to die. As a result of this fear of death, any small act of kindness prompts them to be thankful for the gift of life. This can ultimately lead to them developing Stockholm syndrome.

It is important to understand the interaction between victims and captors in cases of Stockholm syndrome as this knowledge can improve the chances of hostage survival. As such, the FBI is willing to devote resources in order to improve crisis negotiation.

51. People who get kidnapped will eventually develop positive emotions towards their kidnapper.
52. The bank workers hugged and kissed their kidnappers because the criminals forced them to.
53. Stockholm syndrome is useful to understand for crisis negotiation.
54. According to the passage, it is the victims that fear for their life that tend to develop Stockholm Syndrome.
55. The bank robbery in 1973 was the first recorded instance of a positive relationship developing between captors and hostages.

SET 12

Clownfish are a type of fish that live in salt water. They are orange fish that have white stripes. They are capable of growing up to 10-18 cm. They have also been called anemone fish, as they have a symbiotic relationship with certain sea anemones.

The tentacles of sea anemone are capable of stinging fish that come near them, which the anemone then eat. The clownfish have a special mucous covering that protects them from this sting. As a result of this, clownfish that live inside sea anemone are safe from other predators but do not get stung themselves. The sea anemone benefit from the clownfish, as the clownfish eat the algae that grows on the anemone. The bright colour of the clownfish lures in small fish to the anemone, which ultimately get stung. They also receive better water circulation from the action of the clownfish fins.

Many people like keeping clownfish in aquariums because of their bright orange colour and how easy they are to look after. This can be dangerous as the clownfish lifespan is greatly increased by living within an anemone. Even if an anemone is added to the aquarium, only certain species of clownfish are capable of living within certain species of anemone.

56. A clownfish that loses its mucous layer can live inside sea anemone.
57. Clownfish help sea anemone to catch fish.
58. Clownfish will die if they do not have an anemone to live in.
59. Clownfish have a mutually beneficial relationship with all anemone.
60. Anemone protect clownfish from predators.

SET 13

The guillotine was a machine used to kill people by chopping off their head. It consists of a heavy blade attached to a frame. When the blade was released, it would fall down under its own weight and chop off the victim's head, killing them instantly. It was commonly used in France during the French Revolution as it was the only legal method of execution in order to enact the death penalty.

The guillotine was named after a French doctor called Joseph Guillotin. He decided that a more humane way of executing someone was needed, as he realised he was unable to get rid of the death penalty. He decided that using an automatic mechanical device for decapitation would be more humane than by a person with an axe. The first guillotine built was then tested on animals to see if the axe would have enough force to decapitate its victim.

Before the guillotine was used in execution, the criminal would be hanged. This was seen to be less humane, as the victim was supposed to die from the impact of the rope snapping their necks, however this did not happen all the time. The victim could be in agony for up to forty minutes before eventually dying from asphyxiation.

61. Joseph Guillotin agreed with the death penalty.
62. According to the passage, the guillotine was used for execution before the French Revolution.
63. Hanging usually causes death by asphyxiation.
64. The guillotine was seen as being more humane, as it was automatic with the blade falling through its own weight.
65. During the French Revolution, hanging was the common form of execution.

SET 14

"The Gherkin" is a building in the City of London named after – and famous for – its distinctive shape. Its modern architecture was designed by Norman Foster and was built between 2001 and 2003. Norman Foster is famous for utilising the laws of physics in designing many of his buildings. The walls of the Gherkin would allow air to enter the building for passive cooling. As this air warms up, it rises and is then let out of the building.

The site where the Gherkin is built used to belong to the Baltic Exchange, the headquarters of the global marketplace for ship sales. In 1992, the site was damaged by bombs placed by the Provisional IRA. As there were many historic buildings in the area and only a few were damaged, the City of London governing body was insistent that any redevelopment must restore the old historic look. They later discovered that the amount of damage caused was too severe and so removed this restriction.

The building was sold in 2007 for a sum of £630 million, making it the most expensive office building in the UK. The building was then put up for sale in 2014, initially at a lower price, as its owners could not afford to pay loan repayments due to high interest rates and the devaluing of the British pound. It was bought by a Brazilian billionaire for £700 million.

66. According to the passage, The Gherkin is famous because of its passive cooling system.
67. The Baltic Exchange was built with a modern architectural design.
68. The Gherkin was sold in 2014 at a loss.
69. The Provisional IRA intended to destroy the Baltic Exchange.
70. Norman Foster has designed many buildings that incorporated physics in their design.

SET 15

The living wage represents the minimum hourly rate for employment, which allows an individual to cover their basic costs of living. This wage is set at £9.15 per hour in London and £7.85 per hour in the rest of the UK. This difference in living wage between London and the rest of the UK is explained by the significant costs associated with living in London.

The minimum wage is currently £6.50 for employees aged over 21 and £5.13 for employees aged between 18 and 20. This is lower than the living wage values quoted above and represents the legal minimum wage. It would be illegal for an employer to pay less than these values. Although many employers have agreed to pay a living wage, they are not legally obliged to do so.

The introduction of the living wage in companies has been argued to be beneficial for these companies. Many employers found that employees who were paid the living wage were able to work harder with better quality. It has also improved the quality of life for the families of employees, as it has allowed those who are parents to spend more time with their children. However, some employers have argued that the introduction of the living wage would force them to fire some workers, forcing others to work harder.

71. The living cost across UK cities is approximately equal.
72. Companies introduce the living wage to avoid the legal complications of underpaying their employees.
73. A 24-year-old working at minimum wage would be able to live comfortably in Manchester.
74. Introducing a living wage would be beneficial for all employees.
75. Paying someone a living wage will only benefit that individual.

SET 16

The ecological footprint is a simple way to look at how sustainable people are being. It is based on the idea that all the resources taken from the Earth are finite. It is defined by how much land and water would be required to produce the resources that the population consumes within a year. It has been calculated that there are currently 11.2 billion bio-productive hectares available on the Earth.

A study in 2004 has suggested that our ecological footprint is 13.5 billion hectares, meaning that we are using the Earth's resources 20% faster than they are being renewed. This will ultimately result in the loss of all the Earth's resources.

Individual countries can look at their own ecological footprint and compare it to the size of their bio-productive capacity. Some countries are in an ecological deficit - they require more land than their bio-productive capacity to sustain them. Other countries have an ecological reserve, meaning that their bio-productive capacity is greater than their footprint.

It can be difficult for individual countries to reduce their ecological footprint. This can either be performed by reducing that countries reliance on unsustainable resources or by increasing the amount of bio-productive land available. It is important, however, that a global effort is made to increase our sustainability.

76. The ecological footprint of a country directly depends on its population.
77. The combined area of the Earth's land and water mass is 11.2 billion hectares.
78. The ecological footprint can be reduced by using sustainable resources.
79. Only the countries with an ecological deficit are able to tackle the global problem of sustainability.
80. The bio-productive capacity of the Earth is fixed.

SET 17

English punk rock band The Sex Pistols formed in 1975, and sparked the British punk movement, leading to the subsequent creation of multiple punk and alternative rock acts. They produced only one album – 'Never Mind the Bollocks, Here's the Sex Pistols' – in their brief existence. However, despite these, some state The Sex Pistols are one of the most important bands in the history of popular music.

Originally, the band was made up of Johnny Rotten (the singer), Paul Cook (the drummer) and Glen Matlock (the bassist), however the latter was subsequently replaced by Sid Vicious. The band was involved in numerous controversies, due to their lyrics, performances and public appearances. One may argue the band was asking for trouble when they created songs attacking the music industry (such 'EMI') and commenting on controversial topics like consumerism, the Berlin wall, the Holocaust and abortion ('Bodies'). The band did not take kindly to local figureheads, as demonstrated with the release of 'God Save the Queen' in 1977, which was an attack on both conforming to societal norms and also blindly accepting the royalty as an authority.

81. It is believed by some that pop music's most influential act is The Sex Pistols.
82. The Sex Pistols kick-started the punk movement.
83. The Sex Pistols controversially equated the music industry with the Holocaust.
84. The Sex Pistols' songs showed they were staunch royalists.
85. The Sex Pistols had two bassists.

SET 18

Cancer is a disease of the tissues of the body which occurs when cells begin to grow and replicate rapidly. These cells are capable of becoming masses called tumours, which can obstruct the parts of the body in which they are found. Some of these tumours are also able to spread to other parts of the body in a process known as metastasis.

The incidence of cancer has significantly increased recently in the Western developed world. The most common form of cancer in the UK is breast cancer, even though it very rarely affects men. Most cancers seem to have no obvious cause, whilst a few are known to have a specific cause. Mesothelioma, for example, is a type of lung cancer that is caused by exposure to asbestos. People who have worked with asbestos without adequate protection in the past are eligible for compensation from the government.

Before the 19th century, the only way to treat a cancer was to physically remove the tumour from the body. This usually involved amputation or removing a lot of tissue. It was only in the 19th century when improvements in surgical hygiene enhanced the success rates of tumour removal. At this time, Marie and Pierre Curie discovered the first non-surgical treatment, which involved irradiating the tumour.

86. Everyone exposed to asbestos will eventually suffer from mesothelioma.
87. Breast cancer is the most common type of cancer in British women.
88. The surgical success rate for tumour removal in the 19th century was improved by irradiating the tumour.
89. Irradiation is more effective than surgery in removing tumours.
90. Only cells that are capable of spreading cause tumours.

SET 19

The indigenous Australians are the native people of Australia, also known as the Aborigines. It is believed that they arrived in Australia 50,000 years ago from South-east Asia. They lead a traditional life, which involved living in wooded areas and hunting animals with spears and boomerangs. This lifestyle would not harm the environment of Australia, as they believe that the land – with all of its animals and plants – is sacred.

When the British people came to Australia in 1788, there were not many people living in Australia. According to British law, any land could be claimed for the monarchy if they believed that nobody owned it, and so they claimed all of the land. It was later agreed by the Australian government in 1976 that the aboriginal people would have the rights to the land where they were originally located if they could prove that they have been living there.

Nowadays, many of the 517,000 aboriginal people in Australia have chosen to integrate with the modern ways of life. They live in cities and towns and some of them have acquired professional jobs. Others have decided to maintain their traditional aboriginal way of living. Few have been unfortunate in that they haven't been educated enough to benefit from Australian society but have also lost their traditional aboriginal ways.

91. The British people claimed the Australian land because the Aborigines only lived in the wooded areas.
92. There are 517,000 Aborigines currently living in the cities and towns of Australia.
93. The aboriginal people were able to reclaim all their land in 1976.
94. Most Aborigines have received enough education to integrate with Australian culture.
95. The Aborigine lifestyle is similar to that of the south-east Asians from 50,000 years ago.

SET 20

Chilli peppers are a type of fruit grown all over the world. Most of these peppers are spicy and used in cooking. These peppers are believed to initially originate from Bolivia. As they spread throughout Europe, it was found that their spiciness had a similar taste to black peppercorns, which were incredibly valuable in the 15th century. As such, many people began to grow chilli peppers, which spread rapidly to India and China.

These chilli peppers began to be incorporated into the cooking of different cultures, being used more commonly in hotter countries. There are a number of reasons suggested for why these countries would prefer spicy food. One suggestion is that spicy food would help people to sweat in hot conditions, allowing them to cool down. This, however, is unlikely to explain the prevalence of chilli peppers, as it is possible to sweat without eating them. Adding spice to food was also found to be a convenient method of preserving food as it discouraged the growth of bacteria.

Chilli peppers are spicy because they produce the chemical capsaicin. This chemical binds to receptors in the mouth and throat and cause the sensation of heat. This receptor is also capable of responding to heat directly. This is an example of labelled line coding, which suggests that the perception of a stimulus is determined by which receptor it activates, not the nature of the stimulus itself.

96. Chilli peppers became more valuable in the 15th century.
97. Eating chilli peppers in hot conditions causes sweating.
98. All chilli peppers are spicy.
99. An individual lacking the capsaicin receptor would be able to eat the spiciest chillies without any pain.
100. Different methods of activating the capsaicin receptor (TRPV1) cause different sensations.

SET 21

The social determinants of health are factors in which people are born, grow, live, work and age. These factors depend on the social distribution of resources, and can affect the life expectancy and quality of life that people have. These factors refer to the social context that people live in and include characteristics such as level of education, culture, stress and socioeconomic conditions, as well as many others. It can be difficult to see how some of these factors may affect somebody's health, but it is likely to involve a combination of multiple factors.

A number of mechanisms acting together have been described to explain why someone with a poor diet would have a lower life expectancy. One such mechanism is as follows: the individual would be more likely to be malnourished, which would weaken their immune system. This would ultimately increase their likelihood of suffering from infections. Recurrent infections would place strain on the body, which could eventually result in organ failure. On average, the life expectancy in the most deprived areas can be up to 10 years lower than in the least deprived areas.

Many of these health inequalities are avoidable. Understanding how these social determinants affect the health of a population will allow us to improve its care. Knowledge of how social policies impact health can better allow us to monitor changes in health care, and is allowing us to reduce the gaps between those with a more disadvantaged social background from those with a privileged background.

101. Dropping out of school can have an effect on an individual's health.
102. The effects of the social determinants of health are principally measured by life expectancy.
103. The health impact of poor diet can be avoided completely by using multivitamins that supplement the immune system.
104. Nothing can be done to improve the health care of the poor in comparison to the rich.
105. Alan lives in a less deprived area than Henry so Alan will live longer than Henry.

SET 22

J.S. Mill describes S, 'Utilitarianism', and states:

'The creed which accepts as the foundation of morals, Utility, or the Greatest Happiness Principle, holds that actions are right in proportion as they tend to promote happiness, wrong as they tend to produce the reverse of happiness. By happiness is intended pleasure, and the absence of pain; by unhappiness, pain, and the privation of pleasure. To give a clear view of the moral standard set up by the theory, much more requires to be said; in particular, what things it includes in the ideas of pain and pleasure; and to what extent this is left an open question. But these supplementary explanations do not affect the theory of life on which this theory of morality is grounded—namely, that pleasure, and freedom from pain, are the only things desirable as ends; and that all desirable things are desirable either for the pleasure inherent in themselves, or as means to the promotion of pleasure and the prevention of pain.

Now, such a theory of life provokes in many minds, and among them in some of the most estimable in feeling and purpose, dislike. To suppose that life has (as they express it) no higher end than pleasure—no better and nobler object of desire and pursuit—they designate as utterly mean and grovelling; as a doctrine worthy only of swine, to whom the followers of Epicurus were, at a very early period, contemptuously likened; and modern holders of the doctrine are occasionally made the subject of equally polite comparisons by its German, French, and English assailants.

When thus attacked, the Epicureans have always answered, that it is not they, but their accusers, who represent human nature in a degrading light; since the accusation supposes human beings to be capable of no pleasures except those of which swine are capable.'

106. How do the Epicureans answer their critics?
A. By claiming the critics are miserable, in their refusal to embrace pleasure.
B. That the critics do not understand the multiplicity of things contained in the word 'pleasure'.
C. By calling their critics degraded.
D. By suggesting their critics are more susceptible to animalistic pleasures than they.

107. Which of the following actions are NOT in keeping with the theory of utility?
A. Providing a crash mat for a gymnast, to prevent him or her hurting him or herself.
B. Getting a crash mat for yourself, to prevent hurting yourself when performing gymnastics.
C. Not eating a chocolate bar because social pressures deem it wrong.
D. Eating a chocolate bar because it is delicious.

108. Which of the following does the passage suggest about critics of utilitarianism?
A. They are Christians.
B. They are European.
C. They are unintelligent.
D. They are reactionary.

109. Utilitarianism is only concerned with ends.
A. True. B. False. C. Can't tell.

110. The above passage defines:
A. What is included by the term pleasure.
B. What is included by the term pain.
C. What is meant by Epicureanism.
D. What is meant by utility.

SET 23

Geology deals with the rocks of the earth's crust. It learns from their composition and structure how the rocks were made and how they have been modified. It ascertains how they have been brought to their present places and wrought to their various topographic forms, such as hills and valleys, plains and mountains. It studies the vestiges, which the rocks preserve, of ancient organisms that once inhabited our planet. Geology is the history of the earth and its inhabitants, as read in the rocks of the earth's crust.

To obtain a general idea of the nature and method of our science before beginning its study in detail, we may visit some valley, on whose sides are rocky ledges. Here the rocks lie in horizontal layers. Although only their edges are exposed, we may infer that these layers run into the upland on either side and underlie the entire district; they are part of the foundation of solid rock found beneath the loose materials of the surface everywhere.

Take the sandstones ledge of a valley. Looking closely at the rock we see that it is composed of myriads of grains of sand cemented together. These grains have been worn and rounded. They are also sorted, with those of each layer being similar in size. By some means, they have been brought hither from some more ancient source. Surely these grains have had a history before they here found a resting place – a history which we are to learn to read.

The successive layers of the rock suggest that they were built one after another from the bottom upward. We may be as sure that each layer was formed before those above it, as that the bottom courses of stone in a wall were laid before the courses which rest upon them.

111. Based on the passage, each of these statements can be verified, EXCEPT?

A. We can learn about earth's inhabitants through its crust.
B. Individual layers of sandstone form one after another.
C. Rocks are made of sand.
D. Geology does not always demand explicit evidence.

112. Wall-building is used in this passage to help us understand:

A. Mountains. B. Valleys. C. Hills. D. Plains.

113. The sand mentioned in the passage comes from:

A. An ancient beach. B. The sea. C. The earth's crust. D. It is undisclosed.

114. A foundation of rock is **NOT** found underneath:

A. Upland. B. Lowland. C. Nowhere. D. Water.

115. 'Grains of sand' are described as sorted by:

A. Shape. B. Texture. C. Age. D. Measurements.

SET 24

The genus of plants called Narcissus – many of the species of which are highly esteemed by the floriculturist and lover of cultivated plants – belongs to the Amaryllis family (Amaryllidaceæ). This family includes about seventy genera and over eight hundred species that are mostly native in tropical or semi-tropical countries, though a few are found in temperate climates.

Many of the species are sought for ornamental purposes and – on account of their beauty and remarkable odour – they are more prized by many than are the species of the Lily family. In this group is classed the American Aloe (Agave Americana) valued not only for cultivation, but also by the Mexicans on account of the sweet fluid which is yielded by its central bud. This liquid, after fermentation, forms an intoxicating liquor known as pulque. By distillation, this yields a liquid very similar to rum, called mescal by the Mexicans. The leaves furnish a strong fibre – known as vegetable silk – from which, since remote times, paper has been manufactured.

The popular opinion is that this plant flowers but once in a century; hence the name 'Century Plant' is often applied to it, though under proper culture it will blossom more frequently.

116. Which of the following are **NOT** mentioned as potential uses for a narcissus plant?

A. Perfume production.
B. Alcohol production.
C. Visual decoration.
D. Stationary production.

117. Why is the plant known as 'the century plant'?

A. It is sown only once every hundred years.
B. It is only able to be fertilised once a century.
C. It is perceived as blooming centennially.
D. It is only able to flower once within a hundred years.

118. Which of the following statements is most supported by the above passage:

A. Lilies are generally valued less than members of the Narcissus genus.
B. Lilies are famously not as attractive as members of the Narcissus genus.
C. A number are people prefer members of the Narcissus genus over Lilies.
D. Members of the Narcissus genus are a welcome addition to any household.

119. Which of the following statements is NOT true?

A. American Aloe can be used to make rum.
B. The Amaryllis family contains more than six hundred species of Narcissus.
C. Members of the Narcissus genus can be found in all climates.
D. The members of the Narcissus genus have a distinctive smell.

120. Which of the following statements can be verified by the passage?

A. The 'Narcissus' genus is named after the mythical character, famed for his beauty.
B. Agave syrup can be collected by American Aloe.
C. A genus belongs to a family.
D. Members of the Narcissus genus are used for their soothing properties.

SET 25

The following passage is found in a book on nature published in 1899:

Five women out of every ten who walk the streets of Chicago and other Illinois cities, says a prominent journal, by wearing dead birds upon their hats, proclaim themselves as lawbreakers. For the first time in the history of Illinois laws, it has been made an offense punishable by fine and imprisonment, or both, to have in possession any dead, harmless bird except game birds, which may be possessed in their proper season. The wearing of a tern, or a gull, a woodpecker, or a jay is an offense against the law's majesty, and any policeman with a mind rigidly bent upon enforcing the law could round up, without a written warrant, a wagon load of the offenders any hour in the day, and carry them off to the lockup. What moral suasion cannot do, a crusade of this sort undoubtedly would.

Thanks to the personal influence of the Princess of Wales, the osprey plume, so long a feature of the uniforms of a number of the cavalry regiments of the British army, has been abolished. After Dec. 31, 1899, the osprey plume, by order of Field Marshal Lord Wolseley, is to be replaced by one of ostrich feathers. It was the wearing of these plumes by the officers of all the hussar and rifle regiments, as well as of the Royal Horse Artillery, which so sadly interfered with the crusade inaugurated by the Princess against the use of osprey plumes. The fact that these plumes, to be of any marketable value, have to be torn from the living bird during the nesting season induced the Queen, the Princess of Wales, and other ladies of the royal family to set their faces against the use of both the osprey plume and the aigrette as articles of fashionable wear.

121. In 1899:

A. Women across the USA could be prosecuted for owning ornamental dead birds.
B. There was a significant rise of female arrests in America.
C. Possession of a dead gull could lead to trouble.
D. Americans responded to law by citing the use of jays as ornamentation unfashionable.

122. Ostrich feathers were seen as preferable to osprey plums because:

A. Ostriches are less intelligent birds.
B. Ostriches are killed for their meat, so one might as well use their feathers.
C. Queen Elizabeth has an especial love of ospreys.
D. Harvesting osprey feathers was seen as an inhumane process.

123. Games birds could be possessed by citizens of Illinois all year round.

A. True.
B. False.
C. Can't tell.

124. Banning Osprey feathers in the UK's army was difficult because:

A. Many uniforms required them.
B. The Princess did not have the authority to implement the ban.
C. Her ultimate support was predominately female, and thus their concerns seemed to have no relevance from the male domain of the army.
D. It would be hard to differentiate between other regiments within the army, who were already wearing ostrich feathers.

125. Which of the following could NOT be legally owned in Illinois, according to the passage?

A. A live bird intended for personal ornamentation.
B. A dead bird of prey that had violently attacked you.
C. Feathered garments.
D. None of the above.

SET 26

Indie game developer Lucas Pope created 'Papers Please', a video game where the player is an immigration officer processing people attempting to enter Arstotzka, a fictional dystopia. Released in 2013, the game was originally made for Microsoft Windows and OS X platforms. It was subsequently released for Linux and the iPad in 2014.

The game is set in 1982, and gameplay involves the player processing large numbers of applicants attempting to enter the country, by checking various pieces of paperwork. This is intended to keep criminals out, whether they are terrorists or drug smugglers. When looking through the applicant's 'papers', discrepancies may be discovered. The player must then enquire about these and may go on to use other tools, such as a body scanner and finger printing to discover the truth of the candidate's motives. Applicants may attempt to bribe the officer in order to get through. Ultimately, the game player must stamp candidates' passports, either accepting into or rejecting them from the country. Their work is being monitored however: after two false acceptances/rejections, the player will be pecuniarily punished, with their day's wages being decreased in response to their administrative sloppiness. They have a limited amount of time to work – representing each 'day' – during which they will be paid in accordance to the number of people processed.

126. Which of the following statements is best supported by the above passage?
A. Lucas Pope created the 'Papers Please' for a small games company.
B. 'Papers Please' is a multi-platform game.
C. Arstotzka is a fictionalised version of an ex-Soviet block state.
D. The game gained significant media attention in 2014.

127. Which of the following statements best sums up the official job of the player's character?
A. To accept as many applicants into Artstotzka as possible.
B. To reject as many new applicants entering Arstotzka as possible.
C. To avoid making mistakes in processing people.
D. To stamp passports.

128. Discrepancies in information provided by applicants lead to the player:
A. Interrogating and performing a fingerprint check on the suspicious individual.
B. Interrogating and performing a full body scan on the suspicious individual.
C. Asking the suspicious individual for further information.
D. Performing one or multiple physical assessments of the individual.

129. Which of the following statements is true?
A. The game-player solely makes money through processing applicants.
B. The game-player will ultimately be responsible for multiple arrests.
C. The game-player will not be forgiven for their mistakes.
D. The game-player may be subject to fiscal penalisation.

130. Body scanner and finger printing must be used if discrepancies are discovered.
A. True. B. False. C. Can't tell.

SET 27

Emerging in 1970s USA, Blaxploitation, or 'blacksploitation', gives homage to many other genres. Within it, there are western, martial arts films, musicals, coming-of-age dramas and comedies, and the genre has even parodied itself with films like 'Black Dynamite'. Blaxploitation movies may take place in the South, and focus on issues like slavery, or be set in the poor neighbourhoods of the Northeast or West coast, but in any case they will feature a predominately black cast. It is also known to feature soundtracks comprised of soul and funk music, and the common feature of character's using the words 'honky', 'cracker' and other slurs against white people.

Originally, the genre's exports were aimed at city-dwelling black Americans, but their appeal has since grown and is not exclusive to any race. Despite the negative sound of the title 'blaxploitation', the term was coined by ex-film publicist Junius Griffin, the then head of LA's NAACP, National Association for the Advancement of Coloured People. He came up with the name through a play on the word 'sexploitation' describing films which featured pornographic scenes.

The film 'Shaft' and 'Sweet Sweetback's Baadasssss Song' are two of the forerunners of this genre, both released in 1971. The latter has been said, by Variety, to have created the genre.

131. Which of the following statements is supported by the information in the above passage?

A. 'Blaxploitation' was a term coined by porn directors moving into a new genre.
B. 'Blaxploitation' was a term made popular by black audiences.
C. 'Blaxploitation' was a term coined by a civil rights activist.
D. 'Blaxploitation' was a term criticised by white sympathisers.

132. Which of the following statements best describes the most common element of a Blaxploitation film?

A. Characters performing funk songs.
B. Characters coming to terms with the legacy of slavery.
C. Characters performing martial arts.
D. Characters using racial slurs.

133. Which of these statements best describes casting in Blaxploitation films?

A. Primarily white.
B. Primarily black.
C. Exclusively white.
D. Exclusively black.

134. Which of the following best describes the audiences of Blaxploitation films?

A. Originally for all middle-class African-Americans.
B. Originally for all urban-dwellers.
C. Multi-ethnic.
D. Shrinking since the mid-1970s.

135. The legacy of films including soft-core porn is knowingly acknowledged in the name of two Blaxploitation titles, 'Shaft' and 'Sweet Sweetback's Baadasssss song', both of which suggest body parts associated with sex films.

A. True.
B. False.
C. Can't tell.

SET 28

When discussing his famous character Rorschach, the antihero of 'Watchmen', Moore explains, 'I originally intended Rorschach to be a warning about the possible outcome of vigilante thinking. But an awful lot of comic readers felt his remorseless, frightening, psychotic toughness was his most appealing characteristic – not quite what I was going for.' Moore misunderstands his own hero's appeal within this quotation: it is not that Rorschach is willing to break little fingers to extract information – or that he is happy to use violence – that makes him laudable. The Comedian, another 'superhero' within the alternative world of Watchmen, is a thug who has won no great fan base; his remorselessness (killing a pregnant Vietnamese woman), frightening (attempt at rape), psychotic toughness (one only has to look at the panels of him shooting out into a crowd to witness this) is repulsive, not winning. This is because The Comedian has no purpose: he is a nihilist, and as a nihilist, denies any potential meaning to his fellow man, and so to the comic's reader. Everything to him is a 'joke', including his self, and consequently, his own death could be seen as just another gag.

Rorschach, on the other hand, does believe in something: he questions if his fight for justice 'is futile?' then instantly corrects himself, stating 'there is good and evil, and evil must be punished. Even in the face of Armageddon I shall not compromise in this.' Jacob Held, in his essay comparing Rorschach's motivation with Kantian ethics, put forward the postulation 'perhaps our dignity is found in acting as if the world were just, even when it is clearly not.' Rorschach then causes pain in others, not because he is a sadist, but because he feels the need to punish wrong and to uphold the good, and though he cannot make the world just, he can act according to his sense of justice, through the use of violence.

136. Which of the following best describes 'Watchmen'?
A. A book that contains only vicious characters.
B. An expression of despair when contemplating an imperfect world.
C. An example of how an author's intentions are not always realised.
D. A book that accidentally glamorises violence.

137. 'The Comedian' is a misnomer – the character that goes by this title should not, logically, be called this.
A. True. B. False. C. Can't tell.

138. Which of the following best articulates the view put forward by Jacob Held?
A. We find dignity through just actions.
B. If one decides to behave as though the world is fair, this may lead to a discovery of self-worth.
C. It is shameful to view the world as corrupt.
D. Self-value can only be found in madness.

139. What does the passage above argue?
A. Rorschach breaking little fingers is preferable to the Comedian attempting rape.
B. The Comedian's depressing sense of humour has made him unpopular.
C. Rorschach is not actually violent.
D. Rorschach is popular because his aggressive behaviour has a moral intent, and is not just violence.

140. What does the word 'nihilist' mean in the context of the passage?
A. Someone who believes there is no meaning to life.
B. Someone who is full of anger at the corruption of society.
C. Someone who is narcissistic.
D. Someone who hates other people.

SET 29

'The Bechdel Test', also known as the 'Mo Movie Measure' and 'The Bechdel Rule' is named after cartoonist Alison Bechdel, who in 1985 wrote a cartoon containing the original proposal of the 'test'. It depicts one woman telling another that she has 'a rule' that she will only see a film if it satisfies three basic requirements: that it contains at least two women, that they talk to each other and that their conversation is on something other than a man. The second woman states that this is 'pretty strict, but a good idea', to which the first responds the last film she saw that complied with this was 'Alien'. The original notion described in the strip has been attributed to Liz Wallace, and the test is sometimes referred to as the Bechdel/Wallace Test.

Following this, a website entitled 'The Bechdel Test Movie List' has formed an extensive list of cinematic output, showing movies that pass and do not pass the test. One may be surprised at the number of movies that would not be watched by first woman in the Bechdel comic: many blockbusters do not make the mark, and such titles as 'Godzilla', 'The Imitation Game' and 'Robocop' all feature on the list of 'failed' films.

141. According to The Bechdel Test, 'The Imitation Game' is a sexist film.
A. True. B. False. C. Can't tell.

142. Which of the following films would pass the Bechdel test?
A. One where the only conversation between two women is on woman A's brother.
B. One where there are two conversations, one on woman A's son and another on woman B's boss, Mr Smith.
C. One where there are five women, in which at one point they all have a chat about how to lose weight and the best hair removal techniques.
D. One where there is one woman who chats about all manner of things with her male colleagues, including her USA presidential campaign.

143. 50% of horror films, according to the above extract, pass the Bechdel test.
A. True. B. False. C. Can't tell.

144. Which of the following phrases best describes the reaction of the second woman within the comic strip?
A. Ecstatically approving.
B. Condemning.
C. Cautiously approving.
D. Apathetic.

145. The two women in the comic strip are manifestations of Bechdel and Wallace, with the piece of art being a recreation of their original conversation on this matter.
A. True. B. False. C. Can't tell.

SET 30

There are many comic tropes that a comedian or group of comedians may want to employ in their set or act, but for the purpose of this extract, we shall focus on the device of the 'call-back'. A call-back is a reference made to a previous joke, in a different context; for example, a comedian may make the joke 'why did the chicken cross the road? To get to the other side' early on in his or her set, and then later on may reference this again by telling an anecdote and saying 'so then I crossed the road - oh, look, there's a chicken! Strange, I could have sworn he was over there a moment ago'. Though the call-back may appear to simply rely on the idea that repetition is inherently funny, it actually has several desirable effects. Firstly, it means that one joke can provide more than one laugh, as the memory of the previous joke encourages renewed chuckling, and so the original quip's comic potential is increased. It also builds up a relationship between comedian and audience, as it builds up a sense of familiarity with the speaker and his or her subject matter, and this bond also may encourage more laughter - the second joke creates the same feeling as an 'in-joke'. If used at the end of a set – as a call-back often is – it gives a sense of completion, and also may lead to the ending of the act culminating in the largest laugh. In TV, a call-back often refers to a joke made in a previous episode.

146. Repetition is inherently funny.

A. True. B. False. C. Can't tell.

147. Which of the following best explains how a call-back works?

A. Previous understanding of a subject makes it potentially more comic.
B. Doubling a joke makes it potentially twice as funny.
C. Making the audience feel comfortable is more likely to make them laugh.
D. We find people we have a relationship with funny.

148. For a call-back to work, the original joke has to be significantly funny.

A. True. B. False. C. Can't tell.

149. A call-back cannot be used in an un-comic setting.

A. True. B. False. C. Can't tell.

150. Which of the following statements is best supported by the above passage?

A. A call-back is used to create a sense of the circle having fully come to pass.
B. A call-back can be a useful addition to an individual comedian's set.
C. A call-back creates unity through disparate TV episodes.
D. A call-back is an especially important trope to consider.

SET 31

Harriet Beecher (Stowe) was born June 14, 1811, in the characteristic New England town of Litchfield, Connecticut. Her father was the Rev. Dr. Lyman Beecher, a distinguished Calvinistic divine, her mother Roxanna Foote, his first wife. Harriet Beecher was ushered into a household of happy, healthy children, and found five brothers and sisters awaiting her. The eldest was Catherine, born September 6, 1800. Following her were two sturdy boys, William and Edward; then came Mary, then George, and at last Harriet. Another little Harriet was actually born three years before, but died when aged only one month old; the fourth daughter, the subject of this passage, was named in memory of this sister Harriet Elizabeth. Just two years after Harriet was born, in the same month, another brother, Henry Ward, was welcomed to the family circle, and after him came Charles, the last of Roxanna Beecher's children.

The first memorable incident of Harriet's life was the death of her mother, which occurred when she was four years old, and which ever afterwards remained with her as the most tender, sad and sacred memory of her childhood. Mrs Stowe's recollections of her mother are found in a letter to her brother Charles, afterwards published in the 'Autobiography and Correspondence of Lyman Beecher.' She says: —

"I was between three and four years of age when our mother died, and my personal recollections of her are therefore but few. But the deep interest and veneration that she inspired in all who knew her were such that during all my childhood I was constantly hearing her spoken of, and from one friend or another some incident or anecdote of her life was constantly being impressed upon me."

151. Harriet, the main character in the article, was the third daughter of Roxanna Beecher:

A. True. B. False. C. Can't tell.

152. Which of the following statements, according to the passage, are true?

A. Harriet Beecher had a religious father.
B. Harriet Beecher was born in the English town Litchfield.
C. Harriet Beecher was born in the 18th century.
D. Harriet Beecher was born in an average American town.

153. Roxanna Beecher was an admired woman.

A. True. B. False. C. Can't tell.

154. Harriet Beecher Stowe's mother's death is described as:

A. Her saddest memory of her life.
B. The earliest significant event in her life.
C. Her most tender memory of her life.
D. All of the above.

155. Which of the following statements is supported by the above passage?

A. Harriet Beecher was between three and four when her father died.
B. Harriet Beecher had five brothers waiting for her when she was born.
C. Harriet Beecher was a letter-writer.
D. Harriet Beecher was an autobiographer.

SET 32

Gutenberg's father was a man of good family. Very likely the boy was taught to read, but the books from which he learned were not like ours; they were written by hand. A better name for them than books is 'manuscripts,' which means handwritings.

While Gutenberg was growing up a new way of making books came into use, which was a great deal better than copying by hand. It was what is called block printing. The printer first cut a block of hard wood the size of the page that he was going to print. Then he cut out every word of the written page upon the smooth face of his block. This had to be very carefully done. When it was finished the printer had to cut away the wood from the sides of every letter. This left the letters raised, as the letters are in books now printed for the blind.

The block was now ready to be used. The letters were inked, paper was laid upon them and pressed down. With blocks the printer could make copies of a book a great deal faster than a man could write them by hand. But the making of the blocks took a long time, and each block would print only one page.

Gutenberg enjoyed reading the manuscripts and block books that his parents and their wealthy friends had; and he often said it was a pity that only rich people could own books. Finally, he determined to contrive some easy and quick way of printing.

156. Which of the following reasons can be inferred from the above passage to explain Gutenberg's desire to create a new way of printing?

A. It was a lucrative business to go into.
B. He wanted to make text more accessible.
C. He was tired of waiting for each book to be handwritten or block pressed, and wanted quicker access to literature.
D. He found the current books too costly for him to continue his reading habit.

157. Which of the following is **NOT** mentioned as a concern of block printing?

A. It exhausts the carver.
B. It is intricate and demands attention to detail.
C. It is a lengthy process.
D. An individual block has limited utility.

158. Which of the following statements is definitely true according to the above passage?

A. Gutenberg was taught to read as a boy.
B. Gutenberg's father belonged to the aristocracy.
C. Block printing was the predominant book manufacturing process whilst Gutenberg was growing up.
D. Gutenberg's family was somewhat sociable.

159. Printing with the block process was a simple task of inking up the prepared block and pressing it down on a piece of paper, to make one page of the text.

A. True. B. False. C. Can't tell.

160. Which of the following statements are **NOT** supported by the above passage?

A. Manuscripts were beautifully crafted.
B. 'Manuscripts' is an appropriate name for what it describes.
C. Block printing is an appropriate name for what it describes.
D. Having well off friends was a good way to expand your reading.

SET 33

Cassandra may be considered an odd name to give your daughter, when you consider the mythical significance of it. Cassandra was a figure in ancient Greek mythology, a Trojan girl born to King Priam, who had been cursed: she had the gift of prophecy, but no one would believe in her words. She ultimately ends up taken from her homeland, as the sexual slave of Agamemnon. Agamemnon's wife then slaughters the girl, and one might wonder why any parent would name their daughter after such an ill-fated figure.

There are several stories that explain how Cassandra gained her gift and her curse. One narrative states that the god Apollo gave the girl the ability to tell the future, in an attempt to seduce her. When she refused him, he corrupted her gift. Another version tells us that Cassandra originally told Apollo she would have sex with him, in exchange for the gift of prophecy. When she subsequently refused him, having attained this power, he then spat in her mouth during a kiss, and this action made her ever after doomed to be disbelieved.

The figure of Cassandra has been presented in various pieces of classical literature, including Homer's epic poem 'The Iliad', Euripides' 'Trojan Women' and Aeschylus' 'The Agamemnon'. Although the presentation of her character alters in the different manifestation, the tragic fate of the woman is known within the different texts, as it would be known by the different authors and audiences of these works.

161. Throughout mythology, Apollo is always presented as the figure who gives Cassandra prophecy.

A. True. B. False. C. Can't tell.

162. Which of the following statements is best supported by the passage?

A. Parents who call their daughter Cassandra must hate their children.
B. Cassandra prizes chastity higher than her personal comfort.
C. Cassandra had supernatural powers.
D. Cassandra is often seen as a home wrecker.

163. Which of the following statements is **NOT** supported by the passage?

A. Cassandra comes from a royal line.
B. Cassandra had a happy childhood before her horrible fate.
C. Cassandra has been written about for the stage.
D. Homer has been inspired by Cassandra.

164. Cassandra's personality is consistently presented in the different pieces of literature she is included in.

A. True. B. False. C. Can't tell.

165. Which of the following is offered in the above passage to explain Apollo's ire?

A. Cassandra breaking her promise.
B. Cassandra not accepting his gift.
C. Cassandra demanding more gifts.
D. Cassandra not acknowledging his gifts.

SET 34

Despite the fact that some associate musicals with cheesy joy, the genre is not limited to gleeful stories, as can be demonstrated by the macabre musical, 'Sweeney Todd'. The original story of the murderous barber appears in a Victorian penny dreadful, 'The String of Pearls: A Romance'. The penny dreadful material was adapted for the 19th century stage, and in the 20th century was adapted into two separate melodramas, before the story was taken up by Stephen Sondheim and Hugh Wheeler. The pair turned it into a new musical, which has since been performed across the globe and been adapted into a film starring Johnny Depp.

Sondheim and Wheeler's drama tells a disturbing narrative: the protagonist, falsely accused of a crime by a crooked judge, escapes from Australia to be told that his wife was raped by that same man of the court. In response, she has committed suicide, and her daughter – Todd's daughter – has been made the ward of the judge. The eponymous figure ultimately goes on a killing spree, vowing vengeance for the people who have wronged him but also declaring 'we all deserve to die', and acting on this belief by killing many of his clients; men who come to his barbershop. His new partner in crime, Mrs Lovett, comes up with the idea of turning the bodies of his victims into the filling of pies, as a way of sourcing affordable meat. After all, she claims, 'times is hard'.

Cannibalism, vengeance, murder and corruption – these are all themes that demonstrate that this show does not conform to a happy-clappy preconception of its genre.

166. Which of the following statements are best supported by the above passage?

A. Sondheim is a brilliant musician and lyricist.
B. Most musicals deal with morbid themes.
C. Wheeler is an avid penny dreadful fan.
D. Generalisations can be misleading.

167. All the adjectives below are explicitly supported by the passage to describe the crimes described within it, except:

A. Comic. B. Culinary. C. Vengeful. D. Sexual.

168. Mrs Lovett and Sweeney Todd are in a romantic relationship.

A. True. B. False. C. Can't tell.

169. The best way to describe the belief of Todd as mentioned in the above passage:

A. Bad people should die so good can live and prosper.
B. Good people should die because the bad have basically taken over.
C. All men should die.
D. All humans merit death.

170. Which of the following statements is best supported in the above passage?

A. There are four themes in 'Sweeney Todd'.
B. Legal corruption is the predominate theme of 'Sweeney Todd'.
C. Several 'Sweeney Todd' themes are morbid.
D. There is nothing positive in 'Sweeney Todd'.

SET 35

The United States released the following as part of a pamphlet titled 'If Your Baby Must Travel in Wartime', released during the Second World War:

'Have you been on a train lately? The railroads have a hard job to do these days, but one that they are doing well. But before you decide on a trip with a baby, you should realise what a wartime train is like. So, let's look into one.

This train is crowded. At every stop more people get on – more and still more. Soldiers and sailors on furloughs, men on business trips, women – young and not so young – and babies, lots of them, mostly small.

The seats are full. People stand and jostle one another in the aisle. Mothers sit crowded into single seats with toddlers or with babies in their laps. Three sailors occupy space meant for two. A soldier sits on his tipped-up suitcase. A marine leans against the back of the seat. Some people stand in line for 2 hours waiting to get into the diner, some munch sandwiches obtained from the porter or taken out of a paper bag, and some go hungry. And those who get to the diner have had to push their way through five or six moving cars.

You will want to think twice before taking your baby into such a crowded, uncomfortable place as a train. And having thought twice, you'd better decide to stay home unless your trip is absolutely necessary.

But suppose you and your baby must travel. Well then, you will have to plan for the dozens of small but essential things incidental to travelling with a baby and equip yourself to handle them.'

171. First World War passenger trains were exceptionally crowded.

A. True. B. False. C. Can't tell.

172. Which of the following phrases is described by the above passage?

A. A soldier responds to the situation by creating his own seat.
B. A sailor rests against a seat's back.
C. Many people queue for over an hour to get to the diner car.
D. Many go without eating for the duration of a train journey.

173. The pamphlet wishes to increase the number of passengers on trains.

A. True. B. False. C. Can't tell.

174. Every station the described train passes through has passengers wanting to get onto the vehicle.

A. True. B. False. C. Can't tell.

175. Which of the following does the above passage do?

A. Compliment the railroads.
B. Insult passengers who are mothers.
C. Insult passengers who work for the navy.
D. Compliment soldiers.

SET 36

The following extract is from 'Foods That Will Win the War', published in the USA during the First World War:

'A slice of bread seems an unimportant thing. Yet one good-sized slice of bread weighs an ounce. It contains almost three-fourths of an ounce of flour. If every one of the country's 20,000,000 homes wastes on the average only one such slice of bread a day, the country is throwing away daily over 14,000,000 ounces of flour—over 875,000 pounds, or enough flour for over a million one-pound loaves a day. For a full year at this rate there would be a waste of over 319,000,000 pounds of flour—1,500,000 barrels—enough flour to make 365,000,000 loaves.

As it takes four and one-half bushels of wheat to make a barrel of ordinary flour, this waste would represent the flour from over 7,000,000 bushels of wheat. Fourteen and nine-tenths bushels of wheat on the average are raised per acre. It would take the product of some 470,000 acres just to provide a single slice of bread to be wasted daily in every home.

But someone says, 'a full slice of bread is not wasted in every home.' Very well, make it a daily slice for every four or every ten or every thirty homes—make it a weekly or monthly slice in every home—or make the wasted slice thinner. The waste of flour involved is still appalling. These are figures compiled by government experts, and they should give pause to every housekeeper who permits a slice of bread to be wasted in her home.'

176. According to the above passage, a slice of bread:
A. Contains 1/6 lb. of flour.
B. Contains a 1/4-ounce of air.
C. Is 75% flour.
D. Is one fourth salt, butter and yeast.

177. The passage denies that 20,000,000 homes at the point of writing wasted at least a slice of bread a day.
A. True.
B. False.
C. Can't tell.

178. If 20,000,000 homes wasted a slice of bread, this waste would be equal to:
A. One million loaves of bread a week.
B. Over 319,000,000 bushels of flour in 365 days.
C. 1.5 million barrels per annum.
D. Over 365,000 loaves a year.

179. According to the above passage, a slice of bread is an unimportant thing.
A. True.
B. False.
C. Can't tell.

180. Which of the following statements are supported by the above passage?
A. The writer has received much criticism for his views.
B. The government should do more to inform the public about waste.
C. The government has taken responsibility for public waste.
D. Responsibility lies with the person who keeps the house.

SET 37

At the election of President and Vice President of the United States, and members of Congress, in November 1872, Susan B. Anthony and several other women, offered their votes to the inspectors of election, claiming the right to vote, as among the privileges and immunities secured to them as citizens by the fourteenth amendment to the Constitution of the United States. The inspectors, Jones, Hall, and Marsh, by a majority, decided in favour of receiving the offered votes – against the dissent of Hall – and they were received and deposited in the ballot box. For this act, the women – fourteen in number – were arrested and held to bail, and indictments were found against them, under the 19th Section of the Act of Congress of May 30th, 1870, (16 St. at L. 144.) independently charging them with the offense of knowingly voting without having a lawful right to vote. The three inspectors were also arrested, but only two of them were held to bail, Hall having been discharged by the Commissioner on whose warrant they were arrested. All three, however were jointly indicted under the same statute – for having knowingly and wilfully received the votes of persons not entitled to vote.

Of the women voters, the case of Miss Anthony alone was brought to trial, a nolle prosequi having been entered upon the other indictments. Upon the trial of Miss Anthony before the U.S. Circuit Court for the Northern District of New York, at Canandaigua, in June 1873, it was proved that before offering her vote she was advised by her counsel that she had a right to vote; and that she entertained no doubt, at the time of voting, that she was entitled to vote.

181. According to the above passage, how many people in total were arrested due to the group of women voting?

A. Fourteen. B. Three. C. Seventeen. D. Sixteen.

182. Susan B. Anthony was the only person brought to trial because of the incident.

A. True. B. False. C. Can't tell.

183. Which of the following best describes initial opinions of the election officers?

A. United by each member's personal support of the women's votes.
B. Divided in response to the women's actions.
C. Apathetic about the women's actions.
D. United by general disapproval of the women's actions.

184. Which defence for Susan B. Anthony is mentioned above?

A. She did not realise she was not allowed to vote.
B. That all people born in the USA should be able to vote for their president.
C. That gender should not prevent her vote.
D. The election officers accepted her vote, showing the responsibility is not with her.

185. The women were charged jointly under the same indictment.

A. True. B. False. C. Can't tell.

SET 38

The following is taken from a book about Norway published in 1909:

'In a country like Norway, with its vast forests and waste moorlands, it is only natural to find a considerable variety of animals and birds. Some of these are peculiar to Scandinavia. Some, though only occasionally found in the British Isles, are not rare in Norway; whilst others (more especially among the birds) are equally common in both countries.

There was a time when the people of England lived in a state of fear and dread of the ravages of wolves and bears, and the Norwegians of the country districts even now have to guard their flocks and herds from these destroyers. Except in the forest tracts of the Far North, however, bears are not numerous, but in some parts, even in the South, they are sufficiently so to be a nuisance, and are ruthlessly hunted down by the farmers. As far as wolves are concerned civilisation is, fortunately, driving them farther afield each year, and only in the most out-of-the-way parts are they ever encountered nowadays. Stories of packs of hungry wolves following in the wake of a sleigh are still told to the children in Norway, but they relate to bygone times – half a century or more ago, and such wild excitements no longer enter into the Norsemen's lives.'

186. Which of the following is best supported by the above passage?

A. The variety of birds and animals to be found in Norway is unique to that country.
B. The variety of birds and animals to be found in Norway is common to all European countries.
C. By having forests, a country is more likely to have a variety of birds and animals.
D. England and Norway have similar geographical features.

187. English people are described as:

A. Having been anxious of certain animals.
B. Sceptical of bears.
C. Living in fear of wolves.
D. Developmentally behind the Norwegians.

188. Bears are described as:

A. Hunting.
B. Scavenging.
C. Damaging.
D. Man-eating.

189. Bears are also:

A. Numerous in all forest tracts.
B. Numerous throughout the North.
C. Numerous throughout the South.
D. At risk in parts of Norway.

190. The passage suggests:

A. The movement of wolves to the out-of-reach parts of Norway is beneficial.
B. Wildlife currently threats Norwegian children.
C. Regret at the loss of adventures.
D. Norsemen particularly respect their natural surroundings.

SET 39

The following extract is taken from Freud's book 'Dream Psychology: Psychoanalysis for Beginners':

In what we may term pre-scientific days, people were in no uncertainty about the interpretation of dreams. When they were recalled after awakening, they were regarded as either the friendly or hostile manifestation of some higher powers; demoniacal and divine. With the rise of scientific thought, the whole of this expressive mythology was transferred to psychology. Today there is but a small minority among educated persons who doubt that the dream is the dreamer's own psychical act.

But since the downfall of the mythological hypothesis, an interpretation of the dream has been wanting. The conditions of its origin; its relationship to our psychical life when we are awake; its independence of disturbances which, during the state of sleep, seem to compel notice; its many peculiarities repugnant to our waking thought; the incongruence between its images and the feelings they engender; then the dream's evanescence, the way in which, on awakening, our thoughts thrust it aside as something bizarre, and our reminiscences mutilating or rejecting it. All these and many other problems have for many hundred years demanded answers, which up till now could never have been satisfactory. Before all, there is the question as to the meaning of the dream – a question that is in itself double-sided. There is, firstly, the psychical significance of the dream, its position with regard to the psychical processes, as to a possible biological function. Secondly, has the dream a meaning – can sense be made of each single dream as of other mental syntheses?

191. Dreams used to be regarded as having a potentially religious quality.

A. True. B. False. C. Can't tell.

192. According to the passage, at this point of time, amongst the educated:

A. A vocal majority believe that dreams come from somewhere outside the dreamer.
B. A small minority believes that dreams come from the dreamer alone.
C. The majority accepts that a dreamer's dream is his or her own psychical act.
D. A vocal minority believes dreams are the direct products of angels and devils.

193. With a dream:

A. Images seemingly logically dictate feelings.
B. Events happen which are pleasant to waking thought.
C. Only boring things occur that are often too dull to be remembered.
D. There are relationships between images and feelings that would appear illogical to the awake mind.

194. The passage wonders about the significance of individual dreams.

A. True. B. False. C. Can't tell.

195. Which of the following statements is supported by the above passage?

A. There is a definite link between the waking and dreaming self.
B. Human society has never had a hypothesis to explain dreams that has satisfied them.
C. A memory of a dream may be untrustworthy.
D. The origin of the dream has been scientifically sourced.

SET 40

Most of the colonists who lived along the American seaboard in 1750 were the descendants of immigrants who had come in fully a century before; after the first settlements there had been much less fresh immigration than many latter-day writers have assumed. According to Prescott F. Hall, "the population of New England ... at the date of the Revolutionary War ... was produced out of an immigration of about 20,000 persons who arrived before 1640," and we have Franklin's authority for the statement that the total population of the colonies in 1751, then about 1,000,000, had been produced from an original immigration of less than 80,000. Even at that early day, indeed, the colonists had begun to feel that they were distinctly separated, in culture and customs, from the mother-country and there were signs of the rise of a new native aristocracy, entirely distinct from the older aristocracy of the royal governors' courts. The enormous difficulties of communication with England helped to foster this sense of separation. The round trip across the ocean occupied the better part of a year and was hazardous and expensive; a colonist who had made it was a marked man—as Hawthorne said, "the petit maître of the colonies." Nor was there any very extensive exchange of ideas, for though most of the books read in the colonies came from England. The great majority of the colonists, down to the middle of the century, seem to have read little save the Bible and biblical commentaries, and in the native literature of the time one seldom comes upon any reference to the English authors who were glorifying the period of the Restoration and the reign of Anne.

196. Over half of the 1750 colonists that lived on the American seaboard had genetic links to immigrants who had arrived a century ago.

A. True. B. False. C. Can't tell.

197. Which of the following statements is supported by the above passage?

A. According to Hall, America's population at the date of the Revolutionary war could be entirely traced back to 20,000 immigrants.
B. The population in the 1751 colonies was over ten times the original immigration that moved there.
C. According to Hall, in 1751 the population in the American colonies was one million.
D. According to Hall, 80,000 people led to a population of 1,000,000.

198. According to the passage, the new aristocracy that existed in the colonies was:

A. Similar to England's.
B. Similar to European aristocratic systems in general.
C. Not based in royal governors' courts.
D. Not based on genetic lines.

199. Most of the books on board ships were Bibles and Biblical commentaries.

A. True. B. False. C. Can't tell.

200. Which of these is **NOT** given as a reason for poor communications with England?

A. Travel between America and England was costly.
B. The English saw the early colonists as backwards.
C. Travel between America and England was slow.
D. Travel between America and England was dangerous.

SET 41

In discussing Russia's role in the past World War, it is customary to cite the losses sustained by the Russian Army – losses running into many millions. There is no doubt that Russia's sacrifices were great, and it is just as true that her losses were greater than those sustained by any of the other Allies. Nevertheless, these sacrifices are by far not the only standard of measurement of Russia's participation in this gigantic struggle. Russia's role must be gauged, first of all, by the efforts made by the Russian Army to blast the German war plans during the first years of the War, when neither America, nor Italy, nor Romania were among the belligerents, and the British Army was still in the process of formation.

[Secondly], and this is the main thing, the role played by the Russian Army must be considered also in this respect that the strenuous campaign waged by Russia – with her 180 million inhabitants – for three years against Germany, Austro-Hungary and Turkey sapped the resources of the enemy and thereby made the delivery of the final blow possible. This weakening of the powers of the enemy by Russia was already bound – at various stages of the War – to facilitate the various operations of the Allies correspondingly. Therefore, at the end of the War, three years of effort on the part of Russia had devoured the enemy's forces, enabling the Allies to finally crush the enemy. The final catastrophe of the Central Powers was the direct consequence of the offensive of the Allies in 1918. Russia made this collapse possible, to a considerable degree, having effected, in common with the others, the weakening of Germany, and having consumed during the three years of strenuous fighting countless reserves, forces, and resources of the Central Powers.

Could Germany have won the War? A careful analysis of this question brings home the conviction that Germany was very close to victory, and that it required unusual straining of efforts on the part of France and Russia to prevent Germany from "winning out".

201. According to the passage, Russia's greatest contribution to the War was?
A. Contributing more sacrifices than any other ally.
B. Blasting the German war plans during the first years of the War.
C. Consuming countless reserves, forces and resources of the Germans.
D. Sapping the resources of Germany, Austro-Hungary and Turkey for 3 years.

202. How many countries were Russian allies?
A. 2. B. 3. C. 4. D. 5.

203. Russia was the main country fighting against Germany in the early years of the War.
A. True. B. False. C. Can't tell.

204. The War was won by?
A. Germany running out of resources.
B. The offensive drive of the Allies.
C. The arrival of America.
D. Turkey and Austro-Hungary changing sides.

205. If it were not for Russia, Germany would have won the war?
A. True. B. False. C. Can't tell.

SET 42

We freeze some moments in time. Every culture has its frozen moments; events so important and personal that they transcend the normal flow of news.

Americans of a certain age, for example, know precisely where they were and what they were doing when they learned that President Franklin D. Roosevelt had died. Another generation has absolute clarity of John F. Kennedy's assassination. And no one who was older than a baby on 11th September 2001, will ever forget hearing about, or seeing, aeroplanes flying into skyscrapers.

In 1945, people gathered around radios for the immediate news and stayed with the radio to hear more about their fallen leader and about the man who took his place. Newspapers printed extra editions and filled their columns with detail for days and weeks afterward. Magazines stepped back from the breaking news and offered perspective on Roosevelt's death.

11th September 2001 followed a similarly grim pattern. We watched again and again the awful events. Consumers of news learned about the attacks, thanks to the television networks that showed the horror so graphically. Then we learned some of the how's and why's, as print publications and thoughtful broadcasters worked to bring depth to events that defied mere words. Journalists did some of their finest work, and made me proud to be one of them.
But something else, something profound, was happening this time around: news was being produced by regular people who had something to say and show, and not solely by the "official" news organisations that had traditionally decided how the first draft of history would look. This time, the first draft of history was being written, in part, by the former audience. It was possible, it was inevitable – because of new publishing tools available on the Internet.

206. The author of this passage is a journalist.

A. True. B. False. C. Can't tell.

207. Which media outlet tended to share a different point of view to the others?

A. Radios. B. Newspapers. C. Magazines. D. Televisions.

208. Which media outlet had the biggest effect on changing the way news is spread?

A. The Internet. B. Newspapers. C. Magazines. D. Televisions.

209. Which media outlet was mainly responsible for notifying consumers of the news that events had occurred in 1945?

A. Televisions. B. Newspapers. C. Radios. D. Magazines.

210. What was the big news story in 1945?

A. President Franklin D. Roosevelt died.
B. John F. Kennedy was assassinated.
C. An aeroplane exploded into skyscrapers.
D. John. F Kennedy was elected.

SET 43

There is nothing in England today with which we can compare the life of a fully enfranchised borough of the fifteenth century. The town of those earlier days, in fact, governed itself after the fashion of a little principality. Within the bounds which the mayor and citizens defined with perpetual insistence in their formal perambulation year after year, it carried on its isolated self-dependent life.

The inhabitants defended their own territory, built and maintained their walls and towers, armed their own soldiers, trained them for service and held reviews of their forces at appointed times. They elected their own rulers and officials in whatever way they chose to adopt, and distributed among officers and councillors just such powers of legislation and administration as seemed good in their eyes. They drew up formal constitutions for the government of the community, and as time brought new problems and responsibilities, more were made, re-made and revised again. Their ordinances with restless and fertile ingenuity, till they had made of their constitution a various medley of fundamental doctrines and general precepts and particular rules, somewhat after the fashion of an American state of modern times.

In all concerns of trade, they exercised the widest powers, and bargained and negotiated and made laws as nations do on a grander scale today. They could covenant and confederate, buy and sell, deal and traffic after their own will; they could draw up formal treaties with other boroughs, and could admit them to or shut them out from all the privileges of their commerce; they might pass laws of protection or try experiments in free trade. Often, their authority stretched out over a wide district, and surrounding villages gathered to their markets and obeyed their laws; it might even happen in the case of a staple town that their officers controlled the main foreign trade of whole provinces.

211. In the 15th century, towns drew up treaties to defend each other in times of attack.

A. True. B. False. C. Can't tell.

212. How were the leaders of boroughs brought into power?

A. Power was passed down the family.
B. Invaders conquered towns and become the rulers.
C. Inhabitants elected their own rulers.
D. There was a leader of the whole country, with majors in each borough.

213. Town life in the 15th century is more comparable to the American state of modern times than England in modern times.

A. True. B. False. C. Can't tell.

214. The authorities in the 15th century controlled who?

A. Their respective villages only.
B. Their respective towns only.
C. Their respective towns and surrounding villages.
D. The whole country.

215. How might disputes between boroughs have been settled in the 15th century?

A. By war.
B. By banning trading between boroughs.
C. With a treaty.
D. All of the above.

SET 44

Nowhere is the influence of sex more plainly manifested than in the formulation of religious conceptions and creeds. With the rise of male power and dominion, and the corresponding repression of the natural female instincts, the principles that originally constituted the God-idea gradually gave place to a Deity better suited to the peculiar bias that had been given to the male organism. An anthropomorphic God, like that of the Jews, whose chief attributes are power and virile, could have had its origin only under a system of masculine rule.

Religion is especially liable to reflect the vagaries and weaknesses of human nature; and as the forms and habits of thought connected with worship take a firmer hold on the mental constitution than do those belonging to any other department of human experience. Religious conceptions should be subjected to frequent and careful examination in order to perceive, if possible, the extent to which we are holding on to ideas which are unsuited to existing conditions.

In an age when every branch of inquiry is being subjected to reasonable criticism, it would seem that the origin and growth of religion should be investigated from beneath the surface and that all the facts bearing upon it should be brought forward as a contribution to our fund of general information. As well might we hope to gain a complete knowledge of human history by studying only the present aspect of society, as to expect to reach reasonable conclusions respecting the prevailing God-idea by investigating the various creeds and dogmas of existing faiths.

216. Masculine rule has always occurred.

A. True. B. False. C. Can't tell

217. Which god has attributes of power?

A. All gods.
B. The Jewish god.
C. The Christian god.
D. No gods.

218. Why is it a good idea to study the different Gods?

A. It provides an insight to societies of the past.
B. Because it is important to understand and respect other people's religion.
C. To find out which God is the most powerful.
D. To find out about the weaknesses of human nature.

219. Where is the influence of sex most clearly displayed?

A. In the formation of religion.
B. In the rules of religion.
C. By the lack of opposition against religion by women.
D. By the god's attributes.

220. The author is religious.

A. True. B. False. C. Can't tell.

SET 45

"What is a novel?" A novel is a marketable commodity, of the class collectively termed "luxuries," as not contributing directly to the support of life or the maintenance of health. The novel, therefore, is an intellectual artistic luxury in that it can be of no use to a man when he is at work, but may conduce to peace of mind and delectation during his hours of idleness.

Probably, no one denies that the first object of the novel is to amuse and interest the reader. But it is often said that the novel should instruct as well as afford amusement, and the "novel-with-a-purpose" is the realisation of this idea. The purpose-novel, then, proposes to serve two masters. Besides procuring a reasonable amount of bread and butter for its writer and publisher, it proposes to escape from my definition of the novel in general and make itself an "intellectual moral lesson" instead of an "intellectual artistic luxury". It constitutes a violation of the unwritten contract tacitly existing between writer and reader. A man buys what purports to be a work of fiction, a romance, a novel, a story of adventure; pays his money, takes his book home, prepares to enjoy it at his ease, and discovers that he has paid a dollar for somebody's views on socialism, religion or the divorce laws.

221. According to the author, a writer should write a novel with the sole purpose of amusement.

A. True. B. False. C. Can't tell.

222. Which of the following is the best use of a novel?

A. To be of use to a man when he is at work.
B. To spread the author's views on socialism, religion, or the divorce laws to those who otherwise would not listen to them.
C. To make moral lessons more interesting.
D. To pleasure a man during periods of idleness.

223. The writer of the passage regards a novel which has a strong view on socialism as their biggest hate.

A. True. B. False. C. Can't tell.

224. What is the unwritten contract between the author and reader?

A. A novel should provide an intellectual moral lesson.
B. A novel should have a purpose.
C. A novel should afford amusement.
D. A novel should be a work of fiction.

225. What is the most common opinion which the author does not share?

A. A novel should have a purpose.
B. A novel should instruct the reader.
C. A novel should conduce to peace of mind.
D. A novel should afford amusement.

SET 46

What is patriotism? Is it love of one's birthplace, the place of childhood's recollections and hopes, dreams and aspirations? Is it the place where, in child-like naivety, we would watch the fleeting clouds and wonder why we too could not run so swiftly? The place where we would count the milliard glittering stars, terror-stricken lest each one "an eye should be," piercing the very depths of our little souls? Is it the place where we would listen to the music of the birds and long to have wings to fly, even as they, to distant lands? Or the place where we would sit at mother's knee, enraptured by wonderful tales of great deeds and conquests? In short, is it love for the spot, every inch representing dear and precious recollections of a happy, joyous, and playful childhood?

If that were patriotism, few American men of today could be called upon to be patriotic, since the place of play has been turned into a factory, mill and mine, while deafening sounds of machinery have replaced the music of the birds. Nor can we still hear the tales of great deeds, for the stories our mothers tell today are but those of sorrow, tears and grief. What, then, is patriotism? "Patriotism, sir, is the last resort of scoundrels," said Dr. Johnson. Leo Tolstoy, the greatest anti-patriot of our times, defines patriotism as the principle that will justify the training of wholesale murderers; a trade that requires better equipment for the exercise of man-killing than the making of such necessities of life as shoes, clothing, and houses; a trade that guarantees better returns and greater glory than that of the average workingman.

226. The author believes patriotism as being the love for the spot where one grew up and had many happy memories.

A. True. B. False. C. Can't tell.

227. According to the author, are few American's of today patriotic?

A. Yes, because where they grew up has been destroyed.
B. Yes, because the current generation didn't have anywhere where they could listen to the music of the birds when they were children as the sounds of machinery has replaced this.
C. Yes, because not many people do justify the training of wholesale murderers.
D. No, because the definition of patriotism has not been defined and so one cannot say whether few American's of today are patriotic.

228. What is a possible negative of being patriotic?

A. Justifying mass killing.
B. Being depressed when one's birthplace is replaced by factories, mills and mines.
C. Reducing production of necessities such as workplaces.
D. Encouraging migration to distant lands.

229. The most common stories of today when children sit at their mother's knee are what?

A. Wonderful tales of great deeds and conquests.
B. Stories to encourage dreams and aspirations.
C. Stories of sorrow, tears and grief.
D. Tales of flying away to distant lands.

230. What might a young child wonder?

A. What distant lands are like.
B. Whether the conquests of their mother's stories are true.
C. Whether their birthplace will one day be turned into a factory.
D. Why they cannot keep up with clouds.

SET 47

The law of benefits is a difficult channel, which requires careful sailing or rude boats. It is not the office of a man to receive gifts. How dare you give them? We wish to be self-sustained. We do not quite forgive a forgiver. The hand that feeds us is in some danger of being bitten. We can receive anything from love, for that is a way of receiving it from ourselves (hence the fitness of beautiful, not useful things for a gift); but not from anyone who assumes to bestow. We sometimes hate the meat that we eat, because there seems something of degrading dependence in living by it.

He is a good man, who can receive a gift well. We are either glad or sorry at a gift, and both emotions are unbecoming. Some violence, I think, is done, some degradation borne, when I rejoice or grieve at a gift. I am sorry when my independence is invaded, or when a gift comes from such as do not know my spirit, and so the act is not supported; and if the gift pleases me overmuch, then I should be ashamed that the donor should read my heart and see that I love his commodity, and not him.

This giving is flat usurpation, and therefore, when the beneficiary is ungrateful, as all beneficiaries hate all Timons, not at all considering the value of the gift, but looking back to the greater store it was taken from, I rather sympathise with the beneficiary than with the anger of my lord, Timon. For, the expectation of gratitude is mean and is continually punished by the total insensibility of the obliged person.

231. Who is described as a good man?

A. A man who can forgive a forgiver.

B. A man who can give a good gift.

C. A man who can take a gift well.

D. A man who can enjoy the meat he eats.

232. Why do some men not like to receive a gift?

A. Because men wish to maintain themselves by independent effort.

B. They do not wish to depend upon it.

C. They only like to receive gifts of love.

D. They prefer to pick their own gifts.

233. The author of this passage does not like to receive gifts.

A. True.

B. False.

C. Can't tell.

234. When is it most acceptable to give a gift?

A. When you can read someone's heart and present the perfect gift.

B. For those most in need.

C. Never.

D. When the receiver loves you.

235. What is the major negative of enjoying a gift?

A. You have to return the favour.

B. It is going against the desire to self-sustain.

C. Appreciating the item rather than the effort of the giver.

D. All of the above.

SET 48

English writers who have spoken of Goethe's "Doctrine of Colours", have generally confined their remarks to those parts of the work in which he has undertaken to account for the colours of the prismatic spectrum, and of refraction altogether, on principles different from the received theory of Newton. The less questionable merits of the treatise consisting of a well-arranged mass of observations and experiments, many of which are important and interesting, have thus been in a great measure overlooked. The translator – aware of the opposition which the theoretical views alluded to have met with – intended at first to make a selection of such of the experiments as seem more directly applicable to the theory and practice of painting. Finding, however that the alterations this would have involved would have been incompatible with a clear and connected view of the author's statements, he preferred giving the theory itself; reflecting, at the same time, that some scientific readers may be curious to hear the author speak for himself even on the points at issue.

In reviewing the history and progress of his opinions and research, Goethe tells us that he first submitted his views to the public in two short essays entitled "Contributions to Optics." Among the circumstances which he supposes were unfavourable to him on that occasion, he mentions the choice of his title, observing that by a reference to optics he must have appeared to make pretensions to a knowledge of mathematics, a science with which he admits he was very imperfectly acquainted.

236. Mathematics was Goethe's greatest science.

A. True. B. False. C. Can't tell.

237. What was Goethe's most popular work?

A. His paper on 'Contribution to Optics'.
B. His paper on 'Doctrine of Colours'.
C. His ideas of refraction.
D. His ideas of mathematics.

238. What was the main problem the translator faced when writing the paper 'Doctrine of Colours'?

A. He wanted to present the scientific evidence before the theory to the audience, while Goethe did not.
B. He wanted to present the theory and then back it up with scientific evidence to the audience, while Goethe did not.
C. He wanted to wait until there was more scientific evidence before publishing as he knew the opposition would believe Goethe's theory.
D. The translator did not believe Goethe's theory and didn't want to write a paper which may convince others it is true.

239. How many papers did Goethe publish, according to the article?

A. 1. B. 2. C. 3. D. 4.

240. What is considered Goethe's most notable work?

A. About colours of the prismatic spectrum and of refraction.
B. His contribution to optics in general.
C. Disproving Newton's theories.
D. Changing the ways in which theories are presented.

SET 49

That marriage is a failure none but the very stupid will deny. One has but to glance over the statistics of divorce to realise how bitter a failed marriage really is. Nor will the stereotyped Philistine argument that the laxity of divorce laws and the growing looseness of women account for the fact that, first, every twelfth marriage ends in divorce; second, that since 1870 divorces have increased from 28 to 73 for every hundred thousand population; third, that since 1867, adultery – as ground for divorce – has increased 270.8 percent; fourth, that desertion increased 369.8 percent.

Henrik Ibsen, the hater of all social shams, was probably the first to realise this great truth. Nora leaves her husband, not as the stupid critic would have it, because she is tired of her responsibilities or feels the need of woman's rights, but because she has come to know that for eight years she had lived with a stranger and borne him children. The moral lesson instilled in the girl is not whether the man has aroused her love, but rather "how much?". The only importance in practical American life: can the man make a living, and can he support a wife? That is the only thing that justifies marriage. Gradually, this saturates every thought of the girl; her dreams are not of moonlight and kisses, of laughter and tears; she dreams of shopping tours and bargain counters. Can there be anything more humiliating, more degrading than a life-long proximity between two strangers? No need for the woman to know anything of the man, save his income. As to the knowledge of the woman – what is there to know except that she has a pleasing appearance?

241. According to the passage, most women get married for the sake of money.

A. True. B. False. C. Can't tell.

242. The author believes that marriages end due to the "looseness" of women.

A. True. B. False. C. Can't tell.

243. Nora did not want children.

A. True. B. False. C. Can't tell.

244. In America, every twelfth marriage ends in divorce.

A. True. B. False. C. Can't tell.

245. Women always end up dreaming of moonlight kisses later in marriage.

A. True. B. False. C. Can't tell.

SET 50

During the 1960s and 70s, terrorism was a contemporary subject due to the conflict between the UK government and the IRA. 'The Troubles' (the name given to the violence) originated in the 1920s and eventually resulted in bombings on the streets of Northern Ireland and occasionally in England. The government felt that in order to prevent mayhem, their actions needed to be swift and decisive. Thus, a series of temporary measures were initiated; policemen and soldiers all over Ulster were given the right to stop, question, search and arrest members of the public.

In 2000, the Terrorism Act 2000 was passed as a definitive measure following twenty years of temporary measures. Policemen were given wider stop and search powers and enabled to detain suspects for up to 48 hours without charge. The Act was met with strong criticism as it outlawed certain Islamic fundamentalist groups, and this was seen as a portrayal of Islam as a religion that fuels terrorism. This, in turn, made it likely that discrimination would occur in the form of the disproportionate stopping and searching of Asians who were thought to 'look Muslim'.

Although, prior to the September 2001 attacks on Washington D.C., government legislation in the UK had attempted to prevent the occurrence of terrorism; the counter-terrorism strategies had focused a lot of attention on the punishment of terrorists and the criminalisation of new offences following their occurrence. However, the Anti-Terrorism Crime and Security Act 2001 (ATCSA) marked a firmer move towards the 'management of anticipatory risk' (Piazza, Walsh, 2010), which was to characterise the counter-terrorism legislation of the 21st century.

246. In the 1960s, policemen and soldiers all over Ulster were given the right to stop, question, search and arrest members of the public.

A. True. B. False. C. Can't tell.

247. The Terrorism Act 2000 is still implemented today.

A. True. B. False. C. Can't tell.

248. The act in 2000 was passed in an effort to combat the threat of Islamic extremists.

A. True. B. False. C. Can't tell.

249. The act in 2000 targets preventing rather than punishing terrorism acts.

A. True. B. False. C. Can't tell.

250. Terrorism management was a big problem between 1980 and 2000.

A. True. B. False. C. Can't tell.

PROCEDURAL THINKING PRACTICE QUESTION WORKED SOLUTIONS

Q	A	Q	A	Q	A	Q	A	Q	A	Q	A
1	C	26	B	51	A	76	C	101	A	126	A
2	D	27	D	52	E	77	E	102	E	127	B
3	D	28	B	53	C	78	D	103	A	128	C
4	D	29	B	54	E	79	D	104	C	129	C
5	C	30	B	55	C	80	D	105	B	130	D
6	B	31	C	56	A	81	A	106	C	131	C
7	A	32	B	57	D	82	C	107	C	132	A
8	A	33	B	58	D	83	E	108	B	133	C
9	B	34	D	59	C	84	B	109	B	134	B
10	A	35	B	60	D	85	D	110	C	135	C
11	D	36	D	61	C	86	E	111	C	136	B
12	B	37	C	62	A	87	D	112	C	137	C
13	A	38	D	63	E	88	B	113	C	138	A
14	B	39	E	64	E	89	B	114	A	139	B
15	B	40	C	65	D	90	B	115	A	140	B
16	D	41	C	66	B	91	C	116	B	141	D
17	B	42	A	67	C	92	D	117	C	142	C
18	D	43	E	68	D	93	C	118	A	143	B
19	B	44	A	69	E	94	E	119	B	144	D
20	B	45	E	70	B	95	E	120	D	145	B
21	B	46	C	71	C	96	B	121	B	146	C
22	B	47	A	72	E	97	D	122	C	147	B
23	C	48	D	73	D	98	C	123	C	148	B
24	B	49	D	74	A	99	D	124	A	149	B
25	B	50	C	75	E	100	A	125	B	150	D

Q	A	Q	A	Q	A	Q	A	Q	A	Q	A
151	C	176	D	201	E	226	C	251	C	276	D
152	B	177	B	202	B	227	E	252	B	277	B
153	C	178	D	203	C	228	C	253	A	278	E
154	B	179	D	204	D	229	B	254	C	279	A
155	B	180	C	205	C	230	D	255	C	280	A
156	D	181	D	206	B	231	D	256	D	281	C
157	D	182	A	207	C	232	C	257	C	282	C
158	C	183	D	208	A	233	E	258	A	283	E
159	B	184	C	209	C	234	D	259	D	284	C
160	A	185	B	210	C	235	C	260	D	285	A
161	B	186	A	211	B	236	B	261	A	286	D
162	B	187	C	212	C	237	C	262	D	287	C
163	A	188	D	213	D	238	C	263	A	288	E
164	B	189	A	214	B	239	B	264	A	289	E
165	A	190	C	215	D	240	D	265	C	290	C
166	D	191	B	216	A	241	A	266	D	291	A
167	A	192	D	217	B	242	B	267	A	292	D
168	B	193	B	218	C	243	E	268	D	293	E
169	B	194	C	219	A	244	B	269	A	294	A
170	C	195	A	220	B	245	D	270	D	295	D
171	B	196	D	221	C	246	A	271	E	296	C
172	C	197	D	222	B	247	B	272	A	297	D
173	B	198	C	223	E	248	B	273	D	298	B
174	B	199	C	224	B	249	B	274	B	299	D
175	D	200	A	225	D	250	C	275	E	300	E

Q	A	Q	A	Q	A	Q	A	Q	A	Q	A
301	E	311	D	321	B	331	A	341	D	351	C
302	C	312	B	322	A	332	B	342	C	352	C
303	B	313	D	323	D	333	A	343	C	353	C
304	E	314	D	324	B	334	C	344	C		
305	D	315	C	325	C	335	C	345	C		
306	C	316	C	326	B	336	C	346	E		
307	B	317	C	327	D	337	C	347	C		
308	C	318	A	328	F	338	C	348	C		
309	D	319	B	329	C	339	D	349	D & E		
310	A	320	D	330	B	340	C	350	C		

SET 1

Question 1: C

We can work out that the tax rates must fit in the following equation:
($50 x Food tax rate) + ($30 x Clothes tax rate) + $80 = $88. Only the tax rates in Casova fit correctly in this equation.

Question 2: D

To answer this question, we calculate how much the supplier will make for selling the items, by considering the tax rate in each state, and deducting it from the price accordingly.
Thus, in Bolovia, each year the supplier makes 250 x ($40/1.20 + $40/1.15 + $40/1.10 + $40/1.15) = $34,812 a year.
In Asteria, each year the supplier makes 250 x ($40/1.10 + $40/1.15 + $40/1.10 + $40/1.15) = $35,572. (Note that in the case of an item being applicable to 2 tax rates, the higher rate will be charged. Thus, in Bolovia, imported clothes will be charged at the clothes tax rate of 15%, since this is higher than the imports rate).
By moving to Asteria, the supplier will make $760 more each year. Therefore, it will take 26.3 years to recover the purchase cost of $20,000.

Question 3: D

If John spends $88, he will spend £12 on tax. Thus, the tax rate is 12/88 = 13.6%.
If John shops in Asteria, the maximum tax rate he would have to pay is 10%; at Casova it would be 10%. If he spends at least $50 on food in Derivia, he pays no tax on it. Thus, he can spend a maximum of $38 on imported goods (at a maximum tax rate of 15%). This equates to a tax of $5.70 (not $12). Finally, if John spends $10 on imported goods in Bolovia – he would pay $0.50 in tax. Thus, he can spend up to $78 on clothes taxed at 15%. The tax on the clothes is therefore $11.70, giving $12.20 tax in total as the maximum. Since he pays $12 dollars tax, he shops in Bolovia.

Question 4: D

The sum of the basic prices is 100+30+10+100 = $240. Now the highest tax rate on the board is 20% (for imports to Asteria), thus the maximum tax is $240 x 1.20 = $288. However, this is impossible to attain (since if we bought everything in Asteria, the ham would be cheaper, as it is not imported and would only be taxed at the food rate). Therefore, no option allows the overall price to be as high as $288, so this is the answer. Answer 'A' is possible if all products were bought in the state they are produced in. Answer 'C' is the correct answer if all products were bought in Asteria (and accounting for the reduced tax rate for the ham, which is not an import). Answer 'B' is possible if the ham was bought in Asteria, the caviar and orange juice were bought in Casova and the dress was bought in Bolovia.

SET 2

Question 5: C

Firstly, find the pressure it can withstand in Pascals: 200 pounds per square inch x 7,000 Pascals per pound per square inch = 1.4 million Pascals.
Then divide this by 1,000 Pa to get the depth the probe can withstand (we can see from the question that the pressure increases by 1,000 Pa for every metre depth increase):
1,400,000/1,000 = 1,400 metres into the ocean, which is 1.4 km.

Question 6: B

Calculate that the probe can drop 300,000 Pa/1,000 Pa per metre = 300 metres into the ocean before breaking. Now rearrange the equation in the question, to make t the subject, as follows:

$2d = \sqrt{(t^3)}$

$(2d)^2 = t^3$

$t = \sqrt[3]{(2d)^2}$

Then substitute the depth into this supplied equation:

$t = \sqrt[3]{(2d)^2} = \sqrt[3]{(2x300)^2} = 71$ seconds.

SET 3

Question 7: A

Calculate the amount of drug taken for each disease:

Black Trump Virus = 4 mg x 80 kg x 3 times a day x 28 days = 26.88 g

Swamp Fever = 3x80x1x7 = 1.68 g

Yellow Tick = 1x80x2x84 = 13.44 g

Red Rage = 5x80x2x21 = 16.80 g

At a quick glance, the swamp fever dosage is much lower than all the others – you can discount this and use that to save a little time if you need to.

Question 8: A

First calculate that Carol took 20.16 grams of the drug during the two courses for Yellow Tick, using the same method as for John, but using Carol's weight of 60kg. Therefore 20.16 grams (the amount left over) corresponds to the dosage for the unknown disease:

4x60x3x28 = 20.16 g, therefore the unknown disease was Black Trump Virus.

Question 9: B

The first time he takes 3 x 80 x 1 x 7 = 1.68 grams, and the second time he takes 4 x 110 x 3 x 28 = 36.96 grams. Thus, the ratio is 1.68 : 36.96 = 1:22.

Question 10: A

By calculating the dose required in each of the cases, we see that the only one that is above 15.5 grams over 4 weeks is the dosage for Red Rage: 5 x 75 x 2 x 21 = 15.75 g – therefore Danny must be suffering from Red Rage.

Question 11: D

Heavier people need a higher dose. To find the maximum weight, we use the equation: 5 x weight x 2 x 21 = 10 g, where 'weight' represents the maximum weight requiring a dosage of less than 10 g.

So, maximum weight to not need a dosage exceeding 10 g is = 10,000 mg/(21 days x 2 daily doses x 5 mg/kg) = 47.62 kg.

SET 4

Question 12: B

To solve this, divide the flour content by the overall mass. A quick inspection might show you that this is likely to be Madeira, which is confirmed by the calculation (250/825 = 0.3). Thus, 30% of the Madeira's total weight is flour, which is a higher percentage than for any other cake.

Question 13: A

In this question, there must be one cake where: (2,600/mass of cake) = (625/mass of flour in cake). Thus, there is a number that both the mass of the cake and the mass of flour can be multiplied by, in order to get these numbers respectively.

We can see that if we multiply the mass of the sponge cake by 5, we get 2,600 g. Equally, if we multiply the mass of flour in the sponge cake recipe (125g) by 5, then we get 625 g. Thus, Sponge cake is the answer. No other cake recipe can be multiplied by a given number to get an overall weight of 2,600 g and 625 g of flour.

Question 14: B

We use 1.50+1.25+1.10+1 times the ingredients for one cake, so the wedding cake will use 4.85 times as much of the ingredients listed for one cake. We can use this to find which of the possible answers can be the amount of sugar in the cake, i.e. the sugar called for in one recipe multiplied by 4.85.

The quickest way to do this is to divide each possible answer by 4.85 and see if the result matches the weight of sugar in any of the cakes. We see that 970 g/4.85 = 200 g, which is the amount of sugar in the chocolate cake. None of the other amounts are possible. Thus, 'B' is the answer.

Question 15: B

A kilogram of flour costs 55 x 2/3 pence and we are using 0.25 kg, so 9.167 p worth of flour goes into a Madeira cake. For sugar, we have 0.175 kg x 70 p per kg = 12.25 p worth of sugar going into the cake.

The ratio is thus 9.167:12.25 = approx. 0.75:1 = 3:4.

Question 16: D

As before, the flour costs: 55 p per 1.5 kg x 2/3 x 0.2 kg = 7.3 pence.

The milk costs: 44 p per kg x 150 g/1000 g per kg = 6.6 pence.

Thus the ratio is 7.3:6.6 = 1:0.9 = 10:9.

SET 5

Question 17: B

In total, 108 people out of the 200 tested have the disease. This is equal to 108/200 = 0.54. Thus, the answer is 54%.

Question 18: D

As the infection rate is different for men and women, the infection rates must be calculated separately and combined: (231,768 x 0.53 women x 0.63 infected) + (231,768 x 0.47 men x 0.45 infected) = 126,406 to the nearest whole person.

Question 19: B

There are 45 men and 63 women in the test group who have the Kryptos virus, for a total of 180. Thus, 15 of the men and 45 of the women have visited Atlantis. As we now know that 60 people have visited Atlantis, we can see that 108 – 60 = 48 have not visited. Now we simply calculate 48 as a percentage of 108. 48/108 = 0.44. Thus, 44% of people testing positive for the Virus in Test A have *not* visited Atlantis.

Question 20: B

We can see that 20/45 men testing positive in Test A have also tested positive in Test B, so we assume that the rest were false positives stemming from the inaccuracies of Test A. We are told to assume the same proportion of false positives in the women tested, so we simply apply this fraction to the number of women testing positive in Test A. Thus, we simply calculate 63 x (20/45) = 28. Thus, we expect that 28 women actually have Kryptos Virus.

Question 21: B

In total, 108 people tested positive under test A, and 49 of these tested positive under test B (using data in the last question). Therefore the percentage of people positive in Test A also testing positive in Test B is 49 out of 108, which is 45.4%.

SET 6

Question 22: B

The cost of the plan is 190 + 600 + 140 = £930 per day.

Question 23: C

Firstly we need to find the two options that save the most money, aside from the one already stated. The two best options are to send material from Plant A to Store 1, and material from plant B to store 2. We can see from the table that these 2 options will be £30 per day cheaper than sending from Plant A to store 2, and plant B to store 1 (as with the current business plan).

The new total cost is 100 + 180 + 450 = £730. Thus the saving is (930 – 730) = £200. £200 is 22% of £930, so the percentage saving is 22% (to the nearest whole number).

SET 7

Question 24: B

The shop sold 512 books outside of the visit event (sum of sales in the table), and 106 at the event.

Thus, the percentage at the event was 106/(512+106) = 17%.

Question 25: B

Firstly calculate the different revenues:

Non-fiction revenue = (12+30) x£10 = £420

Fiction revenue = (50+45+23+90+103+159) x£6 = £2,820

Then calculate the non-fiction percentage: 420/(2,820+420) = 13%.

Question 26: B

The weekly revenue is seven times the daily revenue.

Daily revenue from Fiction: (50+45+23+90+103+159) x£6 = £2,820.

Daily revenue from Non-fiction 2x(12+30) x£10 = £840.

Therefore, weekly revenue is 7x(£2,820+£840) = £25,620.

Question 27: D

The shop's revenue is now £6 x (100+90+23+90+103+159) + £10 x (12+30) per day.

This income equates to £3,810 per day and £26,670 per week.

Therefore, the percentage difference is 26,670/25,620 = 1.04, giving a 4% increase on the previous week.

SET 8

Question 28: B

2 nights in Venice in a 3-star hotel, 1 room (the children are exempt) = 2x1x3 = 6 euros
2 nights in Rome in a 3-star hotel, 3 people paying (the child aged 9 is exempt) = 2x3x5 = 30 euros
2 nights in Padua in a 3-star hotel, 2 people paying (both children exempt) = 2x2x2 = 8 euros
2 nights in Siena in the high season, 3 paying (child aged 9 exempt) = 2x3x2 = 12 euros
So, the entire cost is the sum of these costs = 6+30+8+12 = 56 euros.

Question 29: B

In Rome, he pays 6 euros x 7 nights = 42 euros.
In Padua, he pays 3 euros x 8 nights = 24 euros.
The ratio of this is equal to 42:24 = 7:4.

Question 30: B

A 3-star hotel in Venice for 2 days costs Alice 6 euros.
3 days in a 4-star hotel in Padua costs 9 euros.
This is 50% more in Padua than in Venice.

Question 31: C

The maximum cost of tax in a 4-star hotel in Rome is 6 euros x 10 nights = 60 euros. Up until this point it will always be cheaper in Padua.
In Padua the cost for a 4-star hotel is 3 euros a night, therefore after 20 days the cost of the Padua hotel is equal to the cost of a stay of equivalent duration in Rome.

SET 9

Question 32: B

First find the wall length: 15m x 0.6 = 9m. Therefore, the area of the room is 9m x 9m = 81 m^2.

Question 33: B

The area of the house is 100 + 4 + (10 x 20) + (3 x 10) + (15 x 15) + 81 = 640 m^2.
The area of the master bedroom is 225 m^2, so the percentage area is 225/640 = 35%.

Question 34: D

The extra wall that is needed is the amount to extend both walls plus the new end wall.
The 20m wall is extended to 25m, and it is of height 3m, thus 5 x 3 = 15 m^2 is required.
Then the same amount of wall is needed for the other side, thus 2 x 15 = 30 m^2.
Then the back wall must be rebuilt, size = 10m x 3m = 30 m^2.
Sum these areas to a total of 60 m^2.

Question 35: B

Builder 1 costs: (15 x 300) + 200 = £4,700
Builder 2 costs: (16 x 300) = £4,800.
Therefore, the requested ratio is 47:48, which is 1:1.02 (to 3 s.f.).

SET 10

Question 36: D

200 SMSs are free, so he pays for 7. £5 monthly fee + 7 SMSs x £0.20 + 15 call minutes x £0.20 = £9.40.

Question 37: C

Plan A SMSs cost 10p each. Plan B minimum cost is £5 monthly fee, but then provides 200 free SMSs. 51 SMSs at £0.10 each cost £5.10, which is more than £5. Thus, sending 51 SMSs would be cheaper on Plan B (sending 50 would be the same price on each plan).

Question 38: D

To answer this question, work out the cost of each plan.

5 minutes x 30 days = 150 minutes.

150 minutes' cost is 150 x £0.10 = £15 on Plan A, 150 x £0.20 = £30 on Plan B, (150-100 free minutes) x £0.20 = £10 on Plan C and 150 x £0.00 = £0 on Plan D.

Including the monthly fee, the cost to call becomes = £15 for plan A, £35 for plan B, £20 for plan C and £15 for plan D.

All SMSs cost on Plan A but not D, so D is cheapest. (Note that we did not have to calculate the cost of texts in order to get the answer. If you like, you could work out the cost of the SMSs on each plan too, but if you notice that after calculating the cost of calls and monthly fees Plan A and Plan D come out at the same price, it is apparent that Plan D will be cheaper as SMSs are free, and this will save time).

Question 39: E

They each send 223 SMSs and make no calls. Option E is cheaper for Evan than Chris: For Plan B (223 SMSs – 200 free SMSs) x £0.20 = £4.60, so with the £5 monthly fee the total cost is £9.60. For Plan C all 223 SMSs are within the free limit, but the monthly fee is £10, so Chris pays more.

In option A, Evan pays £10.80, whilst Chris pays just the £10 monthly fee.

In option B, Evan pays £10.20, whilst Chris still just pays the monthly fee of £10.

In option C, Evan pays £36.80, whilst Chris still pays only the monthly fee of £10 (this is the biggest saving Chris makes relative to Evan out of all the options).

In option D, Evan pays between £27.40 and £29.80, depending on which month (and whether there are 28, 30 or 31 days in it), whilst Chris pays between £12.40 and £14.80, again dependent on which month.

Question 40: C

100 minutes are free on Plan C. Plan D has unlimited minutes and costs £5 more than C per month. At 20p a minute, Rachel can call for 25 minutes for £5, so can exceed her free minutes by 25 %, at which point Plan D is the same price. If she exceeds the free minutes allowance by any more than this, then plan D would be cheaper.

SET 11

Question 41: C

4 tablespoons is 4 x 15 ml = 60 ml. 250 ml is 1 cup, so 4 tablespoons is 60 ml/250 ml = 0.24 cups.

2 cups + 1 cup + ½ cup + 0.24 cups = 3.74 cups.

Question 42: A

First calculate the weight of butter called for by the recipe:
4 tablespoons = 60 ml = 0.06 litres = 0.06 dm^3 (the question states that 1dm^3 = 1 litre).
Weight of butter: 950 grams/dm^3 x 0.06 dm^3 = 57 grams.
Next, calculate the weight of milk called for by the recipe:
½ cup = 1.25 dl = 0.125 litres = 0.125 dm^3.
Weight of milk: 1050 grams/dm^3 x 0.125 dm^3 = 131.25 grams.
Thus, the weight ratio of Milk:Butter is 131.25/57:1 = 2.3:1.

Question 43: E

Any whole number multiple of flour, sugar or milk can be measured with a ½ cup.
4 tablespoons is 60 ml, ½ cup is 125 ml. The least common multiple of 60 and 125 is 1500, representing the smallest possible amount of butter that can be measured with half-cup measures.
1500 grams of butter makes 25 batches of muffins, which would require 25 x 2 cups = 50 cups of flour.

Question 44: A

The recipe will have:
2 cups of milk = 500 ml = 0.5 dm^3
1 cup of sugar = 250 ml = 0.25 dm^3
½ cup of flour = 125 ml = 0.125 dm^3
4 tablespoons of butter = 60 ml = 0.06 dm^3.
Therefore, the volume of the batter is 0.5 dm^3 + 0.25 dm^3 + 0.125 dm^3 + 0.06 dm^3 = 0.935 dm^3.
Now, to calculate the density of the batter, multiply the density of each ingredient by the proportion of the batter it makes up, and then add up these figures, as follows:
(1050 grams/dm^3 milk x 0.5/0.935) + (850 grams/dm^3 sugar x 0.25/0.935) + (600 grams/dm^3 flour x 0.125/0.935) + (950 grams/dm^3 butter x 0.06/0.935)
= 561.5 grams/dm^3 + 227.3 grams/dm^3 + 80.2 grams/dm^3 + 61.0 grams/dm^3
= 930 grams/dm^3.

Question 45: E

10 muffins x 100 grams = 1,000 grams batter required.
The recipe calls for:
2 cups flour = 5 dl = 0.5 dm^3 flour. Weight of the flour is 0.5 dm^3 x 600 grams/dm^3 = 300 grams.
1 cup sugar = 2.5 dl = 0.25 dm^3 sugar. Weight of the sugar is 0.25 dm^3 x 850 grams/dm^3 = 212.5 grams.
From question 42, the weight of the milk as called for by the recipe is 131.25 grams and weight of the butter is 57 grams.
Thus, the overall weight of the batter is 300 + 212.5 + 131.25 + 57 = 700.75 grams.
700.75/1,000 grams batter = 57/B grams butter, where B is the amount of butter required in 1,000g batter.
B = 81.3 grams butter.

Question 46: C

700.75/1,000 grams batter = 300/F grams flour (as per the above explanation), where F is the amount of flour required to make 1,000 grams of muffin. F = 428.11 grams. 428.11 grams/1000 grams = 0.428 = 43% to the nearest whole number.

SET 12

Question 47: A

The trend shows a 10 km^2 decrease in thickness for every 100°C decrease in temperature. 10 km^2 thickness is 1,300°C, so extrapolating the trend gives 0 km^2 thickness at 1,200°C.

Question 48: D

Spreading rate is not affected by temperature, it is an independent variable. So, the rate remains the same as per the table.

This question is designed to test your attention to detail and reinforce the importance of reading questions properly. Ensure you constantly pay attention to what the question is asking.

Question 49: D

Crustal volume per year = 20 km^2 crustal thickness x 20 mm/year spreading rate x 1 year = 20,000,000,000,000 mm^2 x 20 mm = 400,000,000,000,000 mm^3 = 400,000 m^3. (Note: by scanning the options, we can discount 'B' and 'E' due to units).

Question 50: C

In answering this question, it is not necessary to use the same units for crustal thickness and spreading rate, as long as we use the same units for the crustal thickness *from both locations*, and likewise for the spreading rate.

Location A = 10 x 100 = 1,000. Location C = 30 x 150 = 4,500.

Thus, the ratio for A:C = 1:4,500/1,000 = 1:4.5.

Question 51: A

Crustal volume per time = crustal thickness x spreading rate.

Crustal thickness at E is 10 km^2 and at F is 25 km^2 (data taken from the table).

Crustal volume per time is equal, so 10 km^2 x spreading rate for E = 25 km^2 x spreading rate for F.

Therefore, the spreading rate at E = 2.5 times the spreading rate at F. Thus, it is 250% faster.

Question 52: E

Temperature at D is 1,600°C, decreased by 10% it would be 1440°C.

From the trend in temperature and crustal thickness, this corresponds to a crustal thickness of 24 km^2.

Crustal volume per 3 years = 24 km^2 crustal thickness x 50 mm/year x 3 years = 24,000,000,000,000 mm^2 x 150 mm = 3,600,000,000,000,000 mm^3.

SET 13

Question 53: C

A: 9/25, B: 6/23, C: 7/22, D: 8/24.

(9+6+7+8)/(25+23+22+24) = 30/94 = 32% (to the nearest whole number).

Question 54: E

In Group A, drug-takers visual accuracy is 36%/27% = 33.33% improved.

In Group C, drug-takers visual accuracy is 31%/29% = 6.90% improved.

A:C = 33.33%/6.90% : 1 = 4.83:1.

Question 55: C

10 women and 15 men have 45% and unknown (P %) accuracy, respectively.
All 25 have an average of 36% accuracy (based on the data in the table).
(10/25 x 45) + (15/25 x P) = 36.
Therefore, P=30.

Question 56: A

Diabetics with vision problems correspond to Group A. In Group A, 15 of 25 volunteers reported better vision after taking the drug, but 9 of 25 volunteers taking a placebo also reported vision improvement. This suggests only 6 of 25 had reported improvements in their vision thanks to the effects of the drug (as it is assumed that 9 people in the drug group would also have 'spontaneously' improved, i.e. the reason for testing placebo).
6/25 x 100,000 people = 24,000 people.

Question 57: D

The placebo group showed no change, so only the volunteers being affected by the drug compound will see greater improvements to their vision.
15 – 9 = 6 volunteers affected by drug originally.
200% of the dose gave (18-9)/6 = 1.5 = 150 % the number of people with drug-related improvements.
300% of the dose will thus give 300 % / 200 % x 150 % = 225 % the number of people.
6 volunteers x 225% = 13.5 volunteers. (9+13.5)/25 volunteers = 22.5/25 volunteers = 90.0 % of volunteers.

Question 58: D

D is supported, because in all groups taking the placebo, there was an increase in accuracy with reading letters – suggesting better vision – and in many cases this was equivalent to the increase in those taking the drug.
The data suggest that 'A' and 'B' are incorrect. Only one group showed a higher increase in accuracy amongst the placebo group, in all other groups the people taking the drug had a larger % increase in accuracy. In healthy volunteers, there was as much of an increase in accuracy amongst those taking a placebo, suggesting the drug does not have as much of an effect in healthy volunteers. Options 'C' and 'E' are relatively meaningless statements, which are not supported by the data.

SET 14

Question 59: C

5 calories x 200 pounds x 1 hour = 1000 calories running.
Cycling burns 50 calories + (5 calories x -5) for each mile = 25 calories per mile. Cycling 5 miles gives a total burn 125 calories, which is less than the amount burned running.
Thus, the maximum calorie burn comes from running, which will burn 1000 calories.

Question 60: D

Losing 10 pounds requires a 35,000-calorie deficit.
30 min run: 200 pounds x 0.5 hours x 5 calories = 500 calories.
20-mile cycle at 20 mph: 50 calories + (5 calories/mph x 10 mph) = 100 calories/mile for 20 miles = 2,000 calories.
Daily burn is 2500 calories.
35,000/2,500 calories per day = 14 days taken to lose 10 pounds.

Question 61: C

Both their weight loss goal and calories burned running are linearly proportional to weight. Thus, they need to run for the same amount of time in order to achieve their goals. So, the answer is 1:1.

Question 62: A

10% of 140 pounds is 14 pounds of weight, thus this is how much weight she wishes to lose.
At 3,500 calories/pound she needs a 14 pounds x 3500 calories/pound = 49,000 calorie deficit.
Her BMR is 1500 calories and she eats 400+500+250+200=1,350 calories per day.
So, her daily calorie deficit is 1,500 calories–1,350 calories = 150 calories.
It will take her 49,000 calories/150 calories per day = 326.67 days to reach her goal (327 to the nearest day).

Question 63: E

10 miles at 10 mph: 50 calories + (5 calories x 0 mph) = 50 calories/mile for 10 miles = 500 calories.
She requires a 49,000-calorie deficit, as worked out in the previous question. Previously, she had a daily deficit of 150 calories, now she has a daily deficit of 650 calories.
Thus, she now has a calorie deficit which is 4.33 times the previous deficit, so she will reach her goal 4.33 times faster.

Question 64: E

1 chocolate is the least she can eat, which means she eats 3 pieces of chicken and 6 bowls of cereal.
= 1x350 calories + 3x250 calories + 6x400 calories = 3,500 calories.
The lowest calorie arrangement of the 3 other foods is 1 lasagne, 3 vegetables and 6 apples.
= 1x700 calories + 3x200 calories + 6x100 calories = 1,900 calories.
She has 3,500 calories per day – 1500 calorie BMR = 2,000 calorie surplus before
And she has 1,900 calories per day – 1500 calorie BMR = 400 calorie surplus after.
2,000 calories : 400 calories = 5:1.

SET 15

Question 65: D

Price during day with single tickets is 4 coupons x £1 = £4.
Price at night with 10% off coupons is 3 coupons x £0.90 = £2.70.
Thus, the saving is £1.30.
Hence, the % saving is £1.30/£4.00 = 0.325 = 32.5%.

Question 66: B

Price without a wristband is £1 per coupon x 120 % = £1.20 per coupon.
The number of coupons required is: 10 coupons entrance + 40 coupons for roller coaster + 6 coupons for candy floss + 1 coupon for the games + 4 coupons for the fun house + 3 coupons for the swings = 64 coupons.
64 coupons x £1.20 = £76.80.
Price with a wristband: £70 and 6 coupons for candy floss + 1 coupon for the games x £1.20 = £8.40. Thus the total price with a wristband is £78.40.
Therefore, the ratio is 1 : £76.80/£78.40, which is 1:0.98.

Question 67: C

Andy rode the swings 20% more times than he played games. The smallest number of times he could have gone on the swings is 6 times (since he can't have gone on the swings a non-integer number of times) so he played 5 games and went on the rollercoaster 9 times.

At night rates, rollercoaster 9 times x 3 coupons = 27 coupons and swings 6 times x 2 coupons = 12 coupons.

39 coupons at £1 each are worth £39, which is less than the £70 wristband.

If he had played 10 games, ridden the swings 12 times and rollercoaster 18 times, the wristband would have been more cost effective. This is the second cheapest possibility whilst still going on the swings an integer number of times (since 10 is the next multiple of 5). Thus, we know Andy must have played 5 games, been on the swings 6 times and the rollercoaster 9 times.

39 ride coupons + 5 game coupons + 5 entrance coupons = 49 coupons = £49.

Question 68: D

They got 69 coupons each for £69 pounds. They each must have spent 10 coupons at the entrance.

Together the rollercoaster and fun house cost 6 coupons, so Anna took 59/6 = 9 rides on each and had 5 coupons left over, since the question states she went on each ride for *half* her rides, we assume she did not use any of the remaining coupons, since she could only have gone on one more ride, and thus it would not have been exactly half.

The fun house and swings cost 5 coupons together, so James took 59/5 = 11 rides on each and had 4 coupons left which he spent on 1 last ride on the swings.

Anna took 18 rides and James 23 rides. So, Anna : James = 1 : 23/18 = 1:1.28.

Question 69: E

First, we calculate how much candyfloss Erik buys each weekend, using the 100% increase for the first 4 weeks, and the 50% increase thereafter as detailed in the question.

Week 1=1, week 2=2, week 3=4, week 4=8, week 5=16, week 6=24, week 7:=36, week 8=54, week 9=81, week 10=0.

Thus, he bought a total of 226 lots of candy floss.

226 candy floss x 2 coupons x £1 pound each = £452.

Cost with season pass = £1000. Cost without pass = £700 + £452 = £1,152.

Ratio of cost Without : With is £1152/£1000 : 1 = 1.15:1.

SET 16

Question 70: B

2 x (£14.00 + £2.00 + 2x£2.00) + 1 x (£8.00 + 3x£1.00) + 3 x (£10.00) = £40.00 + £11.00 + £30.00 = £81.00.

50% off orders over £50 means he pays £81.00/2 = £40.50.

Question 71: C

£35 is 50% of £70.

£70 buys £70/£14 = 5 large cheese pan pizzas.

Large pizzas have 10 slices: 10 slices x 5 pizzas = 50 slices.

Question 72: E

£60 is 50% off £120.

£120 is evenly divisible by all prices of plain cheese pizzas except the large pan. Dividing £120 by the price of the large pan gives 8.571. Since Joey cannot have bought a non-integer number of pizzas, he cannot have bought this type of pizza which costs £14.00.

Question 73: D

30 slices is 3 large pizzas or 5 small pizzas.

3 large pan pizzas with 2 toppings and stuffed crust cost: 3 x (£14.00 + (2x£2.00) + £2.00) = £60.00.

5 small pan pizzas with 2 toppings and stuffed crust cost: 5 x (£10.00 + 2x£0.50 + £1.00) = £60.00.

Large : Small ratio is 1 : £60.00/£60.00 = 1:1.00

Question 74: A

The lowest price order over £31 is 2 small pizzas and 1 medium pizza costing £32 total. 30% off £32 = £22.40.

They get 20 slices with this order, but we know that they got 25% more than they could eat.

Thus, if we treat 20 slices as 125%, then 100% is the amount that they ate.

20/1.25 = 16, so this is the amount that they could eat.

SET 17

Question 75: E

1 hour at Job A = £10 starter - £5 travel + £10 per hour = £15.

1 hour at Job B = £5 starter - £0 travel + £15 per hour = £20.

1 hour at Job C = £5 starter - £10 travel + £20 per hour = £15.

A:B:C = £15:£20:£15 = 1:1.33:1.

Question 76: C

In her first 50 hours she worked 25 2-hour jobs: 25 x (£10 - £5 + 2x£10) = 25 x £25 = £625.

Her hourly wage was then increased to £10 + £5 = £15 (because she had worked for 50 hours).

She then worked 4 1-hour jobs: 4 x (£10 - £5 + 1x£15) = 4 x £20 = £80.

Then she worked 1 4-hour job: 1 x (£10 - £5 + 4x£15) = 1 x £65 = £65.

Her total earnings were £625 + £80 + £65 = £770.00.

Question 77: E

For Job A, for the first 50 hours she would earn £10 an hour. Thus, for the first 25 2-hour jobs she would earn 25 x (£10 - £5 +2x£10) = £625. After 50 hours, her hourly wage would increase to £15 an hour. Thus, for the second lot of 25 2-hour jobs she would earn 25 x (£10 - £5 + 2x£15) = £875. Thus, in total at Job A she would earn £1,500.

For Job B, for the 50 2-hour jobs, she would earn 50 x (£5 + 2x£15) = £1,750. She does not get the pay increase because she does not work any hours after the pay rise at 100 hours. Thus, in total at Job B she would earn £1,750.

For Job C, for the 50 2-hour jobs, she would earn 50 x (£5 - £10 + 2x£20) = £1,750. Again, she does not get the pay increase because she does not work any hours after the pay rise at 100 hours. Thus, in total at Job C she would earn £1,750.

Therefore, B and C are the same.

Question 78: D
Average job length for Job C is 4 hours.
1 4-hour job earns: £5 starter - £10 travel + 4x£20 per hour = £75 per job.
Maximum earnings £1250/£75 = 17 jobs.
17 jobs x 4 hours = 68 hours.

Question 79: D
Hourly wage has risen twice by £5 to £30 per hour (since it rises £5 for each 100 hours worked).
100 hours/4-hour jobs = 25 jobs.
For a 4-hour job she earns: £5 starter - £10 travel + 4x£30 per hour = £115 per job.
25 jobs x £115 per job = £2,875.
10% of £2,875 = £287.50. This is the amount she pays in income tax.

Question 80: D
Working 50 hours for Job B earns 50 times the hourly rate plus 50 times the fixed starter wage, as jobs average 1 hour in duration. Therefore the income = (50x£15) + (50x£5) = £1,000.00.
The extra 50 hours can be worked at either Job A, B or C (note that Jobs A and B have travel expenses).
The same calculation for Job A gives (10x50) + (10 x 25) – (5x25) = £625.00.
The same calculation for Job C gives (50x20) + (5x12.5) – (10x12.5) = £937.50.
Therefore, she earns most by working 100 hours for Job B.

SET 18
Question 81: A
Monday has the 2nd highest number of passengers, so this will be the 2nd highest grossing day. On Monday the revenue is £5 x 2346 underground passengers = £11,730.00.
On Wednesday the revenue is 3,103 x 0.85 x £5 = £13,187.75.
£13,187.75 – £11,730.00 = £1,457.75.

Question 82: C
Total number of weekday underground passengers = 2346 +1798 +3103 + 2118 + 1397 = 10,762
Total number of weekday car passengers = total passengers – number of drivers. For each day this is:
Monday: 1873-1517=356
Tuesday: 2421-1632=789
Wednesday: 1116-987=129
Thursday: 2101-1465=636
Friday: 2822-2024 =798
Therefore, the total is equal to 356+789+129+636+798 = 2708.
The average ratio is 10,762 : 2,708 = 1:3.97.

Question 83: E
Tuesday: 2,421/1,632 = 1.48
Weekend: 1,339/478 = 2.80
Ratio of Tuesday to Saturday = 1.48/2.8 = 1:1.89.

Question 84: B

This is straightforward: 2,346/576 = 4.07:1 = 1:0.25.

Question 85: D

There are 4,219 commuters each day (as seen by adding the total car passengers and underground passengers on any given day). For every 1 car there are 1.7 passengers and 2 underground riders. Thus, by dividing 1.7 by 3.7 and multiplying this by the total number of passengers (4219), we can calculate how many people are in cars:

1.7/3.7 x 4,219 = 1,938 people drive (to the nearest whole number; there cannot be a non-integer number of people driving).

Now, by dividing the number of people driving (1938) by the number of passengers, we can calculate the number of cars: 1938/1.7 = 1,140 cars.

1,140 cars x £4 = £4,560.

£4,560 + 1,938x£1 = £6,498.

80% of £6,498 is £5,198.40.

SET 19

Question 86: E

First calculate the Superior room cost at night: 3hrs x £26.00/hr = £78.00. Now add 10%: £78 x 1.1 = £85.80.

Question 87: D

Total cost minus deposit = 12hrs x £30/hr = £360

Deposit = £460 - £360 = £100.

Question 88: B

Total deposit = £10 + £25 = £35

6hrs in Standard room = 6hrs x £18/hr = £108

6hrs in Basic Room = £221 – (£108 + £35) = £78

Basic room hourly rate (2-6hrs) = £78 ÷ 6hrs = £13 per hour.

Question 89: B

1.5hrs in Superior room (night session) = 1.5hrs x £30/hr = £45

Decreased by 5% = £45 x 0.95 = £42.75

Total cost = £50 deposit + £42.75 = £92.75.

Question 90: B

Basic room all day cost = 18hrs x £8/hr = £144

All week = 7 days x £144 = £1,008

Three weeks = £1,008 x 3 = £3,024

Deducting the VAT = £3,024/1.25 = £2,419.20.

SET 20

Question 91: C

Total number of people aged under 22 = sum of first two columns = 62

Number aged <22 who spotted >10 differences = 11 + 8 + 3 + 2 = 24

Percentage = 24/62 = 38.7%.

Question 92: D

Valid results for 5-10 spots for ages 16-22 = 0.25 x 12 = 3

Total number of valid results for 16-22 = 10 + 3 + 8 + 2 = 23

Percentage of over 15 spots for 16-22 = 2 ÷ 23 = 8.7%.

Question 93: C

Total who spotted over 10 = sum of bottom two rows = 52. 25% of 52 = 13.

(Note the people who incorrectly spotted differences are not relevant to the question, and the table does not refer to them).

Question 94: E

Total 48+ who spotted less than 5 = 15 + 19 = 34

Total aged 48+ = sum of final two columns = 66

Percentage of 48+ who spotted less than 5 = 34 ÷ 66 = 52% (2 s.f.)

52% of 10,000 = 0.52 x 10,000 = 5,200.

Question 95: E

50% increase in 16-34s who spot 11-15 = 1.5 x (8 + 6) = 21

New total who spot 11-15 = 11 + 21 + 2 + 8 + 9 = 51

Thus, the ratio is equal to 21:51.

SET 21

Question 96: B

Number that play football = 22% of 1300 = 286

Number that play netball = 8 % of 1300 = 104

Thus, the difference = 286–104 = 182 boys and girls.

Therefore, 182/2 = 91 boys (because of the 50:50 split between boys and girls mentioned in the stem).

Question 97: D

Number that play football = 22% of 350 = 77 students

77 ÷ 11 people per team = 7 teams.

Question 98: C

Number of basketball boys = 0.05 x 1,300 = 65. 80% of 65 = 52

Number of netball girls = 0.08 x1, 300 = 104

Total number of netball players = 104 + 52 = 156

Male proportion = 52 ÷ 156 = 33% (2 s.f.).

Question 99: D

Number of *Other* students = 0.12 x 1,300 = 156

Other ball sports = 0.25 x 156 = 39

Total non-ball sports (swimming & athletics) = (0.06 + 0.03) x 1300 = 117

Total "other" non-ball sports = 156 – 39 = 117

Total ball sports = 1,300 – 117 – 117 = 1,066.

Question 100: A

Girls who play hockey = 0.07 x 1,300 = 91

Boys who play cricket = 0.1 x 1,300 = 130

Therefore, the difference = 130-91 = 39.

(Note the tennis info makes no difference, due to the 50:50 split).

SET 22

Question 101: A

Based on the information, human consumption is both edible and passable.

Total apples processed in 1998 = 1,100,547 + 2,983,411 = 4,083,958

Total apples processed in 2003 = 1,931,784 + 2,439,012 = 4,370,796

Ratio for 1998 to 2003 = 4,370,796 ÷ 4,083,958 = 1.07 (i.e. 7% increase).

Question 102: E

Number of No Goods in worst year (i.e. in 2003) = 571,221

Total number of No Goods = sum of bottom row = 2,823,732

Percentage = 571,221 ÷ 2,823,732 = 20.2% (3 s.f.).

Question 103: A

2004 total No Goods = 3 x 571,221 = 1,713,663

70% of edible apples are processed, as are all passable apples.

Difference = (0.7 x 1,931,784 + 2,439,012) – 1,713,663 = 2,077,598.

Question 104: C

Total number of edibles 1998-2003 = sum of top row = 9,201,790

20% increase = 1.2 x 9,201,790 = 11,042,148

30% of these are sold as they come = 0.3 x 11,042,148 = 3,312,644 (to the nearest whole apple).

Question 105: B

Apples processed for cider is 70% of edible apples and all passable apples

= (1,931,784 x 0.7) + 2,439,012 = 3,791,260.8

Litres of cider = 3,791,260.80 ÷ 20 = 189,600 litres (4 s.f.).

SET 23

Question 106: C

Decreased average speed = 0.92 x 5 mph = 4.6 mph

Miles covered = 4.6 x (40 ÷ 60) = 3.07 miles

Km covered = 1.6 x 3.07 miles = 4.9 km.

Question 107: C

Distance per session = 26 miles ÷ 4 = 6.5 miles

Time per session = 6.5 miles ÷ 5 mph = 1.3 hrs = 1hr 18mins.

Question 108: B
New wet average speed = 0.92 x 4.6 mph = 4.232 mph
12 km in miles = 12 km ÷ 1.6 = 7.5 miles
Time taken = 7.5 miles ÷ 4.232 mph = 1.77 hrs = 1hr 46mins.

Question 109: B
Distance of second jog = 4 km x 1.5 = 6 km
Distance of third jog = 6 km x 1.5 = 9 km
Distance of last jog = 9 km x 1.5 = 13.5 km
13.5 km in miles = 13.5 km ÷ 1.6 = 8.4375 miles
Time = 8.4375 miles ÷ 5 mph = 1.69 hrs = 1hr 41mins.

Question 110: C
3hrs 42mins = 3.7 hrs
Average speed = 26 miles ÷ 3.7 hrs = 7.027 mph
7.027 mph ÷ 5 mph = 1.405 (i.e. 41% increase).

SET 24
Question 111: C
Standard price = (£325 + £100) ÷ 2 = £212.50
For two people for one week = £212.50 x 2 = £425
Deducting 20% due to discount = 0.8 x £425 = £340.

Question 112: C
Four weeks rent per person = 4 x £480 = £1,920
Total group rent = 12 x £1,920 = £23,040
Booking fee per person = 0.1 x £480 = £48
Total booking fee = 12 x £48 = £576
Total cost = £23,040 + £576 = £23,616.

Question 113: C
One person for 10 days = £80 x (20÷7) = £228.57
Two people for 10 days = 2 x £228.57 = £457.14
Booking fee = £492.89 - £457.14 = £35.75.

Question 114: A
Total rent = £220 x 2 weeks x 4 people = £1,760
Total discount = £1,760 x 0.2 = £352
Total cost = £1,760 - £352 = £1,408.

Question 115: A
Booking fee = 0.1 x £19,500 = £1,950
Total rental charge = £19,500 - £1,950 = £17,550
Number of people = £17,550 ÷ £325 = 54
Number in each palazzo = 54 ÷ 3 = 18 people.

SET 25

Question 116: B

The price of the food is £3.95 + £2.95 + £3.95 = £10.85. Orders between £10 and £15 are charged £1.50 for delivery. Including delivery, the cost is £12.35. We then add 20%, so multiply this by 1.2. Hence, the cost of the takeaway is £14.82.

Question 117: C

The total price is (3 x £2.95) + (2 x £4.95) + £3.95 = £22.70. Delivery is free above £15. We then add 20% (so we multiply by 1.2), hence the total cost is £27.24.

Question 118: A

The total price is (2 x £2.95) + £3.95 = £9.85. Add £3 for delivery under £10: 9.85 + 3 = 12.85.
Add 20% for VAT: 12.85 x 1.2 = £15.42.

Question 119: B

The total is £3.95 + (3 x £2.95) + £3.95 = £16.75. Delivery is free over £15.
We then add 20% for VAT: 16.75 x 1.2 = £20.10.

Question 120: D

The total price is (2 x £2.95) + (2 x £4.95) + £3.95 = £19.75 (price of only two noodles because of offer)
Delivery is free over £15. We then add 20% for VAT: 19.75 x 1.2 = £23.70.

SET 26

Question 121: B

Divide the profits earned by MediCo by the total profits earned by all suppliers: (15,000 + 30,000 + 25,000 + 35,000) = £105,000. 30,000/105,000 = 28.6%.

Question 122: C

Divide the profits earned by MediCo and Lifecare combined by the total profits earned by all suppliers (as calculated above):
(15,000 + 30,000 + 25,000 + 35,000) = £105000. (30,000 + 35,000)/105,000 = 61.9%.

Question 123: C

Increase the profit of PillPlus by 15% and use value when calculating the new total profit earned by all suppliers (as above):
25,000 x 1.15 = 28,750.
28,750/(15,000 + 30,000 + 28,750 + 35,000) = 26.4%.

Question 124: A

As all profits across suppliers decrease by an equal amount, this is irrelevant and cancels in the division.
0.9(35,000 + 15,000)/0.9(35,000 + 28,750 + 30,000 + 15,000) = 46.0%.

Question 125: B

Take account of the first fall in profits of 10% and then a further fall of 5%: (15,000 + 35,000) x 0.9 x 0.95 = £42,750.

SET 27

Question 126: A

The total value for the Stuntman is £12500 + £345 + £145 + £295 = £13,285.
Adding 20% VAT, this is £13,285 x 1.2 = £15,942.

Question 127: B

Remember to include tax in all calculations:
Saloon: (£21500 + £495 + £245 + £445) = £22,685. Including tax: £22,685 x 1.2 = £27,222.
Pod: (£18000 + £445 + £395 + £495) = £19335. Including tax: £19335 x 1.2 = £23,202.
£27,222 - £23,202 = £4020.

Question 128: C

Racer: (£15,000 x 1.2) = £18,000.
Stuntman: (£12500 + £345 + £145 + £295) = £13,285. Including tax: £13,285 x 1.2 = £15,942.
£18,000 - £15,942 = £2,058.

Question 129: C

The Pod with no optional extras is £18000 x 1.2 = £21,600.
The Racer with all optional extras is £15000 + £395 + £195 + £395 = £15985.
Including tax and discount: £15985 x 1.2 x 0.9 = £17,263.80.
£21,600 - £17263.80 = £4,336.20.

Question 130: D

Saloon with leather seats and easy-park technology = £21500 + £495 + £445 = £22440.
Add 20% taxation = £22,440 x 1.2 = £26,928. Reduced by 20% discount = £26928 x 0.8 = £21,542.40.
Pod = £18,000 x 1.2 = £21600.
£21,600 - £21,542.40 = £57.60.

SET 28

Question 131: C

Emissions increased by 1,000 tonnes from 1,000 to 2,000 tonnes over 5 years, therefore the rate of increase was 200 tonnes per year.

Question 132: A

If there had been no crash, 2010 emissions would have been 3,000 tonnes, as calculated by applying an increase in emissions of 200 tonnes/year from 2005 to 2010.
With the economic crash, 2010 emissions were 2,500 tonnes:
3,000 – 2,500 = 500 tonnes less in 2010 due to the economic crash.

Question 133: C

Percentage increase = (new amount – old amount)/old amount x 100
= (3,000–2,000)/2,000 x 100 = 50%.

Question 134: B

2015 – 2020 the amount would increase from 3,000 tonnes to 3,500 tonnes without any action. This equates to a rate of increase of 100 tonnes per year. With the new act, this is reduced by 50% to 50 tonnes per year, thus over 5 years: Overall saving = 50 x 5 = 250 tonnes.

Question 135: C

The emissions in 2020 = projected rate – rate reduction (50% of the difference between projected total and current total).

Rate reduction = 50 tonnes/year. Projected rate = current emissions (3,000 tonnes) + projected increase without act (5 x 100).

= (3,000+500) – (5 x 50) = 3250 tonnes.

SET 29

Question 136: B

For between 10 and 100 units, single sided black and white printing costs £0.07 per page. 74 x 7p = £5.18.

Question 137: C

£100 will clearly buy more than 100 sheets as all prices are under £1, therefore use the 100+ price:

The price for double sided colour printing over 100 sheets is £0.25.

£100/0.25 = 400 sheets.

Question 138: A

For over 100 sheets of double sided black and white, the cost per sheet is £0.10 each. Hence the total non-discounted price for 150 sheets is 150 x £0.10 = £15. If this is discounted by 10%, this is £15 x 0.9 = £13.50.

Question 139: B

Price for buying separately = 150 x 0.15 = £22.50

Price buying together = 150 x 0.10 x 0.9 (discount) = £13.50

Difference = £9

Number of sheets could buy with £9 = 9/0.15 = 60 sheets.

Question 140: B

The price for 227 sheets of double sided black and white printing is £0.10 each, so the total is £22.70.

The price for 34 sheets of double sided colour printing is £0.30 each, so the total is £10.20.

The total for all the sheets is £32.90.

If this is discounted by 10%, this is £32.90 x 0.9 = £29.61.

SET 30

Question 141: D

We can calculate the number of people who reacted positively in each group and then add up the total:

75% of 300 is 225

65% of 300 is 195

70% of 300 is 210

55% of 300 is 165

Total = 225 + 195 + 210 + 165 = 795.

Question 142: C

In group 2, 30% reacted negatively: 30% of 300 is 90.
In group 3, 15% reacted negatively: 15% of 300 is 45.
Therefore, the difference is 45. So, 45 more people in group 2 reacted negatively than people in group 3.

Question 143: B

We can calculate the number of people who reacted negatively in each group and then add up the total:
20% of 300 is 60
30% of 300 is 90
15% of 300 is 45
25% of 300 is 75
Total = 60 + 90 + 45 + 75 = 270.
270 as a percentage of the total (1200) is 22.5%, or 23% to 2 s.f.

Question 144: D

The overall success rate of the first four groups was = (75 + 65 + 70 + 55)/4 = 66.25%
Therefore, increase in success rate = 82/66.25 = 23.77% increase.

Question 145: B

In the answer to question 143, we calculated that in the first 4 groups, 270 people reacted negatively.
In group 5, 15% of 300 people, which is 45 people, reacted negatively.
Hence, the negative reactions total 315 people.

SET 31

Question 146: C

The total number of views of The Last Chase is 20,000 + 20,000 + 15,000 + 20,000 = 75,000.
The total number of views of The Final Frontier is 15,000 + 20,000 + 25,000 + 35,000 = 95,000.
Hence, the difference is 95,000 – 75,000 = 20,000.

Question 147: B

The difference in viewers is 20,000. If £2,500 is earned per 1,000 viewers, then the difference in advertising revenue will be £2,500 x 20 = £50,000.

Question 148: B

Growth rate is 5,000 per quarter between Q1 and Q3 of 2014. Therefore, the total growth during 2015:
35,000 + (5,000 x 4) = 55,000

Question 149: B

Growth rate is 5,000 per quarter between Q1 and Q3 of 2014. Therefore, the total growth during 2015:
Q1: 35,000 + 5,000 = 40,000
Q2: 40,000 + 5,000 = 45,000
Q3: 45,000 + 5,000 = 50,000
Q4: 50,000 + 5,000 = 55,000
Thus, the total number of views = 40,000 + 45,000 + 50,000 + 55,000 = 190,000.

Question 150: D

Without the show cancellation, there are 35,000 Final Frontier views and 20,000 Last Chase views. With the cancellation, half of the Last Chase views transfer over to Final Frontier, this equates to 10,000 views. Therefore, the Final Frontier now has 45,000 views in this scenario.

SET 32

Question 151: C

55% + 25% = 80% of Scottish patients wait a half an hour or less. 80% of 50,000 patients = 40,000.
Therefore, 40,000 patients waited a half an hour or less for an appointment.

Question 152: B

We can work out how many patients had to wait more than half an hour for an appointment in each part of the UK then find the total:
In England, 10% of 100,000 patients = 10,000 patients had to wait longer than half an hour.
In Scotland, 20% of 50,000 patients = 10,000 patients had to wait longer than half an hour.
In Wales, 25% of 25,000 patients = 6,250 patients had to wait longer than half an hour.
In Northern Ireland, 15% of 25,000 patients = 3,750 patients had to wait longer than half an hour.
The total number of patients that had to wait longer than half an hour is 10,000 + 10,000 + 6,250 + 3,750 = 30,000.
30,000/200,000 = 15%.

Question 153: C

In the previous question we found that 30,000 patients had to wait longer than half an hour, so 40% of 30,000 people complained. 0.4 x 30,000 = 12,000.
No, we can calculate how many had to wait 11-30 minutes:
In England, 30% of 100,000 patients = 30,000 patients had to wait 11-30 minutes.
In Scotland, 25% of 50,000 patients = 12,500 patients had to wait 11-30 minutes.
In Wales, 25% of 25,000 patients = 6,250 patients had to wait had to wait 11-30 minutes.
In Northern Ireland, 25% of 25,000 patients = 6,250 patients had to wait 11-30 minutes.
The total number of patients that had to wait 11-30 minutes is 30,000 + 12,500 + 6,250 + 6,250 = 55,000.
If 20% of 55,000 patients complain, this is 11,000.
Hence, the total number of complaints is 12,000 + 11,000 = 23,000.

Question 154: B

Using answers from the previous questions. Use the total survey size to calculate the proportion as a percentage:
23,000/200,000 = 11.5%.

Question 155: B

We worked out in question 152 and question 153 that 30,000 people had to wait longer than 30 minutes and 55,000 people had to wait between 11 and 30 minutes.
If the targets are met, 15,000 people will wait longer than 30 minutes and 41,250 will wait between 11 and 30 minutes.
If 40% of the 15,000 people complain, this is 0.4 x 15,000 = 6,000 complaints. If 20% of these 41,250 people complain, this is 0.2 x 41,250 = 8,250 complaints.
Hence, there are a total of 14,250 complaints. The previous number of complaints was 23,000.
So, the percentage decrease is (23,000-14,250)/23,000 = 0.38 = 38%.

SET 33

Question 156: D

The decrease in the price of crude oil between January and March is $150-$100 = $50, as can be seen in the first graph.

This fall has occurred over a 2-month period, giving a decrease in price of $25 per month.

Question 157: D

This is a question of estimation; look at the answer options first. The average production across the year is at least 7 million barrels per day. Multiplying this by 365 gives around 2,550 million barrels per year.

All other options require less than 7 million barrels daily production, and it is clear there are at least 7 million barrels per day.

Therefore, the answer is 2,700 million.

Alternatively, we can estimate using 30 days per month, and multiplying the number of barrels produced per day in each month by 30 (this is more accurate but more time consuming, and unnecessary given the different answer options). 6+7+7+7.5+7.5+7+7.5+8+8.5+8.5+8+9 = 91.5, multiplying by 30 gives just over 2,700 million barrels per year.

Question 158: C

Use both graphs. For July, multiply the oil price by the amount sold in the month, and then multiply by the number of days in the month.

July = 7.5 million barrels x $75 per barrel x 31 days = $17,400 million = $17.4 billion.

Question 159: B

If the costs are 40%, the gross profit is 60%.

Oil sales in June 2014 totalled 7 million barrels x $100 per barrel x 30 days = £21,000 million = $21 billion.

Therefore gross profit was 0.6 x $21 billion = $12.6 billion.

Question 160: A

You are given the total sales value of $204 billion, so work with this. Work clearly in stages and this question is not hard.

The profit is 60% of this, which is $122.4 billion.

This is split 5:2 between the oil companies and the oil-producing nation. Thus, the profit for the oil companies is 5/7 of $122.4 billion, which is $87.43 billion.

Corporation tax is then 30% of this profit, which is $26.23 billion.

SET 34

Question 161: B

Calculate the total people with no asthma, and subtract it from the total number of people which is 250 (5 x 50 from passage):
80% of the 50 people aged 0-5 have no asthma, which is 40.
75% of the 50 people aged 5-10 have no asthma, which is 37.5.
85% of the people aged 10-21 have no asthma, which is 42.5.
95% of the people aged 21-30 have no asthma, which is 47.5.
95% of the people aged 30+ have no asthma, which is 47.5.
Hence, the total people who have no asthma is 215.
And the total people with asthma is 250 – 215 = 35.

Question 162: B

Of children aged 0-5, 15% have mild asthma which is 7.5. Hence, 3.75 will develop respiratory problems ('a half chance').
Of children aged 0-5, 5% have severe asthma which is 2.5. Hence, 2.25 will develop respiratory problems (90% in passage).
Of children aged 5-10, 20% have mild asthma which is 10. Hence, 5 will develop respiratory problems ('a half chance').
Of children aged 5-10, 5% have severe asthma which is 2.5. Hence, 2.25 will develop respiratory problems (90% in passage).
3.75 + 2.25 +5 + 2.25 = 13.25.
Therefore, 13.25 children per 100 will develop respiratory problems, so the answer is 13.25%.

Question 163: A

Calculate the average for the 0-5 and 5-10 age groups: (15%+20%)/2 = 17.5% diagnosed.
From the passage, 17.5% x 0.35 = 6.125%. Therefore, 6.125% incorrect diagnoses.

Question 164: B

Taking into account that only 65% of children diagnosed with mild asthma were diagnosed correctly:
17.5% diagnosed (mild); 11.375% correctly diagnosed; 5.69% complications ('half a chance').
5% diagnosed (severe); all are correct diagnoses; 4.5% complications ('90%').
Therefore, 5.69 + 4.5 = 10% overall respiratory complication rate.

Question 165: A

False diagnoses = percent diagnosed x false diagnoses x proportion of population x total population
(0.15x0.35x0.07x50,000,000) 0-5 year olds + (0.2x0.35x0.1x50,000,000) 5-10 year olds = 533,750
Cost per diagnosis: £50 per year = £250 over 5 years
Total money wasted: 533,750 x £250 = £133 million.

SET 35

Question 166: D

Total value of company A = (price per share x number of shares) = £60 x 10 million shares = £600 million
Government holding = 75% of 600 million = £450 million
Disinvestment (50%) = 0.5 x 450 = £225 million
Hence, £225 million is raised from the disinvestment.

Question 167: A

Total value of company B = (price per share x number of shares) = £20 x 50 million shares = 1,000 million
Government holding = 50% of 1,000 million = £500 million
Disinvestment (25%) = 0.25 x 500 = £125 million.

Question 168: B

Government holds 33.33% of the 30 million shares, which is 10 million shares.
It sold each share for £35, which is £5 less than the £40 market price. Hence, the additional revenue for selling at the market price would have been £5 per share x 10 million shares = £50 million.

Question 169: B

Government holds 25% of 40 million shares, which is 10 million shares.
The price of each share fell from £30 to £25, so fell by £5 per share.
If the price of 10 million shares fell by £5, the total fall was £50 million.

Question 170: C

Government holds 12.5% of 50 million shares, which is 6.25 million.
The price has risen by £5 per share, so the total rise is £31.25 million.

Question 171: B

Total value of option A = £10 x 60 million x 75% = £450 million
Total value of option B = £20 x 50 million x 50% = £500 million
Hence, they will fetch difference values, with B fetching more.

SET 36

Question 172: C

In 2011-2012, food grain production was 100, and this was a 25% increase on 2010-2011.
If 100 is 125%, then 100% = 80. Hence, food production in tonnes in 2010-2011 was 80 tonnes.

Question 173: B

Target production (2011-12) = 60 tonnes
Actual production (2010-11) = 50/125% = 40 tonnes
Difference = 60 – 40 = 20 tonnes.

Question 174: B

Difference = Target – Actual = 50 – 40 = 10 tonnes.

Question 175: D

Cotton production (2010-11) = 30/120% = 25 tonnes
Jute production (2010-11) = 20/125% = 16 tonnes
Total of cotton and jute production = 25 + 16 = 41 tonnes.

Question 176: D
Food grain production (2010-11) = 100/125% = 80 tonnes
Oil seeds production (2010-11) = 50/125% = 40 tonnes
Difference = 80 – 40 = 40 tonnes.

Question 177: B
Total production (2011-12) = 100+50+40+30+20 = 240 tonnes
Cotton as a percentage of total = 30/240 = 12.5%.

SET 37
Question 178: D
Sales of product B in Feb = 7,000
Total sales of all products in Feb = 10,250 + 7,000 + 3,750 + 3100 = 24,100
Percentage of product B's sales = 7,000/24,100 = 29%.

Question 179: D
Percentage increase:
Product A = (11,000-10,500)/10,500 = 4.76%
Product B = (7,500-7,250)/7,250 = 3.45%
Product C = (4,250-4,000)/4,000 = 6.25%
Product D = (4,000-3,500)/3,500 = 14.29%
Hence, product D witnessed the highest percentage growth.
However, to answer this question more quickly, look at the numbers – they are giving you a clue. You can visually see that product D's sales' values have gone up the equal maximum amount of £500. But it is also apparent that the absolute value of sales is the lowest, therefore you can deduce that D is the largest percentage increase without any sums.

Question 180: C
Sales of product C in May = 4,250 x 1.2 = 5,100
Therefore, sales of product D in May = 5,100
Percentage increase in sales of D from April to May = (5,100 – 4,000)/4,000 = 27.5%.

Question 181: D
Sale of products (A+C) in January = 9,500 + 3,500 = 13,000
Sale of products (A+C) in April = 11,000 + 4,250 = 15,250
Percentage increase in combined sale from January to April = (15,250 – 13,000)/13,000 = 17.31%.

Question 182: A
Sale of product (A+B) in May = 1.2 x (11,000+7,500) = 22,200
Sale of product (C+D) in May = 1.3 x (4,250+4,000) = 10,725
Total sales in May = 22,200 + 10,725 = 32,925.

Question 183: D

Sale of product A in May = 1.2 x 11,000 = 13,200

Sale of product (B+C+D) in May = 1.1 x (7,500+4,250+4,000) = 17,325

Total sales in May = 13,200+17,325 = 30,525

Percentage of sales of A over total sales = 13,200/30,525 = 43.24%.

SET 38

Question 184: C

Overall profit is 30% of revenue.

Since profit = £2.5 million, overall revenue = 2.5/30 x 100 = £8.3 million.

Question 185: B

Assume cost per article = C; Total number of articles = N.

Cost per consignment:

Rail = 25C/30N = 0.83C/N

Road = 25C/45N = 0.56C/N

Air = 50C/25N = 2C/N

Hence, road has the lowest cost per consignment.

However, if you look at the figures, a shortcut is apparent. Road occupies by far the greatest number of consignments, but the cost is the equal lowest in the business. Therefore, at a glance you can see the answer is road, before doing any sums.

Question 186: A

The ratio will be the same for any number of consignments as the proportions are preserved.

Ratio of total revenue to total cost = £20:£5 = 4:1.

Question 187: C

From the table it is given that 50% of the total costs are associated with air transportation, so 50% of the total costs are due to air travel.

50% x £54,000 = £27,000.

Question 188: D

From the table it is given that 30% are delivered by rail and 45% by road, so 75% of consignments are delivered by rail and road taken together.

75% x 17,145 = 12,859.

SET 39

Question 189: A

This is a difficult question that would be worth "flagging for review".

Set the percentage of lead in alloy A to a, and the percentage of tin in alloy C to b. We can then find the percentage of copper in each as a function of a and b.

Alloy	Zinc	Tin	Lead	Copper	Nickel
A	10%	40%	a%	(40-a)%	10%
B	25%	15%	50%	5%	5%
C	15%	b%	20%	(30-b)%	35%

The key thing here is to use the composition of Alloy G. We can find the composition of Alloy G in terms of a and b and then set the amounts of tin, lead and copper equal to each other to find a and b.

For Alloy G, the percentages will be weighted according to the proportion A:B:C = 2:1:3

$2/6\ (40) + 1/6\ (15) + 3/6\ (b) = 2/6\ (a) + 1/6\ (50) + 3/6\ (20) = 2/6\ (40\text{-}a) + 1/6\ (5) + 3/6\ (30\text{-}b)$

$80 + 15 + 3b = 2a + 50 + 60 = 80 - 2a + 5 + 90 - 3b$

Solving the above equation, we will get values:

$95 + 3b = 2a + 110$

$2a + 110 = 175 - 2a - 3b$

$3b = 65 - 4a$

$2a = 95 - 110 + 65 - 4a$

$6a = 50$

$a = 50/6$

$b = 95/9$

Percentage of Lead in alloy A = a = 50/6% = 8.33%.

Question 190: C

Using the solution from the previous question, we found that the percentage of Tin in alloy C (or b%) was:

$b = 95/9$

Percentage of Tin in alloy C = 95/9 = 10.6%.

Question 191: B

Zinc percentage in alloy X is equal to the average of the percentages of the composite alloys, as they are present in equal proportions. This can be found by adding together and dividing by 3.

$X = (10+25+15)/3 = 50/3 = 16.67\%$.

Question 192: D

To solve, subtract the amounts of the known metals to find the remaining metal, which is equal to the percentage of Tin and Copper combined in alloy C. We know there are no other components as this is stated in the question.

(100% – 15% – 20% – 35%) = 30%.

Question 193: B

We know the percentages of tin in each of the alloys which make up Alloy G, and the composition of Alloy G. Alloy G is made up of alloys A:B:C in the ratio 2:1:3. Alloy A has 40% tin; alloy B has 15%; alloy C has 95/9% tin. Hence, the percentage in Alloy G is (2/6 x 40)+(1/6 x 15)+(3/6 x 95/9) = 21.11%.

Question 194: C

Percentage of elements in alloy G:

We know that Alloy G has 21.11% tin from the last question. We also know from the initial explanation that it has the same concentration of tin, lead and copper. This is 3 elements with the same concentration. We then need to work out how much nickel and zinc there is to check whether there is a 4th.

Alloy G is made up of alloys A:B:C in the ratio 2:1:3. Alloy A has 10% nickel, alloy B has 5% nickel and alloy C has 35% nickel. Hence, the percentage nickel in Alloy G is ((2x10)+(1x5)+(3x35))/6 = 21.6666.

We can also work out from the fact that these 4 elements plus zinc are 100% of the total that zinc is 15%.

Zinc = 15%

Tin = 21.11%

Lead = 21.11%

Copper = 21.11%

Nickel = 21.67%

So, there is still only three elements (tin, lead and copper) that have the same concentration, so the answer is still three.

SET 40

Question 195: A

Number of persons who voted in favour of Hilary Clinton = 60% of 17% of 11,500 = 0.6 x 0.17 x 11,500 = 1173.

Question 196: D

We cannot find the number of people living in New York, as we do not know the proportion of citizens of New York who voted for people other than Robert Guiliani. We can only say that there was a minimum of 460 New York citizens. We cannot determine the actual number.

Question 197: D

0.39 x 11,500 = 4,485 votes for Bush.

4,485/(11,500 x 0.8) gives the proportion of US citizens who voted for Bush, which is equal to 48.8%.

Question 198: C

10% of 40% of people surveyed are in favour of Rumsfield and employees of the federal government, so 10% of 40% of 11,500 = 0.1 x 0.4 x 11,500 = 460 people.

Also from the table, Rumsfield has 5% of 11,500 votes = 575 people who are in favour of him in total.

The number of people who are in favour of Rumsfeld who are not employees of the federal government is 575 – 460 = 115.

Question 199: C

The number of people polled was constant.

The decrease in percentage is from 16% to 2%, which is 14 % of 11,500 = 1,610 people.

Question 200: A

The number of people polled was constant.

The decrease in percentage is from 40% to 39%, which is 1% of 11,500 = 115 people.

SET 41

Question 201: E

15% indicates that only 85% of the total price is to be paid.

50p is the price per unit for premium mugs for quantity below 49 units.

20p is the price per unit for basic mugs for quantity below 49 units.

5p is the price per unit for logo on basic mugs for quantity below 49 units.

Using this information, we can work out:

0.85x(5x50p+4x(20p+5p)) = 297.5p = £2.975 rounded up to £2.98

Therefore, customer A will have to pay £2.98.

Question 202: B

20p is the price per unit for premium mugs for quantity above 500 units.

10p is the price per unit for basic mugs for quantity between 100 and 499 units.

3p is the price to add logos to those mugs.

4p is the price per unit for black and white flyers for quantity between 10 and 99 units.

Combining this information together gives the equation:

750x20p +130x(10p+3p)+80x4p = 17010p = £170.10 rounded down to £170

So, the company will have to pay £170.

Question 203: C

Step I.

10p is the price per unit for colour flyer between 10 and 99 units.

£250 equals 25,000p.

25,000p – (50x10p) = 24,500p.

Step II.

Once the flyers are bought, 24,500p are left and need to know how many medium mugs with logos can be bought.

10p is the price per unit for medium mugs above 500 units.

2p is the price per unit for logo on medium mugs above 500 units.

24,500p/(10p+2p)=2041.667. Therefore, she can buy 2041 medium mugs.

Question 204: D

Step I.

2014: 70x(26p+4p)+150x5p= 2850p

26p is the price per unit for medium mugs below 99 units in 2014.

4p is the price per unit for logo on medium mugs below 99 units in 2014.

5p is the price per unit for colour flyers above 100 units in 2014.

Step II.
2015: 70x(26p+3p)+150x4p=2630p
26p is the price per unit for medium mugs below 99 units in 2015.
3p is the price per unit for logo on medium mugs below 99 units in 2015.
4p is the price per unit for colour flyers above 100 units in 2015.
Step III.
2630/2850 = –0.077 = –8% = 8% cheaper.

Question 205: C
1.2% equals 0.0012.
3 years between 2012 and 2015.
£325,750/(1.012^(3)) = £314,298.9 rounded down to £314,299.

SET 42
Question 206: B
The easiest way to solve this problem is using a Venn diagram. The Venn diagram below shows all possible combinations of the three devices each student can have as well as the number of students with a combination of devices. The sum of the numbers in the Venn diagram must be equal to the total number of students.

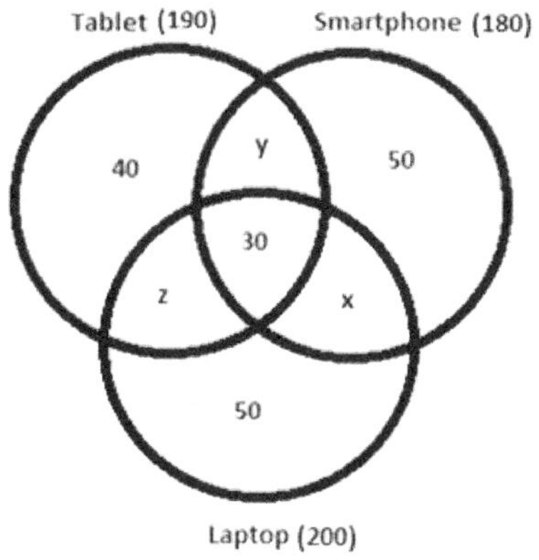

Using the information given in the graphs, we know there are:

- 30 students with all three devices
- 50 students with smartphone only
- 40 students with tablet only
- 50 students with laptop only
- 180 students with smartphone
- 190 students with tablet
- 200 students with laptop

Therefore, we can construct the following Venn diagram.
Laptop: 200 = 50+30+z+x → z = 120-x
Smartphone: 180 = 50+30+x+y → y = 100-x
Tablet: 190 = 40+30+y+z → y = 120-z
So, we see that y = 100-x and y = 120-z and thus z = 20+x
Then, we see that z = 20+x and z = 120-x and thus x = 50
Plus it into the equation to get z = 20+x = 70 and y = 100-x = 50
Now, the total number of students is the sum of the numbers in the Venn diagram, which has a total of 340.

Question 207: C
Using the previously constructed Venn diagram, the total number of students with a smartphone and a laptop is 50.

Question 208: A

180 students have smartphone

100 students have both tablet and laptop

So, 180–100=80. Therefore, the answer is 80 students.

Question 209: C

Total number of students: 340

80 students have both smartphone and laptop.

80/340 = 0.235

Therefore, percentage is 23.5%.

Question 210: C

185 – number of students with smartphone (AFTER)

345 – total number of students (AFTER)

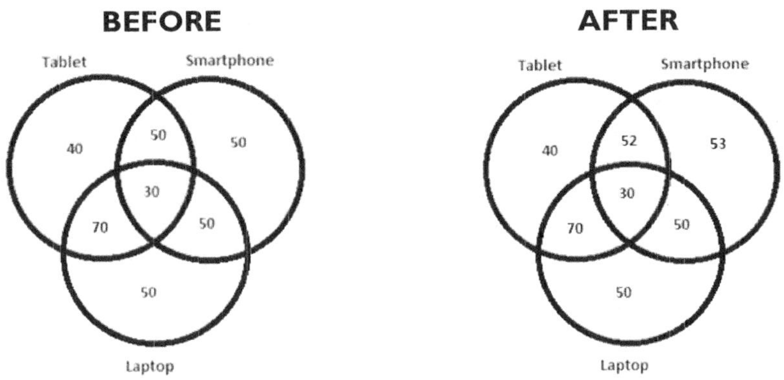

185/345 = 0.536. Therefore the percentage is 54%.

SET 43

Question 211: B

From 7.10am, trains run in every 20 minutes and hence the first one after 2pm will depart at 2.10pm – every 20 minutes. This gives us three trains per hour from 2.10pm which would come to 12 trains before 6.15pm.

Question 212: C

From 8.18am, trains run in every 20 minutes and hence the first one Antonia can catch is the 2.58pm train. As it takes 21 minutes to get to London Liverpool Street station, she can arrive by 3.19pm.

Question 213: D

There are three trains in the morning before 7.10am. Thereafter, 3 trains per hour and the last one departs at 23.10pm. There are 16 hours between 7.10am and 23.10pm, so 3+(16x3) = 51. Therefore, 51 trains run all day.

Question 214: B

The first train after 3pm departs at 3.10pm from Cambridge Station and arrives at Tottenham Hale by 4.28pm.

Question 215: D

Using the equation: velocity = distance/time
7 minutes = 7/60 hour from Audley End to Bishops Stortford
10.5 miles between Audley End and Bishops Stortford
10.5 miles / (7/60) hour = 90 miles per hour.

SET 44

Question 216: A

The top five rivers in the table are the longest.
Take the length in miles from column 2 and add them together.
Total is: 220+215+185+143+134 = 897 miles.

Question 217: B

Firstly, you add the drainage area of all seven rivers from column C. Then you add the increase in drainage area of River Thames (1345.5 square mile). Finally, you can calculate the percentage increase, dividing new by old.
Old: 4,409+4,994+4,029+3,236+1,597+560+431 = 19,256
New: 1345.5+4,409+4,994+4,029+3,236+1,597+560+431 = 20,601.5
Percentage increase: 20,601.5/19,256 = 1.06987.
Therefore, the answer is 7%.

Question 218: C

River Thames: 4,994 square mile
River Wye: 1,597 square mile
Percentage difference: 4,994/1,597 = 3.127.
Therefore, the answer it 313%.

Question 219: A

Lowest average discharge: River Tay has a length of 117 miles
Highest average discharge: River Trent has a length of 185 miles
Difference in length: 185–117 = 68.

Question 220: B

Remember that only the six longest rivers shall be included in the calculation.
Use the figures from column 3 to obtain the equation:
(4,409+4,994+4,029+3,236+1,597+560)/6 = 3137.5.

SET 45

Question 221: C

The largest section on the pie chart for Scottish GDP is Government and Other Services – it accounts for 29% of total.

Question 222: B

Use the figures we are given: 4.2tn pounds and 5% (1.05) growth.
Plug them into the equation: GDP_{2014} x 1.05 = 4.2tn
This can be arranged as: GDP_{2014} = 4.2/1.05 = 4.

Question 223: E

Manufacturing in Scottish GDP is 14%

Business Services and Finance in UK GDP is 28%

Difference is equal to 28–14 = 14.

Therefore, the answer is 14%.

Question 224: B

We can use the figures given to formulate the following equation:

(GDP in 2014) x (3% GDP increase) x (1% share of Agriculture, Forestry and Fishing)

= £1.2tn x 1.03 x 0.01 = 0.01236tn.

Question 225: D

The three largest sections of the UK GDP pie chart are:

Distribution, Hotels and Catering 15%

Business Services Finance 28%

Government and Other Services 24%.

SET 46

Question 226: C

The most-watched TV show is Geordie shore.

Year 1 divided by Year 2 = 9.2/12.5 = 1.35869.

Therefore, the answer is 36%.

Question 227: E

The Voice: 3.4 and 4.1 in year 1 and 2 respectively

Britain's got talent: 5.2 and 5.6 in year 1 and 2 respectively

Year I: 5.2+3.4 = 8.6

Year II: 5.6+4.1 = 9.7

The difference between year II and I is 9.7 – 8.6 = 1.1.

Question 228: C

The show that the fewest percentage of males watched in year 2 was The Voice, with only 2%.

Question 229: B

Year 2 (all five TV shows) / Year 1 (all five TV shows)

= (4.1+5.6+1.4+12.5+3) / (5+9.2+1.3+5.2+3.4) = 1.1037.

Therefore, the answer is 10%.

Question 230: D

Total population of females in year 2: 30 million

Number of females who watched Geordie Shore: 30x0.21 = 6.3 million

Number of males who watched Geordie Shore: 12.5-6.3 = 6.2 million.

SET 47

Question 231: D

Basic plan: 250 free texts and more than 75 free minutes = (300-250) x15 = £7.50.
Therefore, the basic plan costs £45.29 + £7.50 = £52.79.
Premium plan: more than 300 free texts and more than 75 free minutes.
Therefore, the premium plan costs £47.89.
So, the premium plan is cheaper by £52.79 – £47.89 = £4.90.

Question 232: C

Premium plan: £47.89
£60 – £47.89 = £12.11 left.
Cheapest calls are standard calls, which cost 6p.
12.11/0.06 = 201.83 = 201 minutes.

Question 233: E

45 texts free, 125 mins same network free, 100 minutes free with other network.
225 mins other network in both options.
Before: 225 x 0.15 = 33.75
After: 225 x 0.16 = 36
The difference is 36 – 33.75 = £2.25.

Question 234: D

Basic plan: £45.29 + £58.50 = £103.79
150 minutes for free = (800 – 150) x 9p = £58.50.
Premium plan: £47.89 + £45.00 = £92.89
500 minutes for free = (800-500) x15p = 4500p = £45.00.
Therefore, the difference is £103.79 – £92.89 = £10.90.

Question 235: C

Basic plan: £45.29 x 1.15 + (450 – 250) x £0.15 = £52.08 + £30.00 = £82.08.
Premium plan: £47.89 x 1.15 = £55.07.
Therefore, the difference is £82.08 – £55.07 = £27.01.

SET 48

Question 236: B

Davos: 15cm, 15cm, 15cm and 10cm in November, December, January, February respectively.
Chamonix Mont-Blanc: 5cm, 40cm, 15cm, 20cm in November, December, January, February respectively.
We can use these figures to create the following equation:
(15+15+15+10) + (5+40+15+20) / 8 = 16.875 cm.

Question 237: C

Davos: 15cm, 15cm, 15cm and 10cm in November, December, January, February respectively.
Average snowfall in Davos: (15+15+15+10)/4 = 13.75
Chamonix Mont-Blanc: 5cm, 40cm, 15cm, 20cm in November, December, January, February respectively.
Average snowfall in Chamonix Mont-Blanc: (5+40+15+20)/4 = 20
Cortina d' Ampezzo: 5cm, 50cm, 50cm, 40cm in November, December, January, February respectively.
Average snowfall in Cortina d' Ampezzo: (5+50+50+40) / 4 = 36.25
Garmisch Partenkirchen: 10cm, 15cm, 20cm, 35cm in November, December, January, February respectively.
Average snowfall in Garmisch Partenkirchen: (10+15+20+35) / 4 = 20
So, the highest average snowfall was in Cotine d'Ampezzo, with 36.25.

Question 238: C

Inserting figures from all of the places into an equation:
December compared to February = (15+15+50+40) / (35+10+40+20) = 120/105 = 1.14.

Question 239: B

We are told that in November 2014 there is 30cm of snowfall (in all four areas).
To work out November 2015, we need to add all the areas for November 2015:
Garmisch-Partenkirchen is 10cm, Davos is 15cm, Cortina d'Ampezzo is 5cm, Chamonix Mont-Blanc is 5cm.
This is equal to 35cm for November 2015.
Therefore, 2015 vs 2014 = 35/30 = 1.1667 = 17%.

Question 240: D

We need to add the values for November and February for both of these places.
Cortina d' Ampezzo = 5 + 40 = 45
Garmisch Partenkirchen = 10 + 35 = 45
The total of both places is 45 + 45 = 90.

SET 49

Question 241: A

Notice that two expenses relate to HSBC:
Mileage to and from presentation in Cambridge = £16.80
Breakfast with client = £35.90
The sum of both is equal to £35.90 + £16.80 = £52.70.
Remember to check that the sum is greater than any other item on the list.

Question 242: B

Add all of the expenses from each company together.
£35.90 + £16.80 + £15.40 + £20.00 + £49.50 = £137.60.

Question 243: E

Remember to only include meals and train tickets – not all mileage!

Soros Fund Management	Single ticket - Train journey to meeting in London	£15.40	Train
HSBC	Breakfast with client	£35.90	Meal
Black Rock	Return ticket – Train journey to meeting in London	£20.00	Train
MKB	Lunch with client	£49.50	Meal

Meal compared to train: (£35.90+£49.50)/(£15.40+£20.00) – 1 = 1.413 = 141%.

Question 244: B

Mileage paid at £0.25 per mile for the first 100 miles each month and £0.10 thereafter

He paid £16.80.

100 miles x £0.25 per mile = £25, which is higher than £16.80 that Kevin actually paid, so the £0.25 per mile applies.

£16.80/£0.25 = 67.2.

Question 245: D

The total sum of travel expenses = £16.80+£15.40+£20.00 = £52.20.

75% of travel expenses = £52.2 x 0.75 = £39.15.

Difference is £52.2 – £39.15 = £13.05.

Accommodation and meal expenses = £35.90+£49.50 = £85.40.

90% of accommodation and meal expenses = £85.40x0.9 = £76.86.

Difference is £85.40 – £76.86 = £8.54.

The sum of differences is equal to £13.05+£8.54 = £21.59.

SET 50

Question 246: A

£30 per hour and total cost £50.

£50 – £30 = £20.

Question 247: B

Gamma for 6 hours = £25 deposit + (£115 x 6 hours) = 25 + 690 = £715

Beta for 6 hours = £20 deposit + (£90 x 6 hours) = 20 + 540 = £560

The difference is equal to 715 – 560 = £155.

Question 248: B

Using the information from the table:

Alpha: £50

Gamma: £140

Beta: £110

Delta: £250

Aron can afford to rent Alpha, Beta and Gamma for one hour (£300).

Alpha, Beta, Gamma and Delta would cost £550 which is out of his budget.

Question 249: B

Alpha: £30 per half an hour and £90 for three hours plus deposit of £20 is equal to £110
Gamma: 3 hours x £115 (cost per hour) + £25 (deposit) = £370
The sum of these figures is £110+£370 = £480.

Question 250: C

Old: Deposit £100 + (£150x8) = £1300.
New: (£100 x 1.05) + (£150x8) = £1305.

SET 51

Question 251: C

Remember to convert all of the prices into £
Around the World offers a price of 400 €.
Every 1.5€ equals the value of 1£. Thus, 400/1.5 = 266,67 rounded up to £267.
Therefore, Around the World is the cheapest offer to East Asia in pounds (£).

Question 252: B

The differences from the European price in pounds are 190, 175, 180 and 200.
The average of the differences is (190+175+180+200)/4 = 186.25 rounded up to 186.3.

Question 253: A

The discounted price of Take Me There is 560 – 50 = $510, in pounds it is 510/2 = 255.
This discounted ticket is £5 more expensive than the original price of In The Air (£250).
In percentages, this difference is 5/250x100 = 2%.

Question 254: C

The total revenue of Around The World is (10x450) + (5x300) = €6000, which is in pounds 6000/1.5 = £4000.
The total revenue of Good Fly is (25x100) + (12x300) = £6100.
The difference between revenues is £2100.
This is 2100/6100x100 = 34.42% of the higher revenue, which is rounded up to 34.43%.

Question 255: C

The original price in pounds is 610/2=£305, the new price is 610/2.5=£244.
The difference is 305 – 244 = £61.

SET 52

Question 256: D

Looking at the pie chart for Indian GDP, the largest section is for manufacturing, accounting for 24% of total Indian GDP.

Question 257: C

UK: Government and Other Services (24%) / Business Services and Finance (28%) = 86%
India: Government and Other Services (9%) / Business Services and Finance (15%) = 60%
The difference is equal to = UK – India = 26%.

Question 258: A

The three largest sections of the pie chart for Indian GDP are:
Distribution, Hotels and Catering 20%
Business Services Finance 15%
Manufacturing: 24%

Question 259: D

Bottom two performing sectors in the UK: Agriculture, Forestry and Fishing (1%); Other Production (4%)
Their contribution to UK GDP = £4.2tn (total GDP) x 0.05 (1%+4%) = £210 billion.
Bottom two performing sector in India: Other Production (3%); Construction (6%)
Their contribution to Indian GDP = £2tn (total GDP) x 0.12 (9%+3%) = £180 billion.
UK compared to Indian GDP: £210 billion – £180 billion = £30 billion.

Question 260: D

Largest sector in the UK: Business Services and Finance = £4.2tn x 0.28 = £1.176tn
Largest sector in India: Manufacturing = £2tn x 0.2 = £400 billion
Size of Business Services and Finance in the UK is £1.176tn, which is the largest

SET 53

Question 261: A

1500 JPY at 1 JPY = 0.013 USD.
1500 x 0.013 = 19.50.

Question 262: D

1 JPY = 0.022 GBP
1 JPY = 0.015 USD
Average exchange rates = GBP/USD = 0.022 / 0.015 = 1.47.

Question 263: A

% increase: ((JPY/CAD) of 2012 / (JPY/CAD) of 2011) – 1 = (0.119 / 0.115) – 1 = 0.0348 = 3.5%.

Question 264: A

USD 1300 at USD/JPY rate of 0.010 in 2010 = JPY 130,000
USD 1300 at USD/JPY rate of 0.015 in 2013 = JPY 86,667
Therefore, the difference is JPY 130,000 – JPY 86,667 = 43,333.

Question 265: C

Looking at the table it is easy to notice that EUR exchange rate is near constant over the given time period except for one change in 2011 by 0.001.
Therefore, this is smaller than all the other currency changes.

SET 54

Question 266: D

Boston: 4.4 – 4 = 0.4 million
Chicago: 3.3 – 3.5 = -0.2 million
Denver: 2.1 – 2 = 0.1 million
El Monte 1.5 – 0.8 = 0.7 million
El Monte has the highest growth in population, with 0.7 million.

Question 267: A

Boston: 542,000– 235,675 = 306,325
Chicago: 350,685 – 345,526 = 5159
Denver: 249,990 – 231,456 = 18,534
El Monte 62,044 – 54,000 = 8044
Therefore, Boston had the largest growth.

Question 268: D

Boston: 542,000/4.4 million = 0.123
Chicago: 350,685/3.3 million = 0.106
Denver: 249,990/2.1 million = 0.119
El Monte 62,044/1.5 million = 0.041
Therefore, El Monte had the lowest number of cars per person.

Question 269: A

2014 vs 2009:
Boston: 542,000/4.4 million = 0.123 vs. 235,675/4 million = 0.059
Chicago: 350,685/3.3 million = 0.106 vs. 345,526/3.5 million = 0.099
Denver: 249,990/2.1 million = 0.119 vs. 231,456/2 million = 0.116
El Monte 62,044/1.5 million = 0.041 vs. 54,000/0.8 million = 0.068
Difference:
Boston: 0.123 – 0.059 = 0.064
Chicago: 0.106 – 0.099 = 0.007
Denver: 0.119 – 0.116 = 0.003
El Monte: 0.041 – 0.068 = –0.027
Therefore, Boston has the largest change in number of cars per person between 2009 and 2014.

Question 270: D

2009 Boston = 235,675/4 million = 0.059
2014 Boston = 542,000/4.4 million = 0.123
The difference in Boston is equal to 0.123 – 0.059 = 0.064.

SET 55

Question 271: E

Starting rate: 15% of 2,450 = £367.50.

Basic rate: 25% of 2,450 = 33,500.

So, 25% of £31,050 = £7762.50.

Higher rate: 40% of 33,500 = 37,000.

So, 40% of £3500 = £1400.

Overall: £367.5 + £7762.25 + £1400 = £9530.

Question 272: A

They earn the same salary.

So, the difference between their annual income is £0.

Question 273: D

Starting rate: 15 % of 2,450 = £367.5.

Basic rate: 25% of 2,451 = 33,500.

So, 25% of £31,049 = £7762.25.

Higher rate: 40% of 33,500 = 42,000.

40% of £8500 = £3400.

Monthly average: (£367.5 + £7762.25 + £3400)/12 = £960.80.

Question 274: B

<u>Adam's income tax with £37,000 salary</u>

Starting rate: 15 % of 2,450 = £367.50.

Basic rate: 25% of 2,451 = 33,500.

So, 25% of £31,049 = £7762.25.

Higher rate: 40% of 33,500 = 37,000.

So, 40% of £3500 = £1400.

Overall: £367.50 + £7762.25 + £1400 = £9529.75.

<u>Adam's income tax with £41,000 salary</u>

Starting rate: 15 % of 2,450 = £367.50.

Basic rate: 25% of 2,451 = 33,500.

So, 25% of £31,049 = £7762.25.

Higher rate: 40% of 33,500 = 41,000.

So, 40% of £7500 = £3000.

Overall: £367.5 + £7762.25 + £3000 = £11,129.75.

Difference: £11129.75 – £9529.75 = £1600.

Question 275: E

2014-15: £2,450

2015-16: £2,730

Difference: £2,730 – £2,450 = £280 increase.

SET 56

Question 276: D

Follows from the table.

Daniel received 10%, which is the highest bonus.

Question 277: B

Total sales / number of projects

£654,150,000 / 7 = £93,450,000.

Question 278: E

£45,000,000 x 1% + £180,000,000 x 4% = 450,000 + 7,200,000 = 7,650,000.

Question 279: A

Follows from the table.

Adam received 97%, which is the highest satisfaction rate.

Question 280: A

Total sales = £45,000,000 + £150,453,000 + £180,000,000 + £654,150,000 = £1,029,603,000

SET 57

Question 281: C

Previous day share price x (1 + change from previous day) = current share price

Change from previous day is +0.13%

Current share price is £134.432

£134.432 / (1-0.0013) = £134.257.

Question 282: C

British Land highest: 54.934

British Land lowest: 54.914

Difference between daily highest and lowest: 54.934 – 54.914 = 0.02.

Question 283: E

Calculate previous day share price first, then calculate market capitalisation

HSBC current share price: 25.432

HSBC volume: 7,345,321

Market capitalisation: 25.432 x 7,345,321 = 186,806,203.672

Change from previous day: -0.03%

25.432/(1-0.0003) = 25.4396318896

Therefore, the market capitalisation previous day was 186,806,203.672 / (1 + 0.03) = 186,750,178.618. 25.4396318896 x 7,345,321 = 186,862,262.351.

Question 284: C

Follows from the table.

BP had their share price change by '+4.5%', which is the largest change from yesterday.

Question 285: A

Share price x volume

BP market cap: 286.123 x 4,431,748 = 1,268,025,033.004

British Land market cap: 54.923 x 4,999,432 = 274,583,803,736

Difference: 1,268,025,033.004 – 274,583,803,736 = 993,441,229.268.

SET 58

Question 286: D

Psychology: 10/6 = 1.66

To determine the course with a similar ratio of men to women as psychology, we need to calculate the ratios for all of the other courses:

Mathematics: 8/7 =1.14

Physics: 10/15 = 0.66

Programming: 4/5 = 0.8

Literature: 12/8 = 1.5

History: 7/7 =1

From these figures, we can see that Literature has the most similar ratio.

Question 287: C

Physics: 10/15 = 0.66

Similarly to the previous question, we need to calculate the ratios for all other courses:

Psychology: 10/6 = 1.66

Mathematics: 8/7 =1.14

Programming: 4/5 = 0.8

Literature: 12/8 = 1.5

History: 7/7 =1

From these figures, we can see that Programming has the most similar ratio.

Question 288: E

Can't tell, because students can take more than one course.

Question 289: E

As one student can take more than one course and we do not have any information about the total number of students, we can't tell.

Question 290: C

Before ratio is equal to 10:6 = (10/6):1 = 1.66:1

After ratio is equal to 13:6 = (13/6):1 = 2.16:1

Change in ratio of women to men studying psychology = 2.16 – 1.66 = 0.5.

SET 59

Question 291: A

Women in employment: 85.5% (employed) + 5% (self-employed) + 2.7% (employed other) = 93.2%

Men in employment: 81.3% (employed) + 8% (self-employed) + 4.5% (employed other) = 93.8%

Difference between percentage of women and men in employment = 93.8% – 93.2% = 0.6.

Question 292: D

Women self-employed is 5%; women unemployed is 6.8%.
Sum is equal to 11.8%.
Men self-employed is 8%; men unemployed is 6.1% .
Sum is equal to 14.1%.
Ratio of men to women = 14.1% / 11.8% = 1.2.

Question 293: E

21 million (women employed) x 0.05 (5% self-employed) = 1.05 million
If there are 21 million women in employment, 21 million are either employed, self-employed or employed other.
21 million women is 85.5+5+2.7 = 93.2% of the country. This means 6.8% of the country is 1,532,189. So, country population is 22,532,189.
5% of this is 1,126,609 so the answer should be 1.13 million.

Question 294: A

Men unemployed: 6.1% → 31 million x 0.061 = 1.891
Women unemployed: 6.8% → 32 million x 0.068 = 2.176
Difference in number unemployed = 2.176 – 1.891 = 0.285 of 1 million = 285,000 more women.

Question 295: D

Women in employment (as defined above) = 93.2.
Unemployed women: 6.8.
Therefore, proportion of employed to unemployed women = 93.2/6.8 = 13.7.

SET 60

Question 296: C

Gas and Electricity together add up to about ¼ of the total area.
Therefore, 360 pounds x ¼ = 90 pounds.

Question 297: D

Household purchases, travel and gas costs = ½ of the total area = 180 pounds.
Energy costs = ¼ of the total area = 90 pounds.
Ratio is 180 / 90 = 2.

Question 298: B

The largest section of the pie chart is for 'Travel'.

Question 299: D

Household purchases, travel and gas costs = ½ of the total area = 180 pounds.
Energy costs = ¼ of the total area = 90 pounds.

Question 300: E

The smallest section of the pie chart is for 'TV subscription'.

Question 301: E

A. Incorrect. UCL study found eating more portions of fruit and vegetables was beneficial.
B. Incorrect. This is a possible reason but has yet to be fully investigated.
C. Incorrect. Fruit and vegetables are more protective against cardiovascular disease, and were shown to have little effect on cancer rates.
D. Incorrect. Inconclusive – people who ate more vegetables generally had a lower mortality but unknown if this is due to eating more vegetables or other associated factors.
E. Correct. Although this has previously been the case, this study did not find so. 'they recorded no additional decline for people who ate over 5 portions'.
F. Incorrect. The 5% decline per portion was only up to 5 portions and no additional reduction in mortality for 7 than 5 portions.
G. Incorrect. Study only looks at cancers in general and states need to look into specific cancers.

Question 302: C

Deaths in meta-analysis = 56423/800000 = 0.07 or 7%
1% lower in UCL study so 6%
6% of 65,000 = 65000 x 0.06 = 3,900

Question 303: B

A. Eating more fruit and vegetables doesn't particularly lower overall risk but need research into specific cancer risk.
B. The UCL research alone found that increasing the number of fruit and vegetable portions had a beneficial effect, even though this wasn't the overall conclusion when combined with results from the meta-analysis.
C. The results were not exactly the same but showed similar overall trends.
D. Although this may be true, there is no mention of this in the passage.
E. Fruit and vegetables are protective against cardiovascular disease, but not exclusively. They also reduce the rates of death from all causes.
F. The UCL study is in England only and the meta-analysis a combination of studies from around the world.
G. Suggested by the UCL research, but not the meta-analysis, so not an overall conclusion of the article.

Question 304: E

Remember that you don't need to calculate exact values for this question. Thus, you should round numbers frequently to make this more manageable. Work out percentage of beer and wine consumption and then the actual value using the total alcohol consumption figure:

Belarus: 17.3 + 5.2 = 22.5%;
0.225 x 17.5 = 3.94

Lithuania: Missing figure 100 – 7.8 – 34.1 – 11.6 = 46.5
46.5 + 7.8 = 54.3%
0.543 x 15.4 = 8.36

France: 18.8 + 56.4 = 75.2%
0.752 x 12.2 = 9.17

Ireland: 48.1 + 26.1 = 74.2
0.742 x 11.9 = 8.83

Andorra: missing figure 100 – 34.6 – 20.1 = 45.3
34.6 + 45.3 = 79.9%
0.799 x 13.8 = 11.0

Question 305: D

Russia:
2010 – Total = 11.5+3.6 = 15.1. Spirits = 0.51 x 15.1 = 7.7
2020 – Total = 14.5. Spirits = 0.51 x 14.5 = 7.4
Difference = 0.3 L

Belarus:
2010 – Total = 14.4 + 3.2 = 17.6. Spirits = 0.466 x 17.6 = 8.2
2020 – Total = 17.1. Spirits = 0.466 x 17.1 = 8.0
Difference = 0.2 L

Lithuania:
2010 – Total = 15.4. Spirits = 0.341 x 15.4 = 5.3
2020 – Total = 16.2. Spirits = 0.341 x 16.2 = 5.5
Difference = 0.2 L

Grenada:
2010 – Total = 12.5. Spirits % = 100 – 29.3 – 4.3 – 0.2 = 66.2%. Spirits = 0.662 x 12.5 = 8.3
2020 – Total = 10.4. Spirits = 0.662 x 10.4 = 6.8
Difference = 1.5 L

Ireland:
2010 – Total = 11.9. Spirits = 0.187 x 11.9 = 2.2
2020 – Total = 10.9. Spirits = 0.187 x 10.9 = 2
Difference = 0.2 L

Question 306: C

Work out 4.9 as a percentage of total beer consumption in Czech Republic and search other rows for similar percentage.

4.9/13 = 0.38, approx. 38% which is very similar to percentage consumption in Russia (37.6).

Question 307: B

We can add up the total incidence of the 6 cancers in men, which is 94,000. Then we can add up the total incidence in women, which is 101,000. As a percentage of 10 million, this is 0.94% of men and 1.01% of women. Therefore the difference is 0.07%.

Question 308: C

Given there are 1.15 times as many men as women, the incidence of each cancer amongst men needs to be greater than 1.15 times the incidence amongst women in order for a man to be more likely to develop it. The incidence is at least 1.15 higher in men for 3 cancers (prostate, lung and bladder).

Question 309: D

If 10% of cancer patients are in Sydney, there are 10,300 prostate/bladder/breast cancer patients and 9,200 lung/bowel/uterus cancer patients in Sydney. Hence the total number of hospital visits is 10,300 + 18,400, which is 28,700.

Question 310: A

The proportion of men with bladder cancer is 2/3 and women 1/3.

Question 311: D

First we work out the size of each standard drink. 50 standard drinks of vodka is equivalent to 1250ml, so one drink is 25ml or 0.025 litres. 11.4 standard drinks of beer is 10 pints of 5700ml, so one standard drink is 500ml or 0.5 litres. 3 standard drinks of cocktail is 750ml so one is 250ml or 0.25 litres. 3.75 standard drinks of wine is 750ml, so one is 200ml or 0.2 litres.

We can then work out the number of units in each drink. Vodka has 0.025 x 40 = 1 unit, Beer has 0.5 x 3 = 1.5 units, Cocktail has 0.25 x 8 = 2 units and Wine has 0.2 x 12.5 = 2.5 units. Since the drink with the most units is wine, the answer is D.

Question 312: B

We found in the last question that vodka has 1 unit, beer has 1.5, cocktail has 2 and wine has 2.5. Hence in the week, Hannah drinks 23.5 units and Mark drinks 29 units. Hence Hannah exceeds the recommended amount by 9.5 units and Mark by 9 units.

Question 313: D

We found that vodka has 1 unit, beer has 1.5, cocktail has 2 and wine has 2.5. Hence it is possible to make 5 combinations of drinks that are 4 units: 4 vodkas, 2 cocktails, 2 vodkas and a cocktail, 1 vodka and 2 beers, or a wine and a beer.

Question 314: D

The total number of males in Greentown is 12,890. Adding up the rest of the age categories, we can see that 10,140 of these are in the older age categories. Hence there are 2750 males under 20.

Question 315: C

Given that in the first question we found the number of males under 20 is 2,750, we can then add up the totals in the age categories (apart from 40-59) in order to find that 15,000 of the residents of Greentown are in other age categories. Hence 9,320 of the population are aged 40-59. We know that 4,130 of these are male, therefore 5,190 must be female.

Question 316: C

The age group with the highest ratio of males:females is 20-39, with approximately 1.9 males per females (approximately 3800:2000). As a ratio of females to males, this is 1:1.9.

Question 317: C

There are 4 instances where the line for Newcastle is flat from one month to the next per year, hence in 2008-2012 (5 years) there are 20 occasions when the average temperature is the same from month to month. During 2007, there are 2 occasions, and during 2013 there are 3.

Question 318: A

The average temperature is lower than the previous month in London for all months from August to December, which is 5 months. However, in August and November in Newcastle, the average temperature remains the same as the previous month. Hence there are only 3 months where the average temperature is lower in both cities. Hence from 2007 to 2012, there are 18 months where the average temperature is lower than the previous month. During 2013, the only included month where the temperature is lower in both cities than the previous month is September. Hence there are 19 months in total when the temperature is lower in both cities than the previous month.

Question 319: B

Firstly work out the difference between average temperatures for each month (2, 3, 1, 2, 1, 3, 3, 2, 2, 5, 1, 0). Then sum them to give 25. Divide by the number of months (12) to give $2^1/_{12}$, which is 2°C to the nearest 0.5°C.

Question 320: D

There is not enough information to tell which month the highest sales are in. We know it increases up to a point and decreases after it, but as we don't know by how much we cannot project where the maximum sales will be.

Question 321: B

Given that by observation, Q2 and Q3 both account for 1/3 of the sales and Q4 accounts for 1/4, this leaves that Q1 accounts for 1/12 of sales. 1/12 of £354,720 is £29,560.

Question 322: A

Quarter 2 accounts for 1/3 of the sales, which is £60,000 in sales revenue. If a tub of ice cream is sold for £2 and costs the manufacturer £1.50, this means profit is 1/4 of sales revenue. Hence £15,000 profit is made during Q2. Hence the answer is A.

Question 323: D

A. and B – Incorrect. Both *could* be true but neither is *definitely* true as it is dependent on the relative number of families with each number of children, which is not given in the question. Therefore we cannot know for certain whether these statements are true.

C – Incorrect. C is definitely *untrue* as half of the families spend £400 a month on food, which totals £4800 a year.

D – Correct. This option is true as 1/6 of families with 1 child and 1/6 of families with 3 children spent £100 a month on food.

E – Incorrect. This option is definitely untrue as the average expenditure for families with 2 children is actually £400 a month.

Question 324: B

2210 out of 2500 filled in responses, meaning that 290 did not. 290 as a percentage of 2500 is roughly 12% (11.6%) of the school that did not respond.

Question 325: C

The percentage of students that saw bullying and reported it was 35%, so 65% of those who saw it did not which is equivalent to 725 students. Of this 725, 146 which roughly equals 20%, gave the reason that they did not think it was important.

Question 326: B

Of the students who told a teacher, 286 did not witness any action. Of those who did notice action, i.e. 110, only 40% noticed any direct action with the bully involved. 40% of 110 is 44, so the correct answer is B.

Question 327: D

"427 cited fears of being found out" which means about 59% out of the 725 students that did not tell about the bullying, cited that it was because they worried about others finding out.

Question 328: F

North-east: 56 per 100,000 on average. This means that there must be a higher proportion of women than this and a lower proportion of men, such that the average is 56/100,000

We must make the reasonable assumption that there are the same number of men and women in the population as the question asks us to approximate.

Therefore there are 18.6/50,000 men and 37.3/50,000 women

This scales to 74.4/100,000 women which is roughly 74/100,000.

Question 329: C

8 million children – question tells to approximate to 4 million girls and 4 million boys.

Girls: 20% eat 5 portions fruit and vegetables a day. 20% of 4 million: 4 x 0.2 = 0.8 million

Boys: 16% eat 5 portions of fruit and vegetables a day. 16% of 4 million: 4 x 0.16 = 0.64 million

Number of more girls: 800,000 – 640,000 = 160,000.

Question 330: B

A. Incorrect. Women: 13619+10144+6569 = 30332. Men: 16818 + 9726 + 7669 + 6311 = 40524
B. Correct. Flu + pneumonia, lung cancer and chronic lower respiratory diseases = 15361 + 13619 + 14927 = 43907
C. Incorrect. More common cause of death but no information surrounding prevalence.
D. Incorrect. Colon cancer ranking 8 for both.

Question 331: A

The government has claimed a 20% reduction, so we are looking for an assessment criterion which has reduced 20% from 2013 to 2014. We can see that only "Number of people waiting for over 4 hours in A&E" has reduced by 20%, so this must be the criterion the government has used to describe "waiting times in A&E". Thus, the answer is A.

Question 332: B

Rovers must have played 10 games overall as they played each other's team twice. They lost 9 games scoring no points and so must have won 1 game, which scores 3 points.

Question 333: A

To have finished between City and United, Athletic must have got between 23 and 25 points. Hence they must have got 24 points because no team got the same number of points as another. Athletic won 7 games which is 21 points, so they must have also got 3 points from drawing 3 games. This accounts for all 10 games they played, so they did not lose any games.

Question 334: C

United won 8 games and drew 1, which is 25 points. Rangers drew 2 games and won none, which is 2 points. Therefore the difference in points is 23.

Question 335: C

Type 1 departments reached the new target of 95% at least three times since it was introduced. All the other statements are correct.

Question 336: C

Total attendances in Q1 08-9: 5.0 million
Total attendances in Q1 04-5: 4.5 million
The difference = 0.5 million
0.5/5 x 100 = 10% increase

Question 337: C

There are 16 quarters in total since the new target came into effect.
4/16 = 0.25, so the target has been hit 25% of the time i.e. missed 75% of the time.

Question 338: C

Ranjna must leave Singapore by 20:00 to get to Bali by 22:00. The latest flight she can therefore get is the 19:00. Thus, she must arrive in Singapore by 17:00 (accounting 2 hours for the stopover). The flight from Manchester to Singapore takes 14 hours. Manchester is 8 hours behind Singapore so she must leave Manchester 22 hours before 17:00 on Wednesday i.e. by 19:00 on Wednesday. Thus, the latest flight she can get is the 18:00 on Wednesday.

Question 339: D

The 08:00 flight will arrive at Singapore for 22:00 on Monday (GMT) or 06:00 Tuesday Singapore time. She then needs a 2 hour stopover, so earliest connecting flight she can get is 08:30 on Tuesday. The flight lands in Bali at 10:30. She then spends 1 hour and 45 minutes getting to her destination – arriving at 12:15 Tuesday.

Question 340: C

A. Incorrect. The graph is about level, and certainly not the steepest gradient post 2007.
B. Incorrect. Although there has been a general decline, there are some blips of increased smoking.
C. Correct.
D. Incorrect. The smoking rate in men decreased from 51% in 1974 to 21% in 2010. Thus, it decreased by more than a half.
E. Incorrect. The percentage difference between men and women smokers has been minimal in the 21st century.

Question 341: D

For this type of question you will have to use trial and error after you've analysed the data pattern to find the correct answer. The quickest way to do this is to examine outliers to try and match them to data in the table e.g. the left-most point is an outlier for the X-axis but average for the y-axis. Also look for any duplicated results in the table and if they are present on the graph, e.g. Hannah and Alice weigh 68 kg but this can't be found on the graph.

Question 342: C

This is pretty straightforward; the point is at approximately 172-174 cm in height and 164 -166 cm in arm span. Matthew is the only student who fits these dimensions.

Question 343: C

This is straightforward – just label the diagram using the information in the text and it becomes obvious that C is the correct answer.

Question 344: C

Since we do not know whether they went to university or not, we must add the number of women with children who work and those who went to university, 2, to the number of women with children who work but did not go to university, 1 (2 + 1 = 3).

Question 345: C

To work this out we must add up all the numbers within the rectangle, 4 + 6 + 1 + 2 + 11 + 12 + 7 + 15 = 58

Question 346: E

Calculate the number of men + women who have children and work i.e. 11 + 5 + 2 = 18

Question 347: C

To solve this we must work out the total number of people who had children i.e. 3 + 6 + 5 + 11 + 1 + 2 =28. Then we work out the total number of people who went to university, but that do not also have children so that these are not counted twice: 13 + 12 = 25. Then we add these two numbers together, 28 + 25 = 53 and subtract the number of people who fell into both categories i.e. 53 - (5 + 11 + 2) = 35

Question 348: C

To work this out we must add up all the numbers outside the rectangle that also fall within both the circle and the square, which is 5.

Question 349: D & E

This question asks for identification of the blank space, which is the space within the triangle, the rectangle and the square i.e. indicating working women who went to university but did not have children. This also reveals non-working men who did not have children and did not go to university.

Question 350: C

The normal price of these items would be £18.50 (£8 + £7 + £3.50). However, with the 50% discount on meat products, the price in the sale for these items will be £9.25. Thus, Alfred would receive £10.75 of change from a £20 note.

Question 351: C

The number of games played and points scored is a red herring in this question. The important data is 'Goals For' and 'Goals Against'. As this is a defined league and the teams have only played each other, the 'Goals For' column must equal the 'Goals Against' column.

Total Goals For = 16 + 11 + 8 + 7 + 8 + 4 = 54

Total Goals Against = 2 + Wilmslow + 7 + 9 + 12 + 14 = 44 + Wilmslow

For both columns to be equal, Wilmslow must have a total of 54 – 44 = 10 Goals Against.

Question 352: C

Working with the table it is possible to work out that the BMIs of Julie and Lydia must be 21 and 23, and hence their weights 100 and 115 lbs. Thus Emma's weight is 120 lbs, and her BMI must be 22, making her height equivalent to 160 cm.

Question 353: C

Working through the results, starting with the highest and lowest values, it is possible to plot all values and decipher which point is marked.

VISUAL THINKING PRACTICE QUESTION WORKED SOLUTIONS

Q	A	Q	A	Q	A	Q	A	Q	A	Q	A
1	B	26	B	51	Neither	76	A	101	A	126	Neither
2	Neither	27	A	52	B	77	A	102	A	127	A
3	A	28	A	53	A	78	B	103	Neither	128	Neither
4	A	29	B	54	Neither	79	A	104	B	129	Neither
5	Neither	30	B	55	B	80	Neither	105	Neither	130	B
6	B	31	B	56	A	81	B	106	A	131	Neither
7	A	32	Neither	57	Neither	82	Neither	107	Neither	132	Neither
8	A	33	Neither	58	B	83	Neither	108	A	133	Neither
9	Neither	34	A	59	Neither	84	A	109	B	134	A
10	Neither	35	A	60	A	85	A	110	B	135	B
11	A	36	B	61	A	86	Neither	111	B	136	A
12	B	37	A	62	A	87	A	112	Neither	137	B
13	Neither	38	Neither	63	B	88	B	113	Neither	138	Neither
14	A	39	A	64	B	89	Neither	114	B	139	Neither
15	A	40	Neither	65	A	90	B	115	A	140	B
16	B	41	B	66	A	91	Neither	116	A	141	A
17	B	42	Neither	67	A	92	A	117	A	142	Neither
18	A	43	A	68	B	93	Neither	118	Neither	143	B
19	A	44	B	69	Neither	94	A	119	B	144	A
20	A	45	Neither	70	Neither	95	A	120	Neither	145	B
21	A	46	B	71	B	96	B	121	Neither	146	Neither
22	A	47	Neither	72	A	97	B	122	Neither	147	B
23	B	48	A	73	Neither	98	A	123	A	148	Neither
24	B	49	B	74	Neither	99	B	124	A	149	A
25	Neither	50	Neither	75	A	100	B	125	B	150	A

Q	A	Q	A	Q	A	Q	A	Q	A	Q	A
151	A	176	B	201	C	226	B	251	A	276	D
152	Neither	177	Neither	202	A	227	D	252	D	277	A
153	A	178	B	203	A	228	C	253	D	278	B
154	B	179	B	204	D	229	A	254	D	279	C
155	A	180	A	205	D	230	A	255	C	280	B
156	Neither	181	Neither	206	A	231	A	256	B	281	B
157	A	182	Neither	207	C	232	D	257	C	282	A
158	A	183	A	208	A	233	A	258	C	283	A
159	Neither	184	A	209	B	234	C	259	A	284	D
160	B	185	Neither	210	A	235	B	260	B	285	B
161	B	186	Neither	211	D	236	C	261	B	286	C
162	A	187	Neither	212	A	237	C	262	C	287	C
163	A	188	A	213	C	238	C	263	A	288	A
164	B	189	B	214	A	239	B	264	A	289	C
165	A	190	A	215	D	240	A	265	B	290	C
166	A	191	Neither	216	D	241	A	266	A	291	D
167	B	192	A	217	A	242	D	267	C	292	A
168	Neither	193	Neither	218	C	243	B	268	A	293	A
169	A	194	B	219	D	244	A	269	A	294	C
170	B	195	Neither	220	C	245	A	270	D	295	B
171	Neither	196	B	221	A	246	D	271	A	296	D
172	B	197	Neither	222	D	247	C	272	C	297	A
173	B	198	B	223	D	248	C	273	C	298	C
174	A	199	Neither	224	B	249	D	274	C	299	A
175	Neither	200	B	225	C	250	B	275	D	300	A

	Set A Rule	Set B Rule
Set 1	**3** Shapes are white **2** Shapes are black	**2** Shapes are white **3** Shapes are black
Set 2	**2** Shapes are white **1** Shape is black	**1** Shape is white **2** Shapes are black
Set 3	There is always a **triangle** in the **top left corner**	There is always a **quadrilateral** in the **bottom right corner**
Set 4	There are an **even** number of rectangles	There are an **odd** number of rectangles
Set 5	Each circle has at least one tangential line	At least one circle is **intersected** by a line
Set 6	**None** of the shapes intersect with each other	At least **one** of the shapes intersects with another shape/line
Set 7	The total number of dots is **10**	The total number of dots is **9**
Set 8	The four-sided shapes are in **different** sections of the box	The four-sided shapes are in the **same** section of the box
Set 9	All boxes have a **five-pointed star** in the **centre**	All boxes have a **triangle** in the **bottom left corner**
Set 10	The black **circle** is always in the **bottom left corner**	The two small **dots** are always in the **top right corner**
Set 11	The circles **are all tangential to** each other	The circles **intersect** each other
Set 12	There are always **three squares, two triangles** and one circle	There are always **three triangles, two squares** and one circle
Set 13	The sum of the edges is **odd**	The sum of the edges of is **even**
Set 14	The sum of the edges is **twelve**	The sum of the edges is **fourteen**
Set 15	Each box contains **4** right angles	Each box contains **6** right angles
Set 16	Each black shape has a **larger** white counterpart	Each black shape has a **smaller** white counterpart
Set 17	Number of Dots = Number of **Stars**	Number of Dots = Number of **Diamonds**
Set 18	Even-sided polygons are **black** Odd-sided polygons are **white**	Even-sided polygons are **white** Odd-sided polygons are **black**

Set 19	Number of Stars = Number of **Triangles**	Number of Stars = Number of **Diamonds**
Set 20	There are **no** right angles	There is at least **one** right angle
Set 21	There is a **horizontal** line for each rectangle and a **vertical** line for each square	There is a **vertical** line for each rectangle and a **horizontal** line for each square
Set 22	One shape has **2** more edges than the other	One shape has **3** more edges than the other
Set 23	Even-sided polygons are **black** Odd-sided polygons are **white**	Even-sided polygons are **white** Odd-sided polygons are **black**
Set 24	The number of triangles + circles = **3**	The number of triangles + circles = **2**
Set 25	The vector sum of the arrows is **left/right**	The vector sum of the arrows is **up/down**
Set 26	There are **nine** corners in total	There are **ten** corners in total
Set 27	There is one **more** shape outside the circle than inside the circle	There is one **less** shape outside the circle than inside the circle
Set 28	The arrows only form **acute** angles	The arrows only form **obtuse** angles
Set 29	Shapes are made up of arrows all pointing at the same corner	Shapes are made up of arrows all pointing at different corners
Set 30	A central shape is intersected by an **even** number of other shapes	A central shape is intersected by an **odd** number of other shapes
Set 31	There is an **odd** number of corners in total	There is an **even** number of corners in total
Set 32	All **white** shapes are located on the left side	All **black** shapes are located on the left side
Set 33	The number of edges is a prime number	The number of edges is **not** prime number
Set 34	There are an even number of **black** shapes	There are an even number of **white** shapes
Set 35	All shapes contain right angles	All shapes **don't** contain any right angles
Set 36	Every shape is a quadrilateral	Every shape is **not** a quadrilateral
Set 37	There is always a **circle** in the top left-hand corner	There is always a **triangle** in the top left-hand corner

Set 38	**Two** corners are occupied by shapes	**Three** corners are occupied by shapes
Set 39	There is only **one** black shape	There are only **two** black shapes
Set 40	There are always three members of the same colour and shape, **but** different sizes	There are always three members of the same colour, shape **and** size

Question 201: C

As the sequences progresses, the number of objects within each frame increases by two.

Question 202: A

The total number of objects in each panel totals seven. In the bottom half, the number of white circles increases by one each panel. In the top half, the number of black circles alternates between one and three between each panel with the grey circles making up the remainder to total seven.

Question 203: A

The sequence alternates between a 3-edged and 4-edged zig-zag. Within each zig-zag will be a black circle and a grey shape.

Question 204: D

The circle and triangle begin at the bottom-left corner and rotate clockwise throughout the panels and cycle between the colours white-grey-black. Each panel also contains two white stars and a square.

Question 205: D

The top-right and bottom-left shapes are both the same colour and alternate between white and black. The top-left and bottom-right shapes are also both the same colour and alternate between black and white.

Question 206: A

Whilst the curve rotates 180° with each progressing frame, the total number of sides increases by 1. The colours are distracting factors.

Question 207: C

As the sequence progresses, the difference between the number of squares and circles increases by one.

Question 208: A

The shapes within the smaller white squares rotate 90° clockwise within each frame. The total number of white shapes is greater than the total number of black shapes by one.

Question 209: B

The total number of right-angles in each frame increases by one.

Question 210: A

There are a number of distractors in this series – pay attention to only the arrows. Each frame has an arrow that rotates in both the direction it faces (up-right-down-left) and the quadrant in which it is located. The arrow alternates between the colours white and black.

Question 211: D

The total number of sides for white shapes increases by one each frame. This is the same as the number of black shapes.

Question 212: A

Each of the circles in the top row moves to the left once, each of the circles in the bottom row move to the right once. The circles in the middle row flip in the horizontal axis.

Question 213: C

The total number of edges increases by five each time.

Question 214: A

As the sequence progresses, the number of black circles subtract the number of white circles increases by two (6-8-10-12-14).

Question 215: D

The five-pointed star rotates clockwise by 90° in each frame. One of these points will face either up-down-left-right. If the arrow is pointing in the same direction as this, it will be coloured black.

Question 216: D

The total number of sides of all the shapes increases in the sequence 6, 9, 12, 15... When the total number of sides is odd the shapes are black, when the total is even the shapes are white.

Question 217: A

The number of shapes with right-angles increases by one.

Question 218: C

As the sequence progresses, the quadrant in which the black shape sits rotates. The two closest shapes are always grey and the furthest shape is always white.

Question 219: D

Each shape is rotated 90° clockwise, however their position is random.

Question 220: C

The number of arrows pointing directly at another shape alternates between one and three.

Question 221: A

All circles move closer towards each other and the circles in the bottom row cycle between white-grey-black. The other two circles are the same colour as the circle in their column.

Question 222: D
Each frame contains a two or three-sided 'container' that rotates. Shapes with right angles can only be placed within the container whilst shapes without right angles can only be placed outside the container.

Question 223: D
The difference between the number of the most abundant shape subtract the least abundant increases by one each frame.

Question 224: B
As the sequence progresses, the number of edges outside the central square increases by the number of edges within the central square. The colour of all the shapes outside the central square is the same as that of the shape within the central square in the previous frame.

Question 225: C
Every square alternates its colour between white and grey. New squares that are added are grey.

Question 226: B
Each shape is replaced by another shape with one more edge. Instead of a six-sided shape, two triangles are created instead. If there is another shape with the same number of edges, the shape is coloured black.

Question 227: D
As the sequence progresses, an increasing number of circles are added to the frame. Every circle cycles between the colours white-grey-black.

Question 228: C
Every arrow splits into two arrows pointing in opposite directions, the whole frame then rotates 90°. After pointing in both the up/down and left/right direction the arrows change colour.

Question 229: A
As the sequence progresses, every shape is moved to a random location in each subsequent frame. If the shape was intersecting another shape, it alternates colour between white and grey. All collisions are coloured black.

Question 230: A
The number of stars in the top-right corner increases by one and alternates colour between black-grey-white. The circle-triangle pair rotates clockwise 90° but remains in the bottom left corner and alternates between colours white-grey-black.

Question 231: A
Every rectangle/triangle is split into two right-angled triangles. The circles alternate between being white and outside the rectangle, and being black and inside the rectangle.

Question 232: D
The entire frame rotates by 90° clockwise. The triangles alternate between white and grey.

Question 233: A
The central grey shape alternates between a four-point and six-point star. The total number of other shapes will be the same as the number of points on the star. All arrows are coloured black.

Question 234: C
The overall pattern flips vertically every frame. As the pattern progresses, two more triangles are coloured in.

Question 235: B
The total number of circles increases by one each frame. All circles are coloured grey.

Question 236: C
The total number of intersections that are coloured black increases by one each frame. The colours of the large circles alternate between white and grey.

Question 237: C
The arrows in each frame point in different directions. As the series progresses, the direction that is missed rotates between left-up-right-down

Question 238: C
The pentagon rotates 90° anti-clockwise and alternates between white and grey.

Question 239: B
The black central shape alternates between a square and a pentagon. The number of triangles present in the frame is equal to the number of sides of the central shape.

Question 240: A
Black shapes rotate clockwise 90° whilst white shapes rotate anti-clockwise 90° each frame.

Question 241: A
Every circle moves one space to the right.

Question 242: D
The number of circles in the top half increases by one whilst the number in the bottom half decreases by one. The colour of the circles within each half alternates between white and black.

Question 243: B
The triangles in the outer section rotate anti-clockwise every frame whilst the central diamond rotates clockwise.

Question 244: A
The colours in the central diamond alternate between black and white. The triangles in the outer segment rotate their colours clockwise between grey-black-white.

Question 245: A
Each quadrant of the frame is rotated 90° clockwise.

Question 246: D
The black shapes rotate clockwise within the bottom-left quadrant. The white shapes flip vertically.

Question 247: C
Each frame has an increasing number of points touching. All shapes that touch another shape are coloured grey.

Question 248: C
As the sequence progresses, every large shape is converted into a small shape and one new large shape is added to the frame.

Question 249: D
The large square cycles between the colours grey-white-black. The large triangle cycles between black-white-grey. The smaller shapes in the top-left quadrant rotate clockwise whilst the smaller shapes in the bottom-right rotate anti-clockwise.

Question 250: B
The total number of sides for black shapes increases by one each frame.

Question 251: A
The left half of the image is flipped vertically whilst the right half is flipped horizontally. Any shape that is found in the same area in the same orientation is coloured black.

Question 252: D
Shapes with right-angles are rotated by 90° clockwise whilst those without right-angles are coloured black.

Question 253: D
White shapes increase their number of edges by one black shapes are flipped horizontally.

Question 254: D
All triangles are removed. The other shapes move to a random position.

Question 255: C
The white shapes gain a larger black shape.

Question 256: B
If an arrow points at a shape it turns black, if the arrow points away from the shape then the arrow itself turns black. The orientation / organisation of shapes is not significant.

Question 257: C
White shapes rotated 90° anti-clockwise. Grey shapes are rotated 180°. Black shapes are rotated 90° clockwise.

Question 258: C
Shapes that have an identical pair (regardless of rotation) are coloured black.

Question 259: A
The entire image is rotated 90° clockwise and then flipped vertically.

Question 260: B
The left half of the image is flipped horizontally whilst the right half is flipped vertically.

Question 261: B
The entire image is rotated 180°.

Question 262: C
Circles become triangles, triangles become squares and squares become circles. All shapes keep the same size and position.

Question 263: A
The entire image is rotated 90° anti-clockwise.

Question 264: A
Each shape is split in half along one line of reflection with one half being coloured black.

Question 265: B
Black shapes are moved upwards whilst white shapes are moved towards the left.

Question 266: A
Black shapes are moved such that they all touch each other whilst white shapes are moved such that they do not touch.

Question 267: C
The number of edges of the large black shape increases by one. The rest of the shapes are white and each have the same number of sides. The total number of shapes is equal to this same number.

Question 268: A
The stars that are pointing upwards are coloured black whilst the others are kept white.

Question 269: A
Only the shapes touching another shape remain. Position of the shapes can change.

Question 270: D
The colours rotate clockwise whilst the number of sides for each shape increases by one.

Question 271: A
Each individual quadrant is rotated 90° clockwise.

Question 272: C
Each quadrant is rotated 180° and the colours grey and white are switched.

Question 273: C
Every black shape is rotated 90° clockwise and coloured white whilst every white shape becomes black.

Question 274: C
Black shapes move away from each other whilst white shapes get bigger.

Question 275: D
For every shape with the same number of sides, the total decreases by one.

Question 276: D
The total number of white shapes is equal to the number of sides of the large black shape.

Question 277: A
Each shape is split into two shapes of the same colour with the same total number of edges.

Question 278: B
Every triangle is split in half through its right-angle. Grey triangles are replaced by two smaller white and black triangles. The frame is rotated 180°

Question 279: C
Shapes with right-angles get larger. Shapes without right-angles get smaller.

Question 280: B
The shape in each quadrant has twice as many sides as that of the original shape.

Question 281: B
The shape is flipped diagonally and rotated 90° anti-clockwise.

Question 282: A
The entire image is rotated 90° to the right and then the new bottom half of the image is flipped vertically.

Question 283: A
Each quadrant is rotated 180°.

Question 284: D
Increase the number of sides of black shapes by one and decrease the number of sides of white shapes by one.

Question 285: B
The left half of the image swaps between the shapes. The right half is rotated 180° and the colour of the shaped inverted.

Question 286: C
For every shape, there will be another shape that is not necessarily the same size or rotation.

Question 287: C
The total number of shapes within each quadrant are identical.

Question 288: A
Same number of white, grey and black shapes.

Question 289: C
All objects move quadrant in a clockwise direction. Objects within squares also rotate 90° clockwise.

Question 290: C
The total number of sides is the same.

Question 291: D
Every black shape becomes two different black shapes.

Question 292: A
The entire image is flipped vertically but the colours remain the same.

Question 293: A
All shapes with an odd number of sides are removed.

Question 294: C
For arrows pointing towards each other, one arrow will move to touch the other. For arrows pointing away from each other, one arrow will move away from the other.

Question 295: B
The top-left and bottom-right shapes swap whilst the top-right and bottom-left shapes swap. The location of the colours remains the same.

Question 296: D
The image is flipped in the diagonal axis (top-left to bottom-right).

Question 297: A
The shape in the top-left is rotated 90° clockwise; top-right 180°; bottom-right 90° anti-clockwise.

Question 298: C
The number of white shapes divided by the number of black shapes calculates the number of grey shapes in the second box.

Question 299: A
Each shape is split into two shapes with half the number of sides as the original shape.

Question 300: A
Shapes with right-angles are rotated. Those without right-angles are replaced by other shapes.

MATHEMATICAL THINKING PRACTICE QUESTION WORKED SOLUTIONS

Q	A	Q	A	Q	A	Q	A
			SECTION 1A				
1	B	40	C	79	B	117	B
2	C	41	B	80	D	118	A
3	C	42	D	81	B	119	D
4	C	43	C	82	A	120	C
5	E	44	A	83	C	121	D
6	A	45	C	84	E	122	B
7	C	46	C	85	A	123	D
8	E	47	C	86	C	124	D
9	E	48	B	87	C	125	D
10	C	49	D	88	B	126	C
11	E	50	E	89	C	127	B
12	E	51	D	90	C	128	B
13	E	52	D	91	A	129	C
14	B	53	B	92	E	130	C
15	C	54	E	93	C	131	E
16	B	55	E	94	B	132	B
17	B	56	B	95	C	133	B
18	C	57	C	96	B	134	A
19	D	58	A	97	B	135	D
20	C	59	C	98	C	136	C
21	B	60	B	99	C		
22	A	61	B	100	B		
23	F	62	B	101	B		
24	D	63	C	102	F		
25	A	64	C	103	D		
26	B	65	A	104	D		
27	A	66	C	105	E		
28	F	67	D	106	B		
29	D	68	C	107	C		
30	A	69	D	108	E		
31	D	70	A	109	C		
32	D	71	C	110	D		
33	F	72	B	111	B		
34	B	73	B	112	C		
35	C	74	A	113	B		
36	B	75	C	114	A		
37	C	76	B	115	C		
38	A	77	B	116	C		
39	A	78	A				

1. B

Each three-block combination is mutually exclusive, so the probabilities are added. Each block pick is independent of all other picks, so the probabilities are multiplied. There are three possible combinations:

$P(2\ red\ blocks\ and\ 1\ yellow\ block) = P(red\ then\ red\ then\ yellow) + P(red\ then\ yellow\ then\ red) + P(yellow\ then\ red\ then\ red)$

$(\frac{12}{20} \times \frac{11}{19} \times \frac{8}{18}) + (\frac{12}{20} \times \frac{8}{19} \times \frac{11}{18}) + (\frac{8}{20} \times \frac{12}{19} \times \frac{11}{18}) = \frac{3 \times 12 \times 11 \times 8}{20 \times 19 \times 18} = \frac{44}{95}$

2. C

First get rid of the brackets: $3(3x + 5) + 5(2x - 2)$

Thus: $9x + 15 + 10x - 10 = 270$

$9x + 10x = 270 - 15 + 10$

$19x = 265$

$x = 13.95$

3. C

This is a rare case where you need to factorise a complex polynomial: $3x^2 + 11x - 20 = 0$

$(3x \pm ?)(x \pm ?) = 0$, possible pairs: $2 \times 10,\ 10 \times 22,\ 4 \times 5,\ 5 \times 4$

$(3x - 4)(x + 5) = 0$

$3x - 4 = 0$, so $x = \frac{4}{3}$

$x + 5 = 0$ so $x = -5$

4. C

Multiply the numerators through by the corresponding fraction's denominator in order to place the fractions in like terms and solve.

$\frac{5(x-4)}{(x+2)(x-4)} + \frac{3\,(x+2)}{(x+2)(x-4)}$

$= \frac{5x-20+\,3x+6}{(x+2)(x-4)}$

$= \frac{8x-14}{(x+2)(x-4)}$

5. E

$p = k\sqrt[3]{q}$

$p = 12$ when $q = 27$ gives $12 = k\sqrt[3]{27}$, so $12 = 3k$ and $k = 4$

so $p = 4\sqrt[3]{q}$

Now $p = 24$:

$24 = 4\sqrt[3]{q}$, so $6 = \sqrt[3]{q}$ and $q = 6^3 = 216$

6. A

$8 \times 9 = 72$

$8 = (4 \times 2) = 2 \times 2 \times 2$

$9 = 3 \times 3$

$(2 \times 2 \times 2 \times 3 \times 3)^2 = 2 \times 2 \times 2 \times 2 \times 2 \times 2 \times 3 \times 3 \times 3 \times 3 = 2^6 \times 3^4$

7. C

Note that $1.151 \times 2 = 2.302$

Let 1.151 be x

Thus: $\frac{2x \times 10^5 + 2x \times 10^2}{x \times 10^{10}} = 2 \times 10^{-5} + 2 \times 10^{-8}$

$= 0.00002 + 0.00000002 = 0.00002002$

8. E

$y^2 + ay + b$

$(y + 2)^2 - 5 = y^2 + 4y + 4 - 5$

$y^2 + 4y - 1$

So $a = 4$ and $b = -1$

9. E

Take $5(m + 4n)$ as a common factor to give: $\frac{4(m+4n)}{5(m+4n)} + \frac{5(m-2n)}{5(m+4n)}$

Simplify to give: $\frac{4m+16n+5m-10n}{5(m+4n)} = \frac{9m+6n}{5(m+4n)} = \frac{3(3m+2n)}{5(m+4n)}$

10. C

$A = \frac{k}{\sqrt{B}}$.

Substitute the values in to give: $4 = \frac{k}{\sqrt{25}}$.

Thus, $k = 20$.

Therefore, $A = \frac{20}{\sqrt{B}}$.

When $B = 16$, $A = \frac{20}{\sqrt{16}} = \frac{20}{4} = 5$

11. E

Angles SVU and STU are opposites and add up to $180°$, so STU $= 91°$

The angle of the centre of a circle is twice the angle at the circumference so SOU $= 2 x\ 91° = 182°$

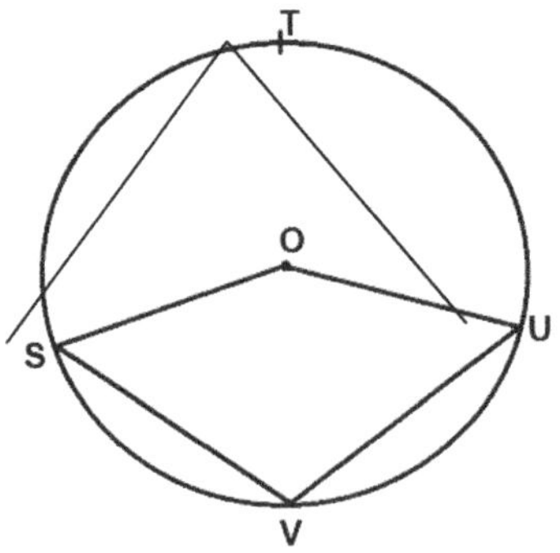

12. E

The surface area of an open cylinder $A = 2\pi rh$. Cylinder B is an enlargement of A, so the increases in radius (r) and height (h) will be proportional: $\frac{r_A}{r_B} = \frac{h_A}{h_B}$. Let us call the proportion coefficient n, where n = $\frac{r_A}{r_B} = \frac{h_A}{h_B}$.

So $\frac{Area\ A}{Area\ B} = \frac{2\pi r_A h_A}{2\pi r_B h_B} = n \times n = n^2$. $\frac{Area\ A}{Area\ B} = \frac{32\pi}{8\pi} = 4$, so, n = 2.

The proportion coefficient $n = 2$ also applies to their volumes, where the third dimension (also radius, i.e., the r^2 in $V = \pi r^2 h$) is equally subject to this constant of proportionality. The cylinder's volumes are related by $n^3 = 8$. If the smaller cylinder has volume 2π cm³, then the larger will have volume $2\pi \times n^3 = 2\pi \times 8 = 16\pi$ cm³.

13. E

$= \frac{8}{x(3-x)} - \frac{6(3-x)}{x(3-x)}$

$= \frac{8-18+6x}{x(3-x)}$

$= \frac{6x-10}{x(3-x)}$

14. B

For the black ball to be drawn in the last round, white balls must be drawn every round. Thus, the probability is given by $P = \frac{9}{10} \times \frac{8}{9} \times \frac{7}{8} \times \frac{6}{7} \times \frac{5}{6} \times \frac{4}{5} \times \frac{3}{4} \times \frac{2}{3} \times \frac{1}{2}$

$= \frac{9\times8\times7\times6\times5\times4\times3\times2\times1}{10\times9\times8\times7\times6\times5\times4\times3\times2\times1} = \frac{1}{10}$

15. C

The probability of getting a king the first time is $\frac{4}{52} = \frac{1}{13}$, and the probability of getting a king the second time is $\frac{3}{51}$. These are independent events, so, the probability of drawing two kings is $\frac{1}{13} \times \frac{3}{51} = \frac{3}{663} = \frac{1}{221}$

16. B

The probabilities of all outcomes must sum to one, so if the probability of rolling a 1 is x, then: $x + x + x + x + 2x = 1$. Therefore, $x = \frac{1}{7}$.

The probability of obtaining two sixes $P_{12} = \frac{2}{7} \times \frac{2}{7} = \frac{4}{49}$

17. B

There are plenty of ways of counting, however the easiest is as follows: 0 is divisible by both 2 and 3. Half of the numbers from 1 to 36 are even (i.e., 18 of them). $3, 9, 15, 21, 27, 33$ are the only numbers divisible by 3 that we've missed. There are 25 outcomes divisible by 2 or 3, out of 37.

In this instance because the range of numbers is quite small it's feasible to simply list numbers divisible by three as the final step. In situations in which the range is large you may want calculate it more systematically. This can be done as follows:

Calculate how many figures between 36 and 1 are divisible by 2, so: $\frac{36}{2} = 18$

Calculate how many figures between 36 and 1 are divisible by 3, so: $\frac{36}{3} = 12$

Find how many numbers are divisible by both 2 and 3 $\frac{36}{3\times2} = 6$

Sum to the total figures divisible by 3, total figures divisible by 2, subtract the total numbers divisible by 2 and 3 (you do not want to double count these numbers). Finally, 1 to account for 0 which is also divisible by 2 and 3.

So $12 + 18 - 6 + 1 = 25$. So, the final answer is $\frac{25}{37}$.

18. C

List the six ways of achieving this outcome: HHTT, HTHT, HTTH, TTHH, THTH and THHT. There are 2^4 possible outcomes for 4 consecutive coin flips, so the probability of two heads and two tails is: $6 \times \frac{1}{2^4} = \frac{6}{16} = \frac{3}{8}$.

As in the prior question because of the limited number of possible combinations listing combinations may be the most time efficient strategy. However, in instances where the number of possible combinations is much larger you may simply want to calculate it using a combinations formula. In this case, we can write the formula as $\frac{n!}{h!t!}$ where n is the number of coin flips and h and t represent the number of heads and tails. In this case $\frac{4!}{2!2!} = \frac{4\times3\times2\times1}{4}$ which would give you 6 (from there you can proceed as above).

19. D

Count the number of ways to get a 5, 6 or 7 (draw the square if helpful). The ways to get a 5 are: 1, 4; 2, 3; 3, 2; 4, 1. The ways to get a 6 are: 1, 5; 2, 4; 3, 3; 4, 2; 5, 1. The ways to get a 7 are: 1, 6; 2, 5; 3, 4; 4, 3; 5, 2; 6, 1. That is 15 out of 36 possible outcomes. Which simplifies down to 5 out of 12.

	1	2	3	4	5	6
1	2	3	4	5	6	7
2	3	4	5	6	7	8
3	4	5	6	7	8	9
4	5	6	7	8	9	10
5	6	7	8	9	10	11
6	7	8	9	10	11	12

20. C

There are $x + y + z$ balls in the bag, and the probability of picking a red ball is $\frac{x}{(x+y+z)}$ and the probability of picking a green ball is $\frac{z}{(x+y+z)}$. These are independent events, so the probabilities are multiplied giving $\frac{xz}{(x+y+z)^2}$ and the probability of picking green then red is the same. These outcomes are mutually exclusive, so are added giving $\frac{2xz}{(x+y+z)^2}$.

21. B

There are two ways of doing it, pulling out a red ball then a blue ball, or pulling out a blue ball and then a red ball. Let us work out the probability of the first by multiplying probabilities of pulling out red $\frac{x}{(x+y+z)}$ by the probability of then pulling out blue $\frac{y}{x+y+z-1}$, and the probability of the second option will be the same. These are mutually exclusive options, so the probabilities may be summed giving $\frac{2xy}{(x+y+z)(x+y+z-1)}$.

22. A

[x: Player 1 wins point, y: Player 2 wins point]

Player 1 wins in five rounds if we get: $yxxxx, xyxxx, xxyxx, xxxyx$.

(Note the case of $xxxxy$ would lead to player 1 winning in 4 rounds, which the question forbids.)

Each of these have a probability of $p^4(1-p)$ Thus, the solution is $4p^4(1-p)$.

Due to the limited number of rounds, we can simply list the possible acceptable rounds, as a above. However, we can also calculate it systematically using a combinations formula $\frac{n!}{y!x!}$ where *n* is the total number of games. In this instance we $\frac{5!}{4!1!} = \frac{5\times4!}{4!}$ which would give us 5. Because $xxxxy$ is not an acceptable combination we would want to subtract 1 leaving us with 4 possible combinations.

23. F

$4x + 7 + 18x + 20 = 14$

$22x + 27 = 14$

Thus, $22x = -13$

Giving $x = -\frac{13}{22}$

24. D

$r^3 = \frac{3V}{4\pi}$

Thus, $r = \left(\frac{3V}{4\pi}\right)^{\frac{1}{3}}$

Now substitute r into the S formula so that, $S = 4\pi\left[\left(\frac{3V}{4\pi}\right)^{\frac{1}{3}}\right]^2 = 4\pi\left(\frac{3V}{4\pi}\right)^{\frac{2}{3}}$

$= \frac{4\pi(3V)^{\frac{2}{3}}}{(4\pi)^{\frac{2}{3}}} = (3V)^{\frac{2}{3}} \times \frac{(4\pi)^1}{(4\pi)^{\frac{2}{3}}}$

$= (3V)^{\frac{2}{3}}(4\pi)^{1-\frac{2}{3}} = (4\pi)^{\frac{1}{3}}(3V)^{\frac{2}{3}}$

25. A

Let each unit length be x.

Thus, $S = 6x^2$. Therefore, $x = \left(\frac{S}{6}\right)^{\frac{1}{2}}$

$V = x^3$. Thus, $V = [\left(\frac{S}{6}\right)^{\frac{1}{2}}]^3$ so $V = \left(\frac{S}{6}\right)^{\frac{3}{2}}$

26. B

Multiplying the second equation by 2 we get $4x + 16y = 24$. We can rearrange this and substitute it into the first equation so $24 - 16y + 3y = 7$ which we can then simplify to $y = \frac{17}{13}$. Then solving for x we get $x = \frac{10}{13}$. You could also try substituting possible solutions one by one, although given that the equations are both linear and contain easy numbers, it is quicker to solve them algebraically.

27. A

Multiply by the denominator to give:	$(7x + 10) = (3y^2 + 2)(9x + 5)$
Partially expand brackets on right side:	$(7x + 10) = 9x(3y^2 + 2) + 5(3y^2 + 2)$
Take x terms across to left side:	$7x - 9x(3y^2 + 2) = 5(3y^2 + 2) - 10$
Take x outside the brackets:	$x[7 - 9(3y^2 + 2)] = 5(3y^2 + 2) - 10$
Thus:	$x = \frac{5(3y^2+2)-10}{7-9(3y^2+2)}$
Simplify to give:	$x = \frac{15y^2}{7 - 9(3y^2 + 2)}$

28. F

$$3x\left(\frac{3x^7}{x^{\frac{1}{3}}}\right)^3 = 3x\left(\frac{3^3x^{21}}{x^{\frac{3}{3}}}\right)$$

$$= 3x\,\frac{27x^{21}}{x} = 81x^{21}$$

29. D

$2x[2^{\frac{7}{14}}\,x^{\frac{7}{14}}] = 2x[2^{\frac{1}{2}}\,x^{\frac{1}{2}}]$

$= 2x(\sqrt{2}\,\sqrt{x}) = 2\,[\sqrt{x}\sqrt{x}][\sqrt{2}\,\sqrt{x}]$

$= 2\sqrt{2x^3}$

30. A

$A = \pi r^2$, therefore $10\pi = \pi r^2$

Thus, $r = \sqrt{10}$

Therefore, the circumference is $2\pi\sqrt{10}$.

31. D

$3.4 = (3 \times 4) + (3 + 4) = 19$

$19.5 = (19 \times 5) + (19 + 5) = 119$

32. D

$$2.3 = \frac{2^3}{2} = 4$$

$$4.2 = \frac{4^2}{4} = 4$$

33. F

This is a tricky question that requires you to know how to 'complete the square'.

$(x + 1.5)(x + 1.5) = x^2 + 3x + 2.25$

$(x + 1.5)^2 - 7.25 = x^2 + 3x - 5 = 0$

Therefore, $(x + 1.5)^2 = 7.25 = \frac{29}{4}$

Thus, $x + 1.5 = \sqrt{\frac{29}{4}}$

Thus $x = -\frac{3}{2} \pm \sqrt{\frac{29}{4}} = -\frac{3}{2} \pm \frac{\sqrt{29}}{2}$

34. B

Whilst you definitely need to solve this graphically, it is necessary to complete the square for the first equation to allow you to draw it more easily:

$(x + 2)^2 = x^2 + 4x + 4$

Thus, $y = (x + 2)^2 + 10 = x^2 + 4x + 14$

This is now an easy curve to draw ($y = x^2$ that has moved 2 units left and 10 units up). The turning point of this quadratic is to the left and well above anything in x^3, so the only solution is the first intersection of the two curves in the upper right quadrant around $(3.4, 39)$.

35. C

The easiest way to solve this is to sketch them (don't waste time solving them algebraically). As soon as you've done this, it'll be very obvious that y = 2 and y = 1-x^2 don't intersect, since the latter has its turning point at $(0, 1)$ and zero points at $x = -1$ and 1. $y = x$ and y = x^2 intersect at the origin and $(1, 1)$, and $y = 2$ runs through both.

36. B

Notice that you're not required to get the actual values – just the number's magnitude. Thus, $897{,}653$ can be approximated to $900{,}000$ and 0.009764 to 0.01. Therefore, $900{,}000 \times 0.01 = 9{,}000$ which is closest to $8{,}764.68$ (answer B).

37. C

Multiply initial equation by the product of the denominators of both fractions (i.e., 70):

$7(7x + 3) + 10(3x + 1) = 14 \times 70$

Simplify: $49x + 21 + 30x + 10 = 980$

$79x + 31 = 980$

$x = \frac{949}{79}$

38. A

Split the equilateral triangle into 2 right-angled triangles and apply Pythagoras' theorem to find height of equilateral triangle.

$x^2 = \left(\frac{x}{2}\right)^2 + h^2$. Thus $h^2 = \frac{3}{4}x^2$

$h = \sqrt{\frac{3x^2}{4}} = \frac{\sqrt{3x^2}}{2}$

The area of a triangle $= \frac{1}{2} \times base \times height = \frac{1}{2} x \frac{\sqrt{3x^2}}{2}$

Simplifying gives: $x \frac{\sqrt{3x^2}}{4} = x \frac{\sqrt{3}\,\sqrt{x^2}}{4} = \frac{x^2\sqrt{3}}{4}$

39. A

This is a question testing your ability to spot 'the difference between two squares'.

Factorise to give: $3 - \frac{7x(5x-1)\,(5x+1)}{(7x)^2(5x+1)}$

Cancel out: $3 - \frac{5x-1}{7x}$

40. C

The easiest way to do this is to 'complete the square':

$(x-5)^2 = x^2 - 10x + 25$

Thus, $(x-5)^2 - 125 = x^2 - 10x - 100 = 0$

Therefore, $(x-5)^2 = 125$

$x - 5 = \pm\sqrt{125} = \pm\sqrt{25}\sqrt{5} = \pm 5\sqrt{5}$

$x = 5 \pm 5\sqrt{5}$

41. B

Factorise by completing the square:

$x^2 - 4x + 7 = (x-2)^2 + 3$

Simplify: $(x-2)^2 = y^3 + 2 - 3$

$x - 2 = \pm\sqrt{y^3 - 1}$

$x = 2 \pm \sqrt{y^3 - 1}$

42. D

Square both sides to give: $(3x+2)^2 = 7x^2 + 2x + y$

Thus: $y = (3x+2)^2 - 7x^2 - 2x = (9x^2 + 12x + 4) - 7x^2 - 2x$

$y = 2x^2 + 10x + 4$

43. C

This is a fourth order polynomial, which you are unlikely to be expected to be able factorise immediately. This is where looking at the options makes your life a lot easier. First notice that all the possible answers have the same basic structure $y = \pm 1 + (\ldots)^{\frac{1}{4}}$. As a result, in all of the possible answers you can start with the same two steps, rearranging the equation and opening up the brackets on the right side.

In doing this the left side becomes $(y \pm 1)^4$, i.e., the answers are hinting that $(y \pm 1)^4$ is the solution to the fourth order polynomial.

Since there are negative terms in the equations (e.g., $-4y^3$) there must be a negative number to create a negative product.

So, of $(y-1)^4$ or $(y+1)^4$ the solution has to be $(y-1)^4$

Now expand the brackets to get $y^4 - 4y^3 + 6y^2 - 4y + 1$ which is 1 off our original equation

Therefore, $(y-1)^4 + 1 = x^5 + 7$

Thus, $y - 1 = (x^5 + 6)^{\frac{1}{4}}$

$y = 1 + (x^5 + 6)^{\frac{1}{4}}$

44. A

Let the width of the television be $4x$ and the height of the television be $3x$.

Then by Pythagoras: $(4x)^2 + (3x)^2 = 50^2$

Simplify: $25x^2 = 2500$

Thus: $x = 10$. Therefore: the screen is 30 inches by 40 inches, i.e., the area is $1{,}200$ inches^2.

45. C

Square both sides to give: $1 + \frac{3}{x^2} = (y^5 + 1)^2$

Multiply out: $\frac{3}{x^2} = (y^{10} + 2y^5 + 1) - 1$

Thus: $x^2 = \frac{3}{y^{10}+2y^5}$

Therefore: $x = \sqrt{\frac{3}{y^{10} + 2y^5}}$

46. C

The easiest way is to double the first equation and triple the second to get:
$6x - 10y = 20$ and $6x + 6y = 39$
Subtract the first from the second to give: $16y = 19$
Therefore, $y = \frac{19}{16}$.
Substitute back into the first equation to give $x = \frac{85}{16}$.

47. C

This is fairly straightforward; the first inequality is the easier one to work with: B and D and E violate it, so we just need to check A and C in the second inequality.
C: $1^3 - 2^2 < 3$ but A: $2^3 - 1^2 > 3$

48. B

Whilst this can be done graphically, it's quicker to do algebraically (because the second equation is not as easy to sketch). Intersections occur where the curves have the same coordinates.
Thus: $x + 4 = 4x^2 + 5x + 5$
Simplify: $4x^2 + 4x + 1 = 0$
Factorise: $(2x + 1)(2x + 1) = 0$
Thus, the two graphs only intersect once at $x = -\frac{1}{2}$

49. D

It's better to do this algebraically as the equations are easy to work with and you would need to sketch very accurately to get the answer. Intersections occur where the curves have the same coordinates. Thus: $x^3 = x$
$x^3 - x = 0$
Thus: $x(x^2 - 1) = 0$
Spot the 'difference between two squares': $x(x + 1)(x - 1) = 0$
Thus, there are 3 intersections: at $x = 0, 1$ and -1

50. E

Note that the line is the hypotenuse of a right-angled triangle with one side unit length and one side of length $\frac{1}{2}$.

By Pythagoras, $\left(\frac{1}{2}\right)^2 + 1^2 = x^2$

Thus, $x^2 = \frac{1}{4} + 1 = \frac{5}{4}$

$$x = \sqrt{\frac{5}{4}} = \frac{\sqrt{5}}{\sqrt{4}} = \frac{\sqrt{5}}{2}$$

51. D

The general principle at hand is to rearrange the equations progressively substituting them into each other to eliminate terms. Below is an example of how we could do this.

First multiply $x + y - z = -1$ (equation 1) by 3 — $3x + 3y - 3z = -3$
Add new equation 1 to equation 2 to get rid of z — $2x - 2y + 3z + (3x + 3y - 3z) = 8 + (-3)$
We can simplify this and call it equation 4 — $5x + y = 5$

Now create a second equation with only two unknowns
As before, start by multiplying equation 1 this time by 2 — $2x + 2y - 2z = -2$
Add new equation 1 to equation 3 to get rid of z — $2x - y + 2z + (2x + 2y - 2z) = 9 + (-2)$
We can simplify this and call it equation 5 — $4x + y = 7$

Now we have two equations with two only unknowns so we can substitute to get the value of x and y
Rearrange equation 4 and substitute it into equation 5 — $4x + (5 - 5x) = 7$
Simplify to obtain x — $x = -2$

Substitute the value of x into equation 4 or 5 to get y — $4 \times -2 + y = 7$
Simplify to obtain y — $y = 15$

Substitute x and y back in to calculate z: — $(-2) + (15) - z = -1$
Simplify to obtain z — $z = 14$

52. D

This is one of the easier questions. Take $3a$ as a factor to give:

$$3a(a^2 - 10a + 25) = 3a(a - 5)(a - 5) = 3a(a - 5)^2$$

53. B

Note that 12 is the lowest common multiple of 3 and 4. Thus:
Multiply the first equation by -3 — $-3(4x + 3y) = -3(48)$
Multiply the second equation by 4 — $4(3x + 2y) = 4(34)$
Add the two equations together to get rid of x — $-(12x + 9y) + 12x + 8y = -144 + 136$
Simplify to find y — $y = 8$

Substitute y back in: $4x + 3(8) = 48$

Simplify to find x $x = 6$

54. E

Don't be fooled, this is an easy question, just obey BODMAS and don't skip steps.

$\frac{-(25-28)^2}{-36+14} = \frac{-(-3)^2}{-22}$

This gives: $\frac{-(9)}{-22} = \frac{9}{22}$

55. E

Since there are 26 possible letters for each of the 3 letters in the license plate, and there are 10 possible numbers (0 to 9) for each of the 3 numbers in the same plate, then the number of license plates would be:
$26 \times 26 \times 26 \times 10 \times 10 \times 10 = 17{,}576{,}000$

Because the range of answers is wide instead of calculating 26^3 you can also save time by realising that to $20^3 \times 10^3 = 8{,}000{,}000$ and $30^3 \times 10^3 = 27{,}000{,}000$ so the correct answer must be between these two figures.

56. B

Expand the brackets to give: $4x^2 - 12x + 9 = 0$.
Factorise: $(2x - 3)(2x - 3) = 0$.
Thus, only one solution exists, $x = 1.5$
Note that you could also use the fact that the discriminant, $b^2 - 4ac = 0$ to get the answer.

57. C

$= \left(x^{\frac{1}{2}}\right)^{\frac{1}{2}} (y^{-3})^{\frac{1}{2}}$

$= x^{\frac{1}{4}} y^{-\frac{3}{2}} = \frac{x^{\frac{1}{4}}}{y^{\frac{3}{2}}}$

58. A

Let x, y, and y represent the rent for the 1-bedroom, 2-bedroom, and 3-bedroom flats, respectively. We can write 3 different equations: 1 for the rent, 1 for the repairs, and the last one for the statement that the 3-bedroom unit costs twice as much as the 1-bedroom unit.

Rent for all three flats $x + y + z = 1240$

Total cost of repairs $0.1x + 0.2y + 0.3z = 276$

Rent of flat 1 relative to rent for flat 3 $z = 2x$

Substitute $z = 2x$ into the other equations to eliminate z.

Call this equation 4 $x + y + 2x = 1240$

Call this equation 5 $0.1x + 0.2y + 0.3(2x) = 276$

Multiply equation 4 by -2, we can call this equation 6. $-6x - 2y = -1480$

Multiply equation 5 by 10, we can call this equation 7. $10x + 2y + 6x = 2760$

Add equations 6 and 7 $10x + 2y + 6x - 6x - 2y = 2760 - 1480$

Now simplify for x $x = 280$

We can now use equations I and 3 to solve for y and z $z = 2(280) = 560$

$$280 + 560 + y = 1240$$

$$y = 400$$

59. C

Following BODMAS:

$= 5\left[5(6^2 - 5 \times 3) + 400^{\frac{1}{2}}\right]^{\frac{1}{3}} + 7$

$= 5\,[5(36 - 15) + 20]^{\frac{1}{3}} + 7$

$= 5\,[5(21) + 20]^{\frac{1}{3}} + 7$

$= 5(105 + 20)^{\frac{1}{3}} + 7$

$= 5(125)^{\frac{1}{3}} + 7$

$= 5(5) + 7$

$= 25 + 7 = 32$

60. B

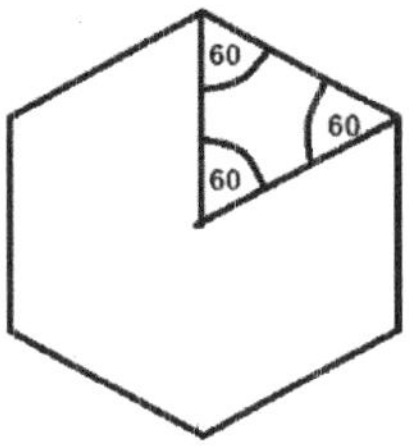

Consider a triangle formed by joining the centre to two adjacent vertices. Six similar triangles can be made around the centre – thus, the central angle is 60 degrees. Since the two lines forming the triangle are of equal length, we have 6 identical equilateral triangles in the hexagon. If this intuition is not clear remember that since the lines are of equal length their opposing angles must be the same and since the other angle is $60°$ then the remaining two angles are also $60°$ (i.e., $\frac{180°-60°}{2} = 60°$).

Now split the triangle in half and apply Pythagoras' theorem:

$1^2 = 0.5^2 + h^2$

Thus, $h = \sqrt{\frac{3}{4}} = \frac{\sqrt{3}}{2}$

Thus, the area of the triangle is: $\frac{1}{2}bh = \frac{1}{2} \times 1 \times \frac{\sqrt{3}}{2} = \frac{\sqrt{3}}{4}$

Therefore, the area of the hexagon is: $\frac{\sqrt{3}}{4} \times 6 = \frac{3\sqrt{3}}{2}$

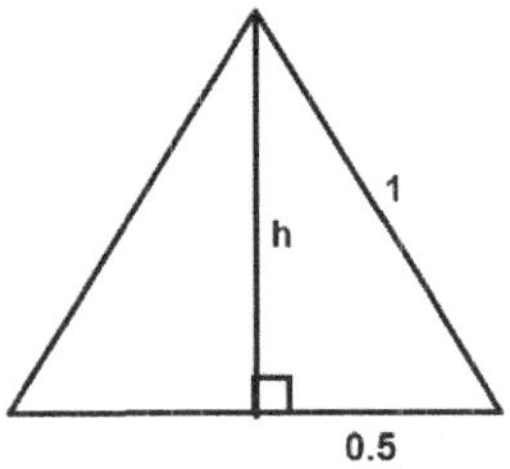

61. B

Let x be the width and $x + 19$ be the length.

Thus, the area of a rectangle is $x(x + 19) = 780$

Therefore:

$x^2 + 19x^2 - 780 = 0$

$(x - 20)(x + 39) = 0$

$x = 20$ or $x = -39$

Since length can never be a negative number, we disregard $x = -39$ and use $x = 20$. So, the width is 20 and the length is 39 metres.

62. B

If you are familiar with Pythagorean triples you should be able to immediately identify the answer as B. The second quickest way to solve is by trial and error, substituting the provided options. However, if you're keen to do this algebraically, you can do the following.

Establish the equation for the perimeter	$2L + 2W = 34$
Establish the equation for the diagonal (using Pythagoras)	$L^2 + W^2 = 13^2$
Simplify and rearrange the equation for the perimeter	$W = 17 - L$
Substitute into the equation for the diagonal	$L^2 + (17 - L)^2 = 169$
Expand the brackets and rearrange	$L^2 + 289 - 34L + L^2 - 169 = 0$
Simplify and factorise	$2L^2 - 34L + 120 = 0$
	$(L-5)(L - 12) = 0$
	$L = 5, L = 12$
	$W = 12, W = 5$

63. C

Multiply both sides by 8:	$4(3x - 5) + 2(x + 5) = 8(x + 1)$
Remove brackets:	$12x - 20 + 2x + 10 = 8x + 8$
Simplify:	$14x - 10 = 8x + 8$
Add 10:	$14x = 8x + 18$
Subtract $8x$:	$6x = 18$
Therefore:	$x = 3$

64. C

Recognise that 1.742×3 is 5.226. Now, the original equation simplifies to: $= \frac{3\times10^6 + 3\times10^5}{10^{10}}$

$= 3 \times 10^{-4} + 3 \times 10^{-5} = 3.3 \times 10^{-4}$

65. A

$$Area = \frac{(2+\sqrt{2})(4-\sqrt{2})}{2}$$

$$= \frac{8 - 2\sqrt{2} + 4\sqrt{2} - 2}{2}$$

$$= \frac{6 + 2\sqrt{2}}{2}$$

$$= 3 + \sqrt{2}$$

66. C

Square both sides:	$\frac{4}{x} + 9 = (y - 2)^2$
Open the brackets and rearrange	$\frac{4}{x} = y^2 - 4y + 4 - 9$
Factorise	$\frac{4}{x} = (y + 1)(y - 5)$
Rearrange	$x = \frac{4}{(y+1)(y-5)}$

67. D

Set up the equation: $5x - 5 = 0.5(6x + 2)$

$10x - 10 = 6x + 2$

$4x = 12$

$x = 3$

68. C

Round numbers appropriately: $\frac{55 + (\frac{9}{4})^2}{\sqrt{900}} = \frac{55 + \frac{81}{16}}{30}$

81 rounds to 80 to give: $\frac{55 + 5}{30} = \frac{60}{30} = 2$

69. D

There are three outcomes from choosing the type of cheese in the crust. For each of the additional toppings to possibly add, there are 2 outcomes: 1 to include and another not to include a certain topping, for each of the 7 toppings.

Thus, the number of different kinds of pizza is: $3 \times 2^7 = 3 \times 128 = 384$

70. A

Although it is possible to do this algebraically, by far the easiest way is via trial and error. The clue that you shouldn't attempt it algebraically is that rearranging the first equation to make x or y the subject leaves you with a difficult equation to work with (e.g., $x = \sqrt{1 - y^2}$) when you try to substitute in the second. Another way to solve is to notice that the equations are symmetric in x and y, i.e., the solution is when $x = y$. Thus $2x^2 = 1$ and $2x = \sqrt{2}$ which gives $\frac{\sqrt{2}}{2}$ as the answer.

71. C

$f(x) = 0 = 16x^4 + 32x^3 + 24x^2 + 8x + 1$

$(2x + 1)^4 = x^4$

This means that $2x + 1 = \pm x \Rightarrow x = -\frac{1}{3}$ or -1

72. B

Rearrange the equation: $x^2 + x - 6 \geq 0$

Factorise: $(x + 3)(x - 2) \geq 0$

You can also do a quick sketch to ensure you don't make a silly mistake with which way the sign is.

Thus, $y = 0$ when $x = 2$ and $x = -3$. y > 0 when $x > 2$ or $x < -3$.

Thus, the solution is: $x \leq -3$ and $x \geq 2$.

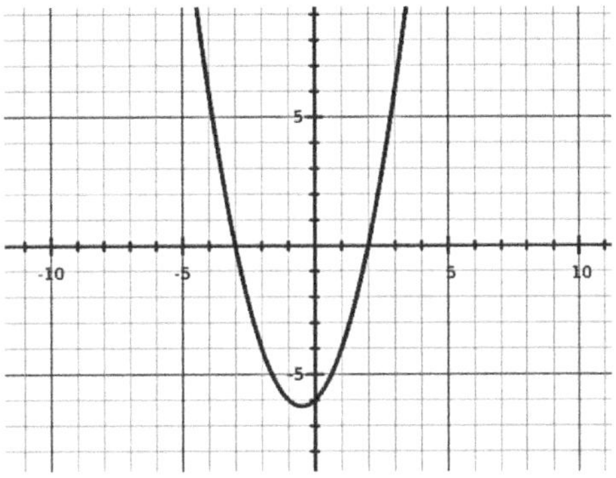

73. B

Using Pythagoras: $a^2 + b^2 = x^2$

Since the triangle is equilateral: $a = b, \ so \ 2a^2 = x^2$

Area $= \frac{1}{2} base \times height = \frac{1}{2}a^2$. From above, $a^2 = \frac{x^2}{2}$

Thus, the area $= \frac{1}{2}x\frac{x^2}{2} = \frac{x^2}{4}$

74. A

If X and Y are doubled, the value of Q increases by 4. Halving the value of A reduces this to 2. Finally, tripling the value of B reduces this to $\frac{2}{3}$, i.e., the value decreases by $\frac{1}{3}$.

75. C

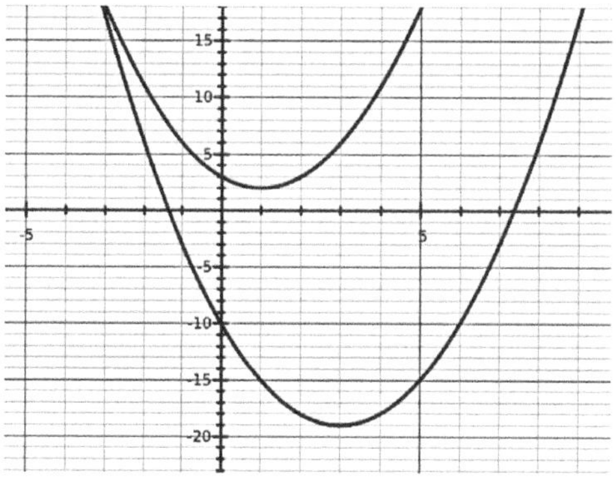

The quickest way to do this is to sketch the curves. This requires you to factorise both equations by completing the square:

$x^2 - 2x + 3 = (x - 1)^2 + 2$

$x^2 - 6x - 10 = (x - 3)^2 - 19$

Thus, the first equation has a turning point at $(1, 2)$ and doesn't cross the x-axis. The second equation has a turning point at $(3, -19)$ and crosses the x-axis twice.

76. B

Let tail $= T$, body and legs $= B$ and head $= H$. We have already been told that $T = 30$kg.

As described in the question $H = T + 0.5B$ and $B = T + H$.

Therefore, substitute the second equation into the first as $H = 30 + 0.5(30 + H)$.

Re-arranging reveals that $0.5H = 45$kg and therefore the weight of the head is 90kg, the body and legs 120kg and as we were told the tail weighs 30kg.

Thus, giving a total weight of 240kg.

77. B

Expand the larger scientific number so that it reads 10 to the power 6 like so: $4.2 \times 10^{10} = 42000 \times 10^6$. Now that the powers are the same across the numerators, a simple subtraction can be performed $(42000 - 4.2) \times 10^6 = 41995.8 \times 10^6$ which can be simplified to 4.19958×10^{10}. Next consider the division which can be competed in a two-step process, first divide the numerator by 2 like so $\frac{4.19958}{2} \times 10^{10} = 2.09979 \times 10^{10}$ and then subtract the powers like so $2.09979 \times 10^{10-3} = 2.09979 \text{ x } 10^7$.

78. A

Note the triangle formed by the right-angle lines and the tangent. Recall that as this is a right-angle triangle then the other two angles must be $45°$. As angles along a straight line add up to $180°$, *a* must equal $180 - 45 = 135^0$. Angles around the origin must add up to $360°$ and therefore $b = \frac{360 - 90}{2} = 135^0$. Therefore, the correct answer is A.

79. B

The probability of drawing a blue ball is $\frac{1}{21}$ and the probability of drawing a black ball once the blue ball has been removed is $\frac{1}{20}$. So, the probability of drawing a blue ball and then a black ball is $\frac{1}{21} \times \frac{1}{20} = \frac{1}{420}$. However, note that it is also possible that these balls could also be drawn out in the opposite order. Therefore, the probability must be multiplied by two giving an answer of $\frac{1}{420} \times 2 = \frac{2}{420} = \frac{1}{210}$.

80. D

To answer this, you need to change one equivalent function to another:

$$y = 9x^{-\frac{1}{3}} = \frac{9}{x^{\frac{1}{3}}} = \frac{9}{\sqrt[3]{x}}$$

81. B

Start by multiplying each term by ax to give: $a(y + x) = x^2 + a^2$

Expand the brackets: $ay + ax = x^2 + a^2$

Subtract ax from both sides $ay = x^2 + a^2 - ax$

Lastly, divide the both sides by a to get: $y = \frac{x^2+a^2-ax}{a}$

82. A

The equation for a circle, with centre at the origin and radius r is $x^2 + y^2 = r^2$

The equation of this circle is therefore $x^2 + y^2 = 25$

Solve the problem using simultaneous equations or by drawing the line onto the graph.

$x^2 + (3x - 5)^2 = 25$

This simplifies to $10x^2 - 30x = 0$

$10x(x - 3) = 0$

So $x = 3$ or $x = 0$ where the two graphs intersect

83. C

$Number\ of\ annual\ flights = Flights\ per\ hour \times Number\ of\ hours\ in\ one\ year \times Number\ of\ airports$

$= 4 \times (24 \times 365) \times 1000$

$= 96 \times 365 \times (1000)$

$\approx 100 \times 365 \times 10 \times 100$

$= 365 \times 10^5 = 36.5$ million

84. E

The way to solve this is to break the calculation down into parts, almost working backwards.

The number of seconds in 66 weeks is given by: $= 60 \times 60 \times 24 \times 7 \times 66$: $(i.e., seconds \times minutes \times hours \times days \times weeks)$.

From there you can break the numbers down by their factors and rearrange them to get the correct factorial.

$= (2 \times 3 \times 10) \times (12 \times 5) \times (4 \times 6) \times 7 \times (11 \times 6)$

Because you know that 11 is a prime number you can infer that it will have to be part of the final factorial – i.e., the final factorial has to be at least 11! To determine whether the answer is 11! or 12! continue to rearrange.

$= 2 \times 3 \times 4 \times 5 \times 6 \times 7 \times 10 \times 11 \times (12 \times 6)$
$= 2 \times 3 \times 4 \times 5 \times 6 \times 7 \times 10 \times 11 \times (3 \times 4 \times 2 \times 3)$
$= 2 \times 3 \times 4 \times 5 \times 6 \times 7 \times 10 \times 11 \times (9 \times 8)$

Because $\times 1$ is a factor of all our numbers and the product will remain the same we can introduce a $\times 1$ to make the factorial complete

$= 1 \times 2 \times 3 \times 4 \times 5 \times 6 \times 7 \times 8 \times 9 \times 10 \times 11 = 11!$

85. A

Write $\frac{\sqrt{20}-2}{\sqrt{5}+3}$ in the form $p\sqrt{5} + q$

When asked to simplify an equation a good place to start is by simplifying any square root functions.

In this case you can write $\sqrt{20}$ as $2\sqrt{5}$ because $\sqrt{20} = \sqrt{4 \times 5}$ and $\sqrt{4} = 2$.

Now you have an equation in the form $\frac{2\sqrt{5}-2}{\sqrt{5}+3}$

To convert this equation from a fraction to you can multiply the term by $\frac{\sqrt{5}-3}{\sqrt{5}-3}$ (i.e., 1) this will make the equation easier to rearrange.

$\frac{(2\sqrt{5}\times\sqrt{5})+(-3\times2\sqrt{5})+(-2\times\sqrt{5})+(-2\times-3)}{(\sqrt{5}\times\sqrt{5})+(3\sqrt{5})-(3\sqrt{5})+(3\times-3)} = \frac{10-6\sqrt{5}-2\sqrt{5}+6}{5-9}$

$\frac{16-8\sqrt{5}}{-4}$

$2\sqrt{5} - 4$

Therefore $p = 2$ and $q = -4$

86. C

ABC and DBE are similar triangles because all of the angles are equal.

Therefore: $\frac{BE}{BC} = \frac{DE}{AC}$

This is the case because the side lengths of the small and large triangles are in proportion to each other. Substitute the side lengths into the expression:

$\frac{4}{6} = \frac{DE}{9}$

$DE = 6$cm

87. C

The formula for calculating compound interest can be given as

$Final\ Amount = Investment \times (1 + \frac{annual\ interest\ rate}{n})^{nt}$

Where n = number of times interest is compounded per unit of time t, and t = the unit of time over which the investment is made. Because in this case the interest compounds annually (i.e., $n = 1$) we can simplify this to $Final\ Amount = Investment \times (1 + annual\ interest\ rate)^{years}$

By substituting the numbers given in the question into this equation we get

$1687.5 = 500 \times (1 + annual\ interest\ rate)^3$

As you can see rearranging this formula to $\sqrt[3]{\frac{1687.5}{500}} = (1 + annual\ interest\ rate)$ does not make it easy for you to find an answer without a calculator. Instead try plugging the answers into $500 \times (1 + annual\ interest\ rate)^3$ and work by a process of elimination starting from the median answer, if the answer is too high, try a lower interest rate, if the answer is too low, try a higher interest rate.
In this instance this tactic would lead you to
$500 \times (1 + 0.5)^3$
$500 \times 3.375 = 1687.5$

88. B

To win one game, Rupert must win one squash game and one tennis game. In order to calculate the probability one winning one game, it is necessary to add the probability of winning one tennis game and losing one squash game to the probability of losing one tennis game and winning one squash game. So $(\frac{3}{4} \times \frac{2}{3}) + (\frac{1}{4} \times \frac{1}{3}) = \frac{7}{12}$

89. C

The formula for the sum of internal angles in a regular polygon is given by: $180(n - 2)$, where n is the number of sides of the polygon.
$180(n - 2) = 150 \times n$
$180n - 360 = 150n$
$3n = 36$
$n = 12$
Each side is 15cm so the perimeter is $12 \times 15\text{cm} = 180\text{cm}$

90. C

Put the numerator and the denominator in like terms: $2.5 \times 10^8 = 2 \times (1.25 \times 10^8)$
$\frac{(1.25 \times 10^{10}) + (1.25 \times 10^9)}{2 \times (1.25 \times 10^8)}$
$\frac{10^2 + 10}{2} = \frac{110}{2} = 55$
Alternatively, if you recognise that all the terms share the common factor of 1.25×10^8 you could let $y = 1.25 \times 10^8$ and solve for $\frac{100y + 10y}{2y} = 55$.

91. A

Equate y to give:
$2x - 1 = x^2 - 1$
$x^2 - 2x = 0$
$x(x - 2) = 0$
Thus, $x = 2$ and $x = 0$
There is no need to substitute back to get the y values as only option A satisfies the x values.

92. E

Firstly, deal with the term in the brackets: $3^3 = 27$.

$(x^{\frac{1}{2}})^3 = x^{1.5}$

$(3x^{\frac{1}{2}})^3 = 27x^{1.5}$

Next, divide by $3x^2$: $\frac{27}{3} = 9$

$\frac{x^{1.5}}{x^2} = x^{-0.5} = \frac{1}{\sqrt{x}}$

Answer $= \frac{9}{\sqrt{x}}$

93. C

The formula for the sum of internal angles in a regular polygon is given by the number of internal triangles in the shape. This can also be expressed as $180°(n-2)$, where n is the number of sides of the polygon. So, the sum of interior angles of a pentagon can be calculated as $180°(5-2) = 540°$.

If the sum of the interior angles is $540°$ then each interior angle in the (regular) polygon is: $\frac{540°}{5} = 108°$

Therefore, angle a is $108°$.

Since angles around a point add up $360°$ we can calculate larger angle in the central quadrilateral by subtracting the two angles of a polygon $2 \times 108°$ from $360°$ this will give us $360° - (2 \times 108°) = 144°$.

Recalling that angles within a quadrilateral sum to $360°$, we can now calculate b. Because the quadrilateral has identical length sides (they are formed from the sides of the polygons) we also know that opposing angles will be of identical sizes.

Therefore, b can be calculated as $\frac{360° - (2 \times 144°)}{2} = 36°$.

The product of $36°$ and $108°$ is $3{,}888°$.

94. B

The ruler and the cruise ship look to be the same size because their edges are in line with Tim's line of sight. His eyes form the apex of two similar triangles. All the sides of two similar triangles are in the same ratio since the angles are the same, therefore:

$\frac{0.3 \text{ meters}}{x \text{ meters}} = \frac{1 \text{ meters}}{1 \text{ meters} + 999 \text{ meters}}$

Thus, $x \text{ meters} = 1000 \text{ meters} \times \frac{0.3 \text{ meters}}{1 \text{ meters}}$

$1000 \times 0.3 = 300 \text{ meters}$

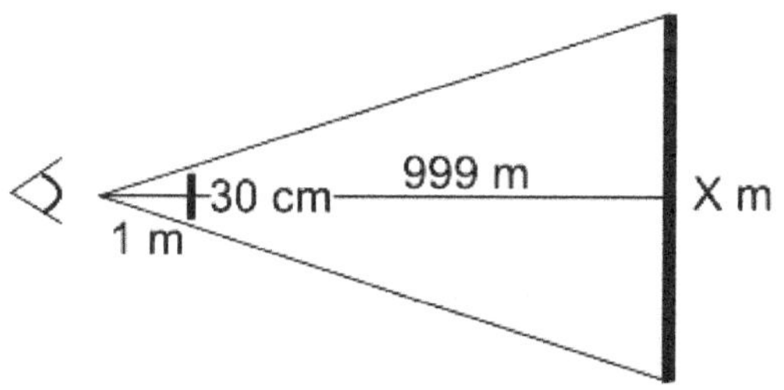

95. C

Let Bob = B, Kerry = K and Son = S.

$B = 2K$, $K = 3S$ and $B + K + S = 50$

$50 = 2K + K + \frac{K}{3} = \frac{6K}{3} + \frac{3K}{3} + \frac{K}{3}$

$50 = \frac{10K}{3}$

Hence: $10K = 150$

$K = 15$

$B = 2 \times 15 = 30$

$S = \frac{15}{3} = 5$

So: Bob's age when his son was born = $30 - 5 = 25$.

96. B

The mean is the sum of all the numbers in the set divided by the number of members in the set. The sum of all the numbers in the original set must be: $11\ numbers \times mean\ of\ 6 = 66$. The sum of all the numbers once two are removed must then be: $9\ numbers \times mean\ of\ 5 = 45$. Thus, any two numbers which sum to $66 - 45 = 21$ could have been removed from the set. 6 and 9 are the only two number option available which does not sum to 21. This answer can also be obtained faster by skipping deriving the correct answer and simply noting that all correct answers will all sum to the same number and only B does not sum to 21.

97. B

Let $y = 3.4 \times 10^{10}$; this is not necessary, but helpful, as the question can then be expressed as:

$\frac{10y + y}{200y} = \frac{11y}{200y} = \frac{11}{200} = \frac{5.5}{100}$

$= 5.5 \times 10^{-2}$

98. C

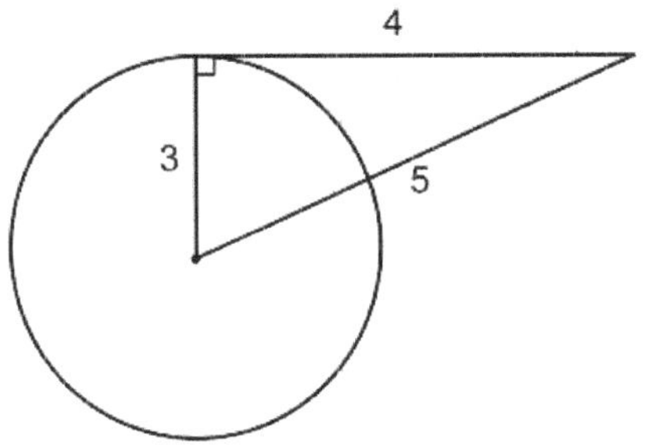

The radius and tangent to a circle always form a right angle, so using Pythagoras:

$3^2 + 4^2 = x^2$

$x = 5$

99. C

Solve as simultaneous equations

Start by rearranging equation A to $x = \frac{y}{3}$ and then substitute it into equation B.

This gives $y = \frac{18}{y} - 7$

Multiply every term by y to give:

$0 = y^2 + 7y - 18$

Factorise this quadratic to give:

$0 = (y + 9)(y - 2)$

Where the graphs meet, y is equal to 2 and -9.

Then $y = 3x$ so the graphs meet when $x = \frac{2}{3}$ and $x = -3$

100. B

Equate the volume with the surface area in the proportion instructed by the question. $3(\frac{4}{3}\pi r^3) = 4\pi r^2$, simplifies to $r = 1$.

101. B

The shortest distance between points A and B is a direct line. Using Pythagoras:
The diagonal of a sports field = $\sqrt{40^2 + 30^2} = \sqrt{1{,}600 + 900} = \sqrt{2{,}500} = 50$.
The diagonal between the sports fields = $\sqrt{4^2 + 3^2} = \sqrt{16 + 9} = \sqrt{25} = 5$.
Thus, the shortest distance between A and B = $50 + 5 + 50 = 105\text{m}$.

102. F

$1 + (3\sqrt{2} - 1)^2 + (3 + \sqrt{2})^2$
$= 1 + (18 - 2(3\sqrt{2}) + 1) + (9 + 2(3\sqrt{2}) + 2)$
$= 31 - 6\sqrt{2} + 6\sqrt{2} = 31$

103. D

It is extremely helpful to draw diagrams to simplify this.

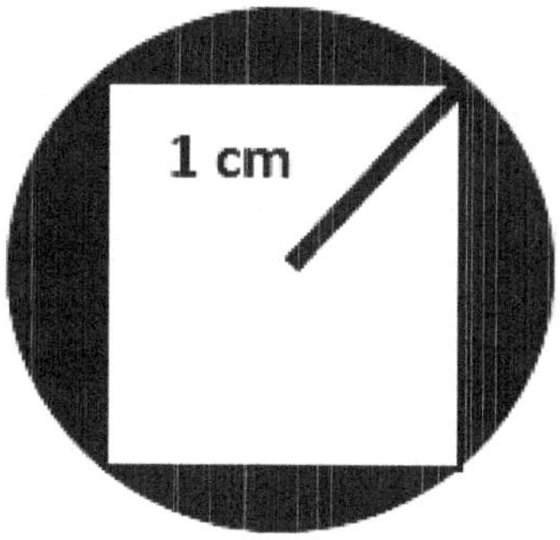

$Shaded\ area = area\ of\ circle - area\ of\ square$
The area of the circle is $\pi r^2 = 3 \times 12 = 3\text{cm}^2$.
We don't know the side length of the square, but we do know the length of the diagonal is 2cm, splitting the shape into two triangles.
The hypotenuse is therefore $= radius \times 2 = 2$
Using Pythagoras' theorem, $2^2 = x^2 + x^2$(where $x = length\ and\ width\ of\ square$)
Hence $2x^2 = 4$
$x^2 = 2 =$ the area of the square
Therefore, the shaded area = $3 - 2 = 1\text{cm}^2$.

104. D

The first step is to multiply out $(3p + 5)^2$
$(3p + 5)(3p + 5) = 24p + 49$
$9p^2 + 30p + 25 = 24p + 49$
$9p^2 + 6p - 24 = 0$
Then put the quadratic into brackets.
$(3p + 6)(3p - 4) = 0$
Therefore, p must equal -6 or 4.

105. E

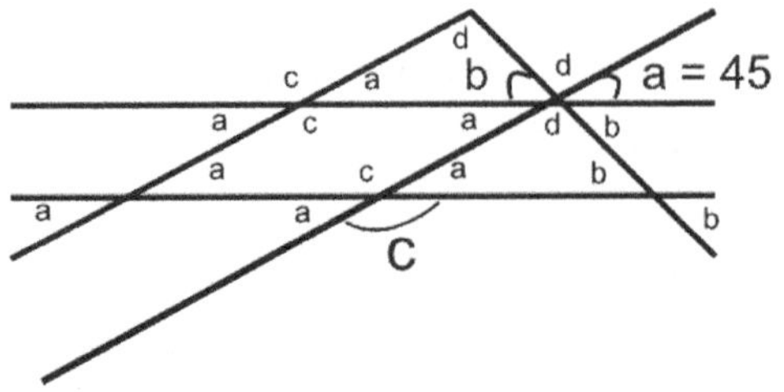

From the rules of angles made by intersections with parallel lines, all of the angles marked with the same letter are equal. There is no way to find if $d = 90°$, only that $b + d = c = 180° - a = 135°$, so b is unknown.

106. B

We know that the product of slopes of perpendicular lines equals -1. Therefore:

$(n + 1)(n + 3) = -1.$

$n^2 + 4n + 3 = -1$

$n^2 + 4n + 4 = 0$

Factorising gives $(n + 2)(n + 2)$, therefore $n = -2$ for the lines to be perpendicular.

107. C

The numerator of the fraction consists of 3 distinct terms all measured in metres (a unit of length). As this shows these 3 terms (all with units of metres) being multiplied together, we can assume the product of them results in a volume. (e.g., the volume of a cube is expressed as xyz)

108. E

Begin by drawing your line of best fit, remembering not to force it through the origin. Begin fitting the general equation $y = mx + c$ to your line. Calculate the gradient as $\frac{\Delta y}{\Delta x}$ and read the y intercept off your annotated graph.

109. C

Rather than converting all the fractions to decimals you just need to figure out the median of 7 numbers. Order the numbers by using their *relative* size to infer their position relative to the decimals.

$$0.25; \frac{7}{36}; 0.\dot{3}; \frac{11}{18}; 0.75; \frac{62}{72}; \frac{7}{7}$$

110. D

Working by orders of magnitude, multiply all the bacteria tested on the numerator and the number of resistances on the denominator. This gives an order of 10^{25}, which is the solution.

111. B

Solve $y = x^2 - 3x + 4$ and $y - x = 1$ as (x, y).

Substitute the quadratic expression into the other non-quadratic. You will get another equation.

$x + 1 = x^2 - 3x + 4$

Rearrange to get a quadratic equation and solve.

$x^2 - 4x + 3 = 0$

$(x - 1)(x - 3) = 0$

Therefore $x = 1$ or $x = 3$

Substitute your x values into the equation, $y - x = 1$ and solve to work out y values.

$y = 2$ or $y = 4$

Therefore, the coordinates are $(1, 2)$ and $(3, 4)$.

112. C

Transform all numbers into fractions then follow the order of operations to simplify. Move the surds next to each other and evaluate systematically:

$$= \left(\left(\frac{6}{8}\times\frac{7}{3}\right)\div\left(\frac{7}{5}\times\frac{2}{6}\right)\right)\times\frac{4}{10}\times\frac{15}{100}\times\frac{5}{100}\times\frac{5}{25}\times\pi\times\left(\sqrt{e^2}\right)\times e\pi^{-1}$$

$$= \left(\frac{42}{24}\div\frac{14}{30}\right)\times\frac{4\times3\times25}{10\times20\times100\times25}\times\pi\times\pi^{-1}\times e^{-1}\times e$$

$$= \left(\frac{21}{12}\div\frac{7}{15}\right)\times\frac{12}{200\times100}\times\frac{\pi}{\pi}\times\frac{e}{e}$$

$$= \left(\frac{21}{12}\times\frac{15}{7}\right)\times\frac{3}{50\,x\,100}$$

$$= \frac{45}{12}\times\frac{3}{5000}$$

$$= \frac{9}{4}\times\frac{1}{1000}$$

$$= \frac{9}{4000}$$

113. B

There are several steps to working out this problem. The first is to work out the area of the entire floor, minus the fish tank and the cut out corner. The length of the room is 8m and the width is 4m. So, the area of the entire room is 32m².

The cut out corner is a square with the dimension 2×2m. Thus, the area of the cut out corner is 4m².
The fish tank is a circle, and thus its area can be worked out using πr^2. π is taken to be 3 and thus $3 \times 1^2 = 3$m².
Therefore, the floor area, Bill needs to cover is $32-(4+3) = 25$m².

We then need to work out the area of one plank. The dimensions of this are in cm and so we need to convert to m. 1m is 100cm and so we can say that the length of the plank is 0.6m and the width is 0.1m. Thus, the area is $0.6 \times 0.1 = 0.06$m².

To work out the number of planks, required, we need to divide the area of the floor space by the area of the plank. A quick way of doing this would be rounding the area of the room down to 24 and multiplying the area of the plank by 100 so it becomes 6. $24 \div 6 = 4$, then because we multiplied the area of the plank by 100, we then multiply the answer by 100 which gives us 400 planks. The closest answer to our solution is 417, which is listed as B.

114. A

$$\frac{(16x+11)}{(4x+5)} = 4y^2 + 2$$

$$16x + 11 = (4y^2 + 2)(4x + 5)$$

$$16x + 11 = 4x(4y^2 + 2) + 5(4y^2 + 2)$$

$$16x - 4x(4y^2 + 2) = 5(4y^2 + 2) - 11$$

$$x(16 - 4(4y^2 + 2)) = 20y^2 - 1$$

$$x = \frac{20y^2 - 1}{[16 - 4(4y^2 + 2)]}$$

115. C

The question asks about the probability of getting at most 2 heads, with 4 coins. There are 16 total outcomes, with the distribution 1,4,6,4,1.

Therefore, the total probability is the sum of the following probabilities:

$\mathrm{P}(0 \text{ heads}) = \frac{1}{16}$

$\mathrm{P}(1 \text{ heads}) = \frac{1}{16} \times 4 = \frac{4}{16}$

$\mathrm{P}(2 \text{ heads}) = \frac{1}{16} \times 6 = \frac{6}{16}$

$\mathrm{P}(2 \text{ at most heads}) = \frac{1}{16} + \frac{4}{16} + \frac{6}{16} = \frac{11}{16}$

116. C

The probability of any 3 given throws giving the same given number is $\left(\frac{1}{6}\right)^3$. Now any number can be repeated 3 times, giving us $\left(\frac{1}{6}\right)^3 \times 6$. Now we count the ways we can place these 3 throws in the 5, this is just 5 choose 3, 10, giving $\left(\frac{1}{6}\right)^3 \times 6 \times 10 = \frac{10}{36}$. Now we have to discount the times that the other two numbers are the same as our given number. Fix a number n. The probability that in two throws, at least one of those yields n is just $\frac{11}{36}$, by counting the possibilities. (say n is 1, we get 11,12,13,14,15,16,21,31,41,51,61) for instance. So, the probability it is not is $\frac{25}{36}$, which we multiply our previous probability by, so our answer is $\frac{10}{36} \times \frac{25}{36} = \frac{125}{648}$

117. B

Obviously, this question could be done by brute force, but there is a much quicker way. $301^5 = (1 + 3 \times 10^2)^5$. If we treat this like a binomial expansion, we are looking for the coefficient of 10^5. If we look at the first few terms, $(301)^5 = 1 + 5 \times 3 \times 10^2 + 10 \times 9 \times 10^4 + 10 \times 27 \times 10^6 + \cdots$. The later terms will be too large, and it is clear here the only 10^5 term here will have coefficient 9.

118. A

This question relies on noticing the reason for not combining the constant terms inside each large square root: they are both square numbers. The expression is equal to $\sqrt{\left(5 - 2\sqrt{5}\right)^2} + \sqrt{\left(\sqrt{5} - 4\right)^2}$. As $\sqrt{}$ implies taking the positive root, we do have to determine whether these are positive or negative; $\sqrt{5} < \sqrt{9} = 3 < 4$, so it is clear that $4 - \sqrt{5} > 0$ but for the first, it is slightly closer. However, $2 < \sqrt{5}$ which means that $2\sqrt{5} < \left(\sqrt{5}\right)^2 = 5$, so $5 - 2\sqrt{5} > 0$. This means our sum is equal to $5 - 2\sqrt{5} + 4 - \sqrt{5} = 9 - 3\sqrt{5}$.

119. D

Possibly the simplest way to consider this problem is to look at the number of patients who will survive. From splitting the wards up, we know that the number of patients who will survive is $\frac{3p}{5} + \frac{q}{9}$. We also know it is $\frac{p+q}{4}$ by taking the number of people in the whole hospital, and the overall survival rate. By rearranging the fractions, we get $108p + 20q = 45p + 45q;\ 63p = 25q; q = \frac{63p}{25}$.

120. C

The first thing to notice is these events are not mutually exclusive, so we cannot find their independent probabilities and multiply them. The easier to work with is the latter; the probability that we get 2 heads in the last three tosses is simply the probability the last three tosses come up as one of HHT, HTH or THH. Each of these is equally likely, with probability $\frac{1}{8}$, so the probability of this is $\frac{3}{8}$. If we know that both events occurred, then we must have gotten more than $(4-2)=2$ heads in the first 4 tosses. This just means getting $2, 3$ or 4 heads in 4 tosses.

Each sequence is equally likely (with probability $\frac{1}{16}$) and the sequences which we care about are $HHHH$, $HHHT, HHTH, HTHH, THHH$, $HHTT, HTTH, HTHT, TTHH, THTH, THHT$. There are 11 of these.

Now, with this event described as "getting more than 2 heads in the first 4 tosses and 2 in the last 3 tosses", the events are independent, because there is no dependence of any 1 toss on any other. This means we can multiply probabilities, and we get the answer to be $\frac{11}{16} \times \frac{3}{8} = \frac{33}{128}$.

121. D

This is a problem about counting. The boxes are indistinguishable, which means we only care about how the balls are distributed, not specifically which boxes they are in. A good way to approach this is to have an order to the counting. We shall do it based on how many boxes are empty at the end:

No empty boxes– This is only true if there is 1 ball in each box, and there is only one way to do this.

One empty box – There must be two balls in 1 box and 1 in the other 3. The two balls could both be blue, both be red, or be 1 of each. (3 possible combinations).

2 – There are two possibilities here, a $3, 1, 1$ split, or a $2, 2, 1$ split. In the former case, the 3 balls could be all red, 2 red 1 blue, or all blue. Either way they uniquely determine the other balls. In the latter case, we consider where the two blue balls are; they could be in the same box, one could be in each of the boxes with 2 balls in, or one could be in a 2 box and the other in the 1 box. As there are no other ways to distribute the blue balls, this is an exhaustive list (6 possible combinations).

3 – All balls being only in 2 boxes means they are split $1, 4$ or $2, 3$. In the former, there are 2 possibilities, the single ball is red, or it is blue. In the latter, there are 3 possibilities for the box with two balls in, RR, BB or RB, but no matter what this also determines what is in the other box (5 possible combinations).

4 – Only one way, all the balls are in the same box (1 possible combination). Summing these possibilities, we have 16 ways.

122. B

The time between 08:34 am and 11:12 am is 158 minutes. For each minute that passes, the minute hand turns an angle of $360 \div 60 = 6°$. Therefore, the total angle turned is 158 mins $\times 6° = 948°$, and the answer is B.

123. D

The inflated football is spherical, so its volume is given by $\frac{4}{3}\pi r^3$ whilst the volume of the box containing the football is given by $(2r)^3 = 8r^3$. The ratio of the volume of the football to the volume of the box is therefore $(\frac{4}{3})\ \pi r^3 : 8r^3$. This simplifies to $\frac{\pi}{6}$: 1, so the answer is D.

124. D

First, the scaling factor between the similar triangles must be calculated which is given by $24\text{m} \div 14\text{m}$. The length of the base of the larger triangle, x, can then be calculated by multiplying the length of the smaller triangle's base by the scaling factor: $4\text{m} \times 24\text{m} \div 14\text{m}$. Therefore, $x = 96 \div 14$ which is simplified to $48 \div 7$ or $6\frac{6}{7}$ m, so the answer is D.

125. D

The external angle of a pentagon is $360° \div 5 = 72°$. Which means that the internal angle is $180° - 72° = 108$. Drawing a line from point 4 to point 2 creates an isosceles triangle. The small opposite angles are therefore $\frac{180°-108°}{2} = 36°$. From point 4 to point 3 is due east (or $90°$ degrees), point 4 to 2 is $36°$ degrees less than this $(90° - 36°) = 54°$degrees. To find the opposite bearing on a compass (point 2 to point 4) simply add $180°$degrees to give $234°$degrees. Therefore, the answer is D.

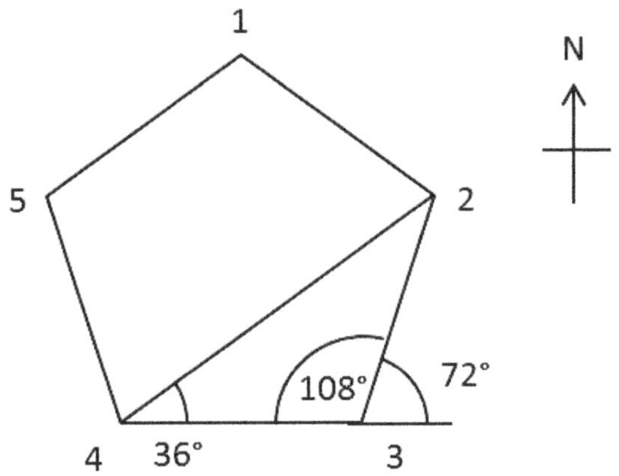

126. C

First x must be found:

$(7x)^2 = (3\sqrt{6})^2 - (2\sqrt{10})^2$

$7x = \sqrt{54 - 40}$

$x = \dfrac{\sqrt{14}}{7}$

Thus, the triangles base is:

$9x = \dfrac{9\sqrt{14}}{7}$

Therefore, to calculate the area, use $\frac{1}{2} \times base \times height$:

$= \dfrac{9\sqrt{14}}{7} \times 2\sqrt{10} \times \dfrac{1}{2}$

$= \dfrac{18\sqrt{140}}{14}$

$= \dfrac{9 \times \sqrt{4} \times \sqrt{35}}{7} = \dfrac{18\sqrt{35}}{7}$

Therefore, C is the correct answer.

127. B

First, the total area of the garden must be determined, and is calculated by $30\text{m} \times 20\text{m} = 600\text{m}^2$. The total white space is then calculated by calculating the area of each of the white rectangles and adding them together. The area of the larger rectangle is $8\text{m} \times 10\text{m} = 80\text{m}^2$, and the area of the smaller rectangle is $(20\text{m} - 8\text{m}) \times 4\text{m} = 48\text{m}^2$. The area of the grey space is then determined by subtracting the white area from the total area: $600\text{m}^2 - (80\text{m}^2 + 48\text{m}^2) = 472\text{m}^2$. The number of rolls of grass is then determined by dividing the grey area by 10m^2 (as the rolls are 1m wide and 10m long so the area of each roll is 10m^2): $472\text{m}^2 \div 10\text{m}^2 = 47.2$. As it is not possible to buy 0.2 rolls, 47.2 must be rounded up. Therefore, 48 rolls are required to cover the garden, and the answer is B.

128. B

There are $(3 + 2) \times 2 \times 4 = 40$ single shoes, half of which are left and half of which are right. After a left size 11 has been removed, there are 39 left. There are still $3 \times 4 = 12$ right size 11 shoes in the bag. Therefore, the probability of picking a size 11 right shoe is $\frac{12}{39}$ and the answer is B.

129. C

First, the surface area of a cylinder with radius 'r' and length '$3r$' is calculated by summing the surface area of each end and the middle section: $(2 \times \pi r^2) + (\pi \times 2r \times 3r) = 8\pi r^2$. The volume is given by the area of the cylinder end multiplied by the length: $(\pi \times r^2) \times 3r = 3\pi r^3$. Therefore, the surface area to volume ratio is $8\pi r^2 : 3\pi r^3$, which simplifies to $8 : 3r$. The answer is C.

130. C

The volume of a cylinder of radius r, height h, is $\pi r^2 h$. The surface area is made up of two circles of area πr^2 each and the curved surface area, which is equivalent to a rectangle of side lengths h & $2\pi r$. Thus, from the question, we know that $2 \times (2\pi r^2 + 2\pi rh) \leq \pi r^2 h \leq 3 \times (2\pi r^2 + 2\pi rh)$. We can cancel some terms here which are positive to get $2 \times 2(r + h) \leq rh \leq 3 \times 2(r + h)$. By substituting in the value known for h, we know that $4(r + 8) \leq 8r \leq 6(r + 8)$. By splitting this up into two inequalities, we can get two conditions for r; $4(r + 8) \leq 8r$ implies that $32 \leq 4r; r \geq 8$ and $8r \leq 6(r + 8)$ implies that $2r \leq 48; r \leq 24$. These must both be true simultaneously so $8 \leq r \leq 24$.

131. E

A tree diagram is very helpful in this situation.

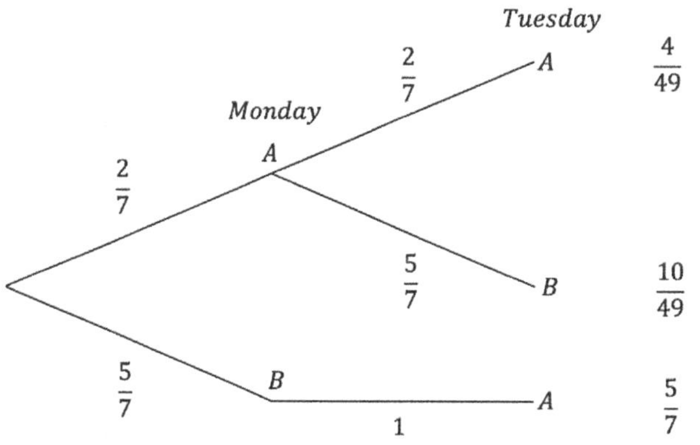

It can be seen that we have a $\frac{39}{49}$ chance of picking A on Tuesday. We also know we have a $\frac{4}{49}$ chance of picking A on Monday and picking it on Tuesday.

Because we know we picked A on Tuesday, we are only concerned with the outcomes AA and BA, as we know the other two did not occur. The probability that it was AA out of these two is then $\frac{P(AA)}{P(AA)+P(BA)} = \frac{\frac{4}{49}}{\frac{39}{49}} = \frac{4}{39}$.

132. B

For the man to walk his dog "at least once every two days", we know he never had two consecutive days which he <u>did not</u> walk the dog. So, representing going for a walk as W, and not going as N, the possible ways he spent his 4 days are $WWWW$, $WWWN$, $WWNW$, $WNWW$, $NWWW$, $NWNW$, $NWWN$, $WNWN$. These are not all equally likely as each W has $\frac{1}{3}$ chance of appearing, and each N has a $\frac{2}{3}$ chance. Thus, the probability that each set of 4 days occurred is $\frac{1}{81}, \frac{2}{81}, \frac{2}{81}, \frac{2}{81}, \frac{2}{81}, \frac{4}{81}, \frac{4}{81}, \frac{4}{81}$. As we only want to know the probability any one of these occurred, we can sum them, to get $\frac{1+2\times4+3\times4}{81} = \frac{21}{81} = \frac{7}{27}$.

133. B

The maximum straight line distance is from the front-bottom-left corner to the back-top-right corner (or another symmetrical orientation). The hypotenuse along the bottom face is calculated as $\sqrt{(3^2+4^2)} = 5$. The hypotenuse corresponding to the longest stick is $\sqrt{(5^2+5^2)} = \sqrt{50}$. This simplifies to $5\sqrt{2}$, so the answer is B.

134. A

Having already thrown a 6 is irrelevant. A fair die has equal probability $P = \frac{1}{6}$ for every throw.

For three throws: $P(6 \cap 6 \cap 6) = \left(\frac{1}{6}\right)^3 = \frac{1}{216}$

135. D

Total probability is sum of all probabilities:

$= P(Y \cap Y \cap Y) + P(Y \cap Y \cap N) + P(Y \cap N \cap Y) + P(N \cap Y \cap Y)$

$= \frac{1}{60} + \frac{2}{60} + \frac{3}{60} + \frac{4}{60} = \frac{10}{60} = \frac{1}{6}$

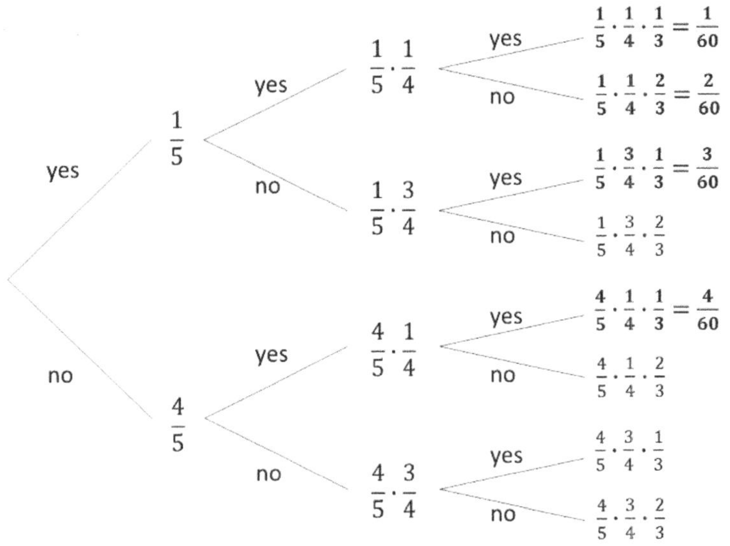

136. C

$P[(A \cup B)'] = 1 - P[(A \cup B)]$

$= 1 - \{P(A) + P(B) - P(A \cap B)\}$

$$= 1 - \frac{2 + 6 - 1}{8} = \frac{3}{8}$$

ACADEMIC LITERACY WORKED SOLUTIONS

Q	A	Q	A	Q	A	Q	A	Q	A
1	False	26	False	51	False	76	False	101	True
2	False	27	True	52	False	77	False	102	False
3	True	28	False	53	True	78	True	103	False
4	Can't tell	29	Can't tell	54	True	79	False	104	False
5	Can't tell	30	False	55	Can't tell	80	False	105	Can't tell
6	False	31	Can't tell	56	False	81	Can't tell	106	B
7	False	32	False	57	True	82	Can't tell	107	C
8	Can't tell	33	False	58	False	83	Can't tell	108	B
9	Can't tell	34	False	59	False	84	False	109	B
10	True	35	False	60	True	85	True	110	D
11	False	36	False	61	False	86	Can't tell	111	C
12	False	37	Can't tell	62	Can't tell	87	True	112	B
13	Can't tell	38	Can't tell	63	False	88	False	113	D
14	False	39	False	64	True	89	Can't tell	114	C
15	Can't tell	40	True	65	False	90	False	115	D
16	False	41	True	66	False	91	False	116	A
17	Can't tell	42	Can't tell	67	False	92	False	117	C
18	True	43	False	68	False	93	False	118	C
19	Can't tell	44	False	69	Can't tell	94	True	119	A
20	True	45	True	70	True	95	Can't tell	120	C
21	Can't tell	46	Can't tell	71	False	96	True	121	C
22	Can't tell	47	False	72	False	97	True	122	D
23	True	48	True	73	False	98	False	123	B
24	False	49	True	74	False	99	True	124	A
25	True	50	Can't tell	75	False	100	False	125	D

Q	A	Q	A	Q	A	Q	A	Q	A
126	B	151	B	176	C	201	D	226	C
127	C	152	A	177	C	202	D	227	D
128	C	153	A	178	C	203	C	228	A
129	D	154	B	179	B	204	B	229	C
130	B	155	C	180	D	205	A	230	D
131	C	156	B	181	C	206	A	231	C
132	D	157	A	182	C	207	C	232	A
133	B	158	D	183	B	208	A	233	B
134	C	159	B	184	A	209	C	234	D
135	C	160	A	185	B	210	A	235	C
136	C	161	C	186	C	211	A	236	B
137	B	162	C	187	A	212	C	237	C
138	B	163	B	188	C	213	A	238	A
139	D	164	B	189	D	214	C	239	C
140	A	165	A	190	A	215	D	240	A
141	B	166	D	191	A	216	B	241	A
142	C	167	A	192	C	217	B	242	B
143	C	168	C	193	D	218	A	243	C
144	C	169	D	194	A	219	A	244	C
145	C	170	C	195	C	220	C	245	B
146	C	171	C	196	A	221	A	246	B
147	A	172	A	197	B	222	D	247	C
148	C	173	B	198	C	223	C	248	C
149	C	174	A	199	C	224	C	249	A
150	B	175	A	200	B	225	B	250	A

Set 1:

False – In paragraph 2, the passage says that only the countries that signed the protocol were legally bound.

False – In 2004, the condition that over 55% of emissions were accounted for was met without Australia and the US.

True – In paragraph 2, the passage states that 'each country that signed the protocol agreed to reduce their emissions to their own specific target'.

Can't tell – We know this is when the Kyoto Protocol was enforced but there is no information to suggest whether emissions actually decreased.

Can't tell – Paragraph 4 says that a 60% emission reduction would have a 'significant impact', but we cannot tell if the remaining effects would be harmful or not. The passage is also talking about a global reduction of 60% – there is no mention of each individual country needing reduce their emissions by 60%.

Set 2:

False – From paragraph 1, we can see that the Soviets were mainly concerned with showing off their economic power and technological superiority.

False – Paragraph 3 says that Project Apollo was tasked with landing the first man on the moon.

Can't tell – The passage does not tell us why the Soviets did not land a man on the moon.

Can't tell – We do not know the state of the American space efforts prior to the launch of Sputnik – we just know that its launch 'prompted urgency'.

True – The Soviets had just sent Yuri Gagarin into space and it wasn't expected that the US would beat the Soviets in landing a man on the moon; therefore, the US was behind the Soviets at this stage.

Set 3:

False – Paragraph 1 says Pheidippides was the fastest runner.

False – Paragraph 2 says that they were standardised from 1921 but using the 1908 distance.

Can't tell – Paragraph 1 says the Greeks were not expecting to beat the Persians, but we do not know if the Persians were expecting to beat the Greeks, despite their larger army.

False – Paragraph 2 says that to be an IAAF marathon, the distance must be 26.2 miles. The original route was 25 miles.

Can't tell – We know that the Persian soldiers outnumbered the Greeks and had superior cavalry, but we are not told about their training.

Set 4:

False – From paragraph 1, we can see that birds would not survive if they did not migrate.

Can't tell – Whilst there is only mention here of migrating in flocks, nowhere does it specifically state that either all migrating birds do so or that any migrating birds do not.

True – Although the leading bird does not benefit at the time, they continually change position within the flock according to paragraph 3. The passage says, 'each individual bird benefits.'

Can't tell – Paragraph 3 shows that the Northern bald ibis does not behave in this way so it is not known what would happen.

True – Paragraph 1 states they migrate north in the spring, and south in the winter.

Set 5:

Can't tell – We know the number of wildflowers has decreased by this amount, but we can't tell if the bee population fell by a proportional amount. The 50% reduction mentioned in Paragraph 1 only refers to honey bees.

Can't tell – Whilst the UK have experienced a significantly greater decline than the European average, there is no data from the rest of the world.

True – Paragraph 2 tells us modern techniques produce more food.

False – As well as pollination, bees are also involved in complex food chains (stated in Paragraph 3) and cannot be replaced.

True – From paragraph 1, we see that pesticides are one of the causes of bee population decline. Therefore, reducing pesticide usage would reduce this rate of decline.

Set 6:

False – This would affect the thinking distance, not the braking distance.

True – From paragraph 2, we see that the increased traction of winter tyres is because the softness of their material allows better traction.

False – From paragraph 4, we are told it is not safe to run the engine when the exhaust pipe is blocked because of the risk of carbon monoxide production.

Can't tell – There is not sufficient information in the passage to suggest whether the softer tyres are dangerous to use in hot conditions.

False – Paragraph 3 says it is safer to steer out of the way than to brake.

Set 7:

Can't tell – In Paragraph 1, we are told the method is named after Socrates, but we are not told whether he was the first person to use it or whether he simply adapted and/or popularised the Socratic method.

False – The Socratic method challenges the statements and opinions that a person makes, not their wisdom.

False – Although Socrates was trialled with these charges, the Socratic method as described was not the cause.

False – We can see from the final paragraph that he chose to die defending knowledge and wisdom, rather than fleeing in fear.

False – From paragraph 2 we see that Socrates did not provide answers to these difficult questions.

Set 8:

False – Paragraph 1 says the dialects of the Saxon, Angle and Jute tribes formed the Anglo-Saxon language.

Can't tell – Paragraph 2 says English speakers would struggle to understand Old English, but we do not know about German speakers.

Can't tell – The story of Beowulf only mentions that he kills Grendel and his mother, not about his strength compared to other warriors.

False – The Friesian dialect is similar to Old English, but they are not the same.

True – The Celtic Britons were originally living in England before being forced into Wales.

Set 9:

True – Paragraph 1 says that stars in the constellation Cassiopeia are visible only in the northern hemisphere; therefore, they are not visible in the southern hemisphere.

Can't tell – The passage does not tell us if Cassiopeia rises and falls in the sky or not.

False – Paragraph 3 says the star sign represents the position of the sun, not the visible constellations.

False – Paragraph 2 says Polaris is used for navigation as its position is constant in the sky.

True – Paragraph 1 mentions different constellations being visible from different places on the Earth.

Set 10:

Can't tell – The passage tells us about maple tree sap, but we don't know about other trees.

False – He was angered because of the laziness of the village people.

True – Paragraph 1 says that the process is similar, although different equipment is used.

True – Paragraph 1 says the sap is only harvested during March.

Can't tell – Although the laziness associated with drinking maple syrup suggests hunting is harder than syrup drinking, the people may just have not hunted because they did not need to – not because it was harder.

Set 11:

False – Paragraph 1 says Stockholm syndrome happens sometimes, not always.

False – The passage suggests that the hugging and kissing occurred due to the positive relationship formed between the captors and hostages.

True – Paragraph 4 says the FBI is willing to devote resources to understanding Stockholm syndrome in order to aid crisis negotiation.

True – The explanation given in paragraph 3 suggests that the hostages fearing for their life is a step in the development of Stockholm syndrome.

Can't tell – Although this incident is the origin of the name 'Stockholm syndrome', it is not mentioned whether this phenomenon has happened before.

Set 12:

False – It is this mucous layer that offers protection from the anemone tentacles.

True – Paragraph 2 mentions that the bright colour of the clownfish lures in fish which the anemone eventually stings and catches.

False – Paragraph 3 mentions that anemones increase the lifespan of clownfish but are not essential for clownfish to live.

False – Paragraphs 1 and 3 mention that only certain anemone form this mutually beneficial relationship.

True – Paragraph 2 says the anemone sting protects the clownfish from predators.

Set 13:

False – Paragraph 2 indicates he was opposed to the death penalty.

Can't tell – The passage only tells us that the guillotine was commonly used during the French Revolution, it doesn't tell us what was used for execution before the French Revolution.

False – Although it can cause death by asphyxiation, the common cause of death is snapping of the neck (paragraph 3).

True – This was Joseph Guillotin's explanation.

False – Paragraph 1 tells us the guillotine was the common form of execution, as it was the only legal method of execution.

Set 14:

False – The Gherkin is famous for its distinctive shape, and although this forms part of a cooling system it is not famous for that reason.

False – The City of London governing body wanted redevelopment to restore the old historic look – implying the Baltic Exchange had this look before the bombing, and was not built with a modern architectural design.

False – The Gherkin was bought for £630m and sold for £700m, so a profit was made on the sale.

Can't tell – We are told the building is damaged by bombs, but we are not told what the intention of the attack was.

True – It is stated in paragraph 1 that Norman Foster is famous for this.

Set 15:

False – The passage tells us London is significantly more expensive.

False – There are no legal implications for paying below the living wage as it is the minimum wage that is legally binding.

False – This individual would be earning less than the living wage and so would not be able to live comfortably according to the definition in paragraph 1.

False – Some employees will be fired and others will have to work harder; some employees may already be earning more than the living wage and so would not benefit.

False – The family of that individual will also benefit from the living wage, as well as the company they work for.

Set 16:

False – Although a country with more people will likely have a greater ecological footprint, it is through their increased usage of resources, not a direct consequence of the population. There can be significant discrepancies.

False – This is the bio-productive capacity of the Earth, not the total space available.

True – The final paragraph mentions that reducing use of unsustainable resources will reduce the ecological footprint.

False – The final paragraph says that a global effort is needed.

False – The final paragraph says that we can increase the bio-productive space available.

Set 17:

Can't tell – Paragraph one states that some believe them to be 'one of the most important', which does not necessarily mean they are the most influential.

Can't tell – The passage states it started the UK punk movement, but this does not necessarily mean it began the global movement.

Can't tell – The passage tells us that some songs attacked the music industry and that controversial topics such as the Holocaust were commented on, however we do not know if these two topics were said to be related.

False – They attacked 'blindly accepting royalty as an authority', and so attacked a royalist standpoint.

True – Not at the same time, but The Sex Pistols had two individual bassists over the course of their existence.

Set 18:

Can't tell – The passage doesn't mention what proportion of people exposed to asbestos will get mesothelioma.

True – As breast cancer is the most common cancer in the UK and very rare in men, it must be very common in women.

False – The success rates of tumour removal procedures were improved by surgical hygiene.

Can't tell – The passage doesn't mention the relative success rates between the two methods.
False – The passages states that some tumours are able to metastasise, meaning that there are also tumours that do not.

Set 19:
False – The land was claimed because the British people did not believe that anybody actually owned the land.
False – Not all of the 517,000 Aborigines are living in cities and towns.
False – They were only able to reclaim the land that they could prove they originally owned.
True – Only a few Aborigines lack the education to integrate with modern Australian life, as is stated in paragraph 3.
Can't tell – We do not know what the south-east Asian lifestyle involved.

Set 20:
True – It was discovered that chilli peppers had similar taste to black peppercorn and so became valuable worldwide.
True – Paragraph 2 says that spicy food allows people to sweat.
False – Paragraph 1 says 'most' peppers are spicy, but not all.
True – Paragraph 3 states that the capsaicin receptor is responsible for the pain associated with spicy chillies.
False – The description of labelled line coding says these different methods of activating this receptor will cause the same sensation.

Set 21:
True – Dropping out of school will affect the level of education, which is a social determinant of health.
False – They can also be measured by the quality of life.
False – Although this would prevent the described mechanism from happening, many other mechanisms are acting at the same time. This was just one example of many possible mechanisms.
False – The final paragraph says we are reducing the gap between those more privileged and those who are more disadvantaged, which suggests that things can be done to improve health care.
Can't tell – The life expectancy described in paragraph 2 is an average and so can't reliably be used in specific examples.

Set 22:
B – The passage suggests that the critics suppose 'human beings to be capable of no pleasures except those of which swine are capable', and so suggest the potential of higher pleasures. They do not call their critics degraded (but suggest that the critics degrade human nature), nor do they accuse critics of being either miserable or indulgent.
C – This action does not see happiness as its justification, but conforming to social norms. It does not seek to increase pleasure or reduce pain, just follow dogma, which is not according to the principle of utility.
B – Mill does not describe the religious views of his critics, or explicitly call them reactionary, and in fact describes them 'some of the most estimable in feeling and purpose'. He does mention the countries of origin for some of his critics, and they are all in Europe.
B – The passage also states 'desirable things' could be 'means' to pleasure.
D – Utility is defined as the foundation of the system, and a belief that the increasing of happiness/decreasing of happiness is good. The passage specifically states that it has not given an exhaustive definition of things that are pleasurable/painful, and it does not specifically define Epicureans, simply suggests a link between them and utilitarians – which is not an exhaustive explanation of the term.

Set 23:

1. **C –** Though sandstone is made from sand, the passage does not state that ALL rocks are made from this material.
2. **B –** The passage discusses the valley when implementing the wall-building analogy.
3. **D –** 'Some ancient source' is all we are told, and so the source is undisclosed (Paragraph 3).
4. **C –** This rock is said in paragraph 2 to be found 'everywhere', so not 'nowhere'.
5. **D –** Paragraph 3 states that the grains are said to be sorted in groups 'of a size', i.e. measurements. They are all described as 'worn and rounded', and no mention is made of differentiation through age/shape.

Set 24:

6. **A** – Though the flowers smell pleasant, no mention is made of this scent being used to manufacture perfumes.
7. **C** – The passage states that the flower could bloom more than once a century, precluding 'D', but that it is thought to only do so in a century, providing evidence for 'C'.
8. **C** – The passage claims that Narcissus plants are 'prized by many' over Lilies, but this does not mean that all people – or even the majority of people – think the Narcissus plants is more attractive/better than Lilies, or that all homeowners enjoy the plant.
9. **A** – Paragraph 2 states that it 'yields a liquid very similar to rum', not rum itself.
10. **C** – The genus 'belongs' to the family, as stated in paragraph 1.

Set 25:

11. **C** – Women in Illinois, not across USA, were subject to the law, and the passage does not state either a change in fashion or actual arrests, only the potential for arrests.
12. **D** – The pulling out of feathers from live birds was seen as the negative to using osprey feathers.
13. **B** – They could be possessed only 'in their proper season'.
14. **A** – The problem cited is that the article was already in use in the clothing of numerous military men. The authority of the princess or political support does not feature in the passage, and 'D' is patently false.
15. **D** – None of those are precluded, as only 'harmless' and 'dead' birds (in their entirety) were prohibited. Wearing a living bird was not explicitly banned.

Set 26:

16. **B** – Nothing in the above passage provides evidence for 'C', 'D' or 'A' – in fact, the 'indie' description of Pope opposes the idea of him working for a games company at all. 'B' is supported by the fact the game is available on a number of devices and system operators.
17. **C** – The immigration officer's job is to process people correctly – not to grow or limit the number of immigrants, as in 'A' and 'B'. 'D' is vague, as 'to stamp passports' does not necessarily mean to stamp them correctly, and false stamps would be counter to the purpose of the border guard's position.
18. **C** – Though the game player may perform either a body scan or fingerprint check when something is amiss in the candidate's documents, they will not necessarily do either of these. First, they will 'enquire', which is synonymous with 'C', 'asking…for further information'. The only statement that will be universally true for discrepancies therefore is 'C'.
19. **D** – The game-player may accept 'bribes', so 'A' is not true. The game player 'may' arrest candidates, but the passage does not state he or she must, so 'B' is false. The game-player is allowed two mistakes, so to an extent, can be forgiven - making 'C' incorrect. As further mistakes will lead to being 'pecuniarily punished', 'D' is the only accurate statement.

20. **B** – While the passage says that 'the player must enquire about these [discovered discrepancies]', they 'may go on to use other tools, such as a body scanner and finger printing'. The use of 'may' would mean their use is not a 'must' as suggested by the statement, so the answer is false (B).

Set 27:

21. **C** – The term was coined by the head of LA NAACP, who is a civil rights activist.
22. **D** – The other aspects may appear in films, but only racial slurs were cited as 'the common feature' in the passage.
23. **B** – 'Primarily' means the same as 'predominately' in this case, and the cast has been described as 'predominately' black – meaning most, but not all, cast members are black.
24. **C** – Original intended audiences were 'city-swelling black Americans' (Paragraph 2): 'B' is too broad and 'A' is too narrow. 'D' is not at all supported in the passage. 'C' describes the growing audience, and how the genre is now 'not exclusive to any race' (Paragraph 2).
25. **C** – It is possible, but nothing in the statement suggests the potentially racy titles are a nod towards sexploitation genre. The innuendo may be incidental, or the choice of words completely divorced from the pornographic films of the past.

Set 28:

26. **C** – It would be a massive assumption to state that just because two characters in a book are 'vicious', all of them will be, so 'A' is not necessarily correct. 'B' also believes in a despair that is described to belong to the Comedian, but not Rorschach. The argument of the passage is that 'D', which Moore may believe, is not the case - the beloved character is not simply worshipped for his violence, but for his belief in justice. 'C' is correct, as Moore describes how he wished Rorschach not to be a favourite character, but a warning.
27. **B** – False. The fact he finds things a 'joke' is what makes him the Comedian. He may not be funny, but the joke is there.
28. **B** – He does not mention madness ('D'), or invoke shame ('C'), or simply state it is good to be good ('A') – specifically, he states we must act as if the world is 'just', even when not, to attain dignity, so the answer is 'B'.
29. **D** – No value judgment is made comparing violent actions or on the Comedian's jokes so 'A' and 'B' are false. The passage also acknowledges Rorschach's violence, so 'C' is wrong. The passage states that his actions are due to the fact he believes he is acting in the name of justice, which lends him an ethical justification to his actions, so 'D' is right.
30. **A** – The lack of meaning in anything is what leads him to treat everything as a joke – it is not hatred, but the inability to see 'purpose' in himself or his fellow man.

Set 29:

31. **B** – The passage's explanation of The Bechdel Test does not state that the test is used to show 'sexism', so a film that fails the test does not equate to a sexist one.
32. **C** – This is the only film that shows a female-female conversation not about a man. 'A' and 'B' only feature conversations focused on males and 'D' does not have two women speaking to one another.
33. **C** – Of the two horror films mentioned in the extract, one passes it and another one fails. However, the passage does not use this to make any claims on the genre as a whole.
34. **C** – Her comment that it is 'strict' shows she has a reservation, but her general agreeing that it is a 'good idea' shows she approves of the notion. Her statement is too qualified to be described by 'A', too positive to be understood by 'B', and contains a judgement precluding 'C' as a correct statement.

35. **C** – The two women are not named within the comic strip - though two women are behind the idea (one in suggesting it, the other in illustrating it), that is not to say that the two depicted women are the same.

Set 30:

36. **C** – The possible 'idea' that repetition is inherently funny is mentioned, but neither confirmed nor denied.
37. **A** – This is the only statement actually mentioned above. Laughing twice at the same joke does not make it 'twice as funny', that is a logical fallacy; being 'comfortable' is not cited as encouraging laughter; it does not state that all relationships dictate that the two parties find themselves funny (this is too vague).
38. **C** – There is no mention of a humour requirement for the first joke.
39. **C** – Though the call-back here is described as a comic trope, this does not necessarily preclude the same device being used in something un-comic. In the same way wordplay or alliteration can be used to achieve a multitude effects, not all humorous.
40. **B** – Though 'A' is a potential, it is not a requirement of the call back, and 'C' is not supported through the passage's material. At no point is the call-back named significant compared to other tropes, it is simply one that the passage focuses on. It does, however, state that it can be used by a comedian, and used for comedy, so 'B' is correct.

Set 31:

41. **B** – She was the fourth, after Catherine, Mary and her namesake Harriet Elizabeth, who died as an infant.
42. **A** – He was a 'Rev', a reverend, and a 'divine'. She was born in the USA, not UK, and in the 19th century. Her town is said to be 'characteristic', and so not 'average'.
43. **A** – She is said to have 'veneration' in all who knew her.
44. **B** – It is only described as the 'most sad' and 'most tender' memory of her childhood, not her life. It is, however, described as 'the first memorable incident' and thus the earliest one of her life.
45. **C** – She wrote her Charles, so at least wrote one letter, which is in support of 'C'. The autobiography mentioned belonged to her brother, not her. She had five brothers and sisters waiting for her when she was born, not only brothers. The passage refers to the death of her mother when she was a child, and not her father.

Set 32:

46. **B** – He thought it was 'a pity that only rich people could own books', and from this he 'finally determined to contrive' of a new way of printing. The passage does not state that he wished to make money, found books too expensive to get a hold of or was impatient himself when it came to the production of books.
47. **A** – The need to be careful is mentioned, as is the fact that the process takes a long time both in creating the block and due to the fact one block can only print one page. That it may tire a carver to make the block is possible, but it is not cited in the passage.
48. **D** – The statement says it is 'very likely' he was taught to read, but is not definite. That his father comes from a 'good family' does not mean he is necessarily a member of the aristocracy. Though block printing was used as the boy grew up, it does not state this was the most popular process. The mention of Gutenberg's family's 'wealthy friends' indicates they were sociable.
49. **B** – The paper was laid on top of the block, not underneath.
50. **A** – There is nothing written in the passage praising the craftsmanship of manuscripts. The appropriateness of the titles for both book production processes is explained, and the 'wealthy friends' are described as a source to borrow books from, thus a way of expanding your reading.

Set 33:

51. **C** – In both examples given above, Apollo is the giver – but these are only two of 'several' versions, and it is possible others exist.
52. **C** – The gift of prophecy is supernatural, therefore this is the best answer. There is no mention that parents use the name to express hate – they may just like the sound, and not care about its history, or not know the history at all. There is no evidence to suggest that she knew chastity would lead to her tragic fate, nor that she is 'often' seen as a home wrecker (though she is killed by Clytemnestra, this does not prove Cassandra, the slave, is perceived as a vindictive 'other woman').
53. **B** – Nothing is said about the state of Cassandra's childhood. The fact her father was a king proves she was from a royal line; it is mentioned that plays are written about her; and that Homer has written about her – suggesting 'A', 'C' and 'D' are true.
54. **B** – The passage states the 'presentation of her character alters'.
55. **A** – It is not said that she ignores or refuses to accept the gift, or demands more presents, even in the first story – just that she refuses to sleep with him. Only the broken promise, as described in the second version of the myth, is mentioned above.

Set 34:

56. **D** – The passage attacks a generalisation, and shows an example that refutes one given to the 'musical' genre. Nothing is mentioned of Sondheim's talents, or what his role was in creating the musical, nor are there claims made to Wheeler's literary tastes (he may just like ONE penny dreadful). This musical may deal with morbid themes, but that's not to say that most do – it could be only a select few that do.
57. **A** – The pies make the crimes 'culinary' in nature, the mention of revenge shows Todd's illegal acts to be 'vengeful' and the judge's rape is a 'sexual' crime. There is nothing explicitly suggesting the crimes of any party are funny, or to be considered funny.
58. **C** – Though the original title 'A String of Pearls: A Romance' may appear to suggest a romantic relationship within the narrative, nothing in the passage states the two are a couple.
59. **D** – 'D' is essentially synonymous with the quoted belief, 'we all deserve to die', which include both bad and good people and makes no significant reference to gender exclusion/inclusion.
60. **C** – There are four mentioned themes, but that does not mean there are only four themes, nor does 'legal corruption' get named as the central theme. As the entirety of Sweeney Todd is not discussed in the passage, only a central plot line, one could not exclude the potential of something positive happening in the play – even a minor incident. The themes mentioned are, however, indeed macabre (i.e. morbid).

Set 35:

61. **C** – The above passage is about WWII trains, not WWI ones.
62. **A** – The soldier makes a chair by using a tipped-up suitcase. It is a marine, not a sailor, learning on the back of a chair, and the passage states 'some', not 'many' queue for two hours to go to the diner car, whilst similarly 'some' (not necessarily 'many') go hungry.
63. **B** – The passage discourages mothers from going on trains with a baby, stating they should only do it as a necessity.
64. **A** – 'At every stop' more people come on the train.
65. **A** – The passage does not insult anyone, but it does say the railroads are doing their job 'well'.

Set 36:

66. **C** – The passage states the slice of bread is an ounce, and contains 3/4 ounce of flour, making it 75% flour.
67. **C** – It says it is possible that they do, but also possible that they don't. There is no emphatic claim, so we can't tell.
68. **C** – It is over a million loaves a day (not week); 319 million pounds (not bushels) a year; 365,000 loaves (not over) a year.
69. **B** – False. It may seem unimportant, but the passage goes on to explain how a single slice of bread has value.
70. **D** – There is no information about the response to this piece (A). The government have researched waste, but not taken responsibility for it, nor is it said they should do more to combat this (B and C). The final sentence confirms that housekeepers are responsible for their own food wastage (D).

Set 37:

71. **C** – Fourteen women and three men are described to be arrested, so the answer is 17 people.
72. **C** – She was the only woman, but it does not state whether or not either man was brought to trial.
73. **B** – The majority ultimately rule, but Hall 'dissented' (or disagreed) with the other two originally.
74. **A** – It is said that it was proved upon trial that she was informed of a right to vote and had no doubt over her entitlement at the time of voting.
75. **B** – They were charged independently.

Set 38:

76. **C** – Nowhere does it state that all European countries have similar creatures (though certain types can be found in both British Isles and Norway), nor does it state the array of animals is limited to this one nation. Sharing animals and birds does not necessitate sharing geographical features, but it is said a country with forest and moorlands is likely to have a variety of birds and animals, so one can see the link between forests and creatures.
77. **A** – There was a time when the English dreaded wolves and bears, but that indicates the past, or at least does not include the present. Norwegians being superior is not suggested here.
78. **C** – Bears are called destroyers, which is sufficient to conclude they cause damage.
79. **D** – They are ruthlessly hunted by farmers in country districts, but numerous only in the forest tracts in the Far North.
80. **A** – The use of the word 'fortunately' implies that it is good the wolves are no longer central. The children are under no threat, as the threat of wolves belongs to a bygone time; there is no mention of regret that such a time is gone; Norsemen are not demonstrated in the above passage to have respect for nature, but instead they are said to interfere with it through hunting and driving wolves farther afield from their current homes.

Set 39:

81. **A** – They were seen as the 'friendly or hostile manifestation of some higher powers; demonical and divine.' The 'manifestation' of the 'divine' could be interpreted as a religious quality.
82. **C** – A small minority believe that dreams are not the dreamer's own psychical act, meaning the majority believe that they are.
83. **D** – There is incongruity between feelings and images, suggesting a lack of a logical link between the two. Waking thoughts are said to find some dreams repugnant, and though dreams are described as forgotten, that is not necessarily due to them being dull.
84. **A** – The passage questions whether sense of each single dream can be made.

85. **C** – A link between the psychical sleeping and waking self is suggested, but not definitively proved. Pre-scientific communities were 'in no uncertainty about the interpretation'. The 'origin of the dream' remains a question in Freud's writing that is left without a satisfactory answer. That 'our reminiscences' may 'mutilate' a dream is mentioned (C).

Set 40:

86. **A** – 'Most' requires over half by definition, and 'most' of the people living in this area were the descendants of immigrants who moved to the country a 'full century ago'.
87. **B** – Hall only makes a claim for New England, not the entirety of America, being the descendants of 20,000 immigrants. The 'one million' figure comes from Franklin, not Hall. Less than 80,000 ('under' 80,000) people led to the population boom of one million. One million is over ten times (under) 80,000, so 'B' is correct.
88. **C** – It is said to be 'distinct' to older aristocracy 'of the royal governor's courts'. It is not similar to any European aristocracy. There is no specific reference to it not being a system based on lineage.
89. **C** – It says that these were the texts read by the most people, but that does not mean they were the most plentiful – other books may have outnumbered the Bibles, even if they received fewer readers.
90. **B** – 'A', 'C' and 'D' are cited in the passage (the journey took 'the better part of the year', it was 'hazardous' and 'expensive'), whereas 'B' is not referenced at all.

Set 41:

201. **D** – Paragraph 2 states that the 'main thing' which must be considered when assessing Russia's role is the sapping of the German, Austro-Hungarian and Turkish resources.
202. **D** – America, Italy, Romania and Britain are mentioned at the end of paragraph 1, and France in paragraph 3.
203. **C** – Russia certainly had a greater role when compared to America, Italy, Romania and Britain (paragraph 1). However, there are no details of France's efforts throughout the war.
204. **B** – A and C contributed, but the final catastrophe of the Central Powers was the direct consequence of the offensive of the Allies in 1918 (paragraph 2). Thus, as this was the final catastrophe, this can be concluded to be what won the war.
205. **A** – The final paragraph states that both Russia's and France's efforts were required to stop Germany from the winning the war, which they came very close to.

Set 42:

206. **A** – At the end of paragraph 4, the passage says, 'Journalists did some of their finest work and made me proud to be one of them'.
207. **C** – Paragraph 3 states magazines offered perspective, rather than necessarily the facts.
208. **A** – Paragraph 4 states that the Internet was responsible for allowing the former audience to write the news.
209. **C** – In paragraph 3 it states, 'people gathered around the radio for the immediate news'.
210. **A** – A or B are the 2 most likely answers, as paragraph 2 states about a fallen leader. However, since paragraph 2 only mentions D Roosevelt as being a president (and not John F. Kennedy), this is the best answer.

Set 43:

211. **A** – Paragraph 2 states inhabitants defended their own territory. While paragraph 3 states towns drew up formal treaties with other boroughs, which may include laws of protection, indicating they did draw up treaties to defend each other, in addition to defending their own territory.

212. **C** – Paragraph 2 states that inhabitants elected their own rulers and officials in whatever way they themselves chose to adopt.
213. **A** – The first sentence concludes that the 15th century town life is nothing like England today. The last sentence in the second paragraph states there is some comparison with modern America. Therefore, this statement is correct.
214. **C** – The final paragraph states that 'often their authority stretched out over a wide district, and surrounding villages gathered to their markets and obeyed their laws'.
215. **D** – There is mention of war (arming soldiers), of banning trading between boroughs (shutting down privileges of commerce) and treaties in the text – so the answer is all of the above (D).

Set 44:

216. **B** – The second sentence states that male power has risen and thus has not always occurred.
217. **B** – At the end of paragraph 1, it is stated that the Jewish God has attributes of power, thus D is wrong. There is no mention of the Christian God, therefore C and A cannot be the answer.
218. **A** – The final sentence talks about how faiths may give an insight into past society.
219. **A** – The first sentence states that 'nowhere is the influence of sex more plainly manifested than in the formulation of religious conceptions and creeds.' Answers B and D could have been right if the question was not 'most clearly'.
220. **C** – There is never any mention of the author's own beliefs, there are only discussions of others' beliefs.

Set 45:

221. **A** – The writer says that a 'novel with a purpose' constitutes a violation of the unwritten contract existing between writer and reader.
222. **D** – At the end of the first paragraph, the passage states that a novel may conduce to delectation (pleasure and delight) during hours of idleness in man. The passage states the opposite for all the other statements.
223. **C** – The author does not agree with novels which portray the author's views on socialism, religion or divorce laws. However, there is no indication to which the author dislikes the most.
224. **C** – The only plausible answers are C and D (the author argues against A and B). It states that the unwritten contract is that a novel should be an 'intellectual artistic luxury', which is earlier described as being able to delectate (to please) – a synonym of amusement. There is no mention of a good novel needing to be fiction.
225. **B** – C and D are beliefs of the author. A novel should instruct the reader is the opinion, while "novel with a purpose" is the answer ('realisation') to this opinion. Therefore, the answer is B rather than A.

Set 46:

226. **C** – While the first paragraph talks of these happy memories, all are asked as questions rather than being presented as fact, so the answer is can't tell.
227. **D** – The passage is based on different opinions on what patriotism is, thus it cannot be deduced that the author can quantify how many American's are patriotic without an agreed definition.
228. **A** – Paragraph 3 states that one proposed definition of patriotism is the training of wholesale murders, i.e. mass killing. There is not mention of depression or workplaces. Children fantasising about having wings to fly to distant lands is not a sufficient reason for D to be the correct answer over A.
229. **C** – While paragraph 1 talks of wonderful tales of great deeds and conquests, this is insinuated to be of the past. The author then in paragraph 2 says that the stories mothers tell today are those of sorrow, tears and grief.

230. **D** – This is the only answer where the author specifically says children wonder. The others could be inferred but are not as factually correct.

Set 47:

231. **C** – The start of paragraph 2 states that a good man can receive a gift well.
232. **A** – In paragraph 1, it states 'we wish to be self-sustained' when referring to some men's opinions.
233. **B** – In paragraph 2, the author states that he can rejoice (i.e. like) to receive gifts as well as sometimes grieving upon the presentation of a gift. He later goes on to say he is ashamed of being pleased by gifts. However, despite this, for certain periods, he does sometimes like gifts.
234. **D** – In paragraph 1, it states 'we can receive anything from love, for that is a way of receiving it from ourselves.'
235. **C** – Paragraph 2 states 'if the gift pleases me overmuch, then I should be ashamed that the donor should read my heart, and see that I love his commodity, and not him.' In this situation, the author feels bad that he does not appreciate the unique effort and insight of the giver as much as the physical gift. Answer B could be inferred; however, the answer C is stated. A is not true, so D cannot be the answer.

Set 48:

236. **B** – False. The final sentence states that mathematics was a science which Goethe was imperfectly acquainted with.
237. **C** – Having writers speak about a paper indicates this is the most popular (the first sentence). But it is specific parts of this paper (prismatic spectrum and refraction) which were mostly spoke about. Therefore, C rather than A is correct.
238. **A** – The translator was aware of the opposition which the theoretical views alluded to conflict with and wanted to first select the experiments which showed evidence to support Goethe's view. It says this was incompatible with the author's view.
239. **C** – "Doctrine of Colours" and two short essays entitled "Contributions to Optics" are mentioned.
240. **A** – This is stated in the first sentence. While his views are different from the received theories of Newton, it does not say it disproves Newton's theories.

Set 49:

241. **A** – In paragraph 2 the passage says 'gradually' (but surely) the thoughts of money takes over the thoughts of a girl so that income is the most important thing. Therefore, based on the information solely in the passage, this is true.
242. **B** – In paragraph one, the passage states that this is the view of stereotypical Philistine's and not the author's view.
243. **C** – Nowhere does the passage mention Nora's opinion of wanting a child (be it with anyone).
244. **C** – The first paragraph states every twelfth marriage ends in divorce, but nowhere does it say what population of people this statistic was calculated from. In paragraph 6, it talks of American life, but this does not necessarily mean the statistic is from America.
245. **B** – In the second paragraph, it states that over time, a married woman's mind strays from these thoughts.

Set 50:

246. **B** – In paragraph 1, it states a series of temporary measures were initiated (sometime in the 1960s/70s). However, in paragraph 2 it says the Terrorism Act 2000 was passed as a definite measure following twenty years of temporary measures, therefore the temporary measures in Ulster could not have been implemented in the 60s, as this would be over thirty years.
247. **C** – The text does not mention anything supporting or contradicting its implementation at present.
248. **C** – Paragraph 2 would suggest so, but there is no definitive description of why the acts were passed (like there is in paragraph 1).
249. **A** – Paragraph 3 states that the ATCSA marked a firmer move towards the 'management of anticipatory risk', which was to characterise the counter-terrorism legislation of the 21st century.
250. **A** – The second paragraph states that the 2000 Terrorism Act was passed 'following twenty years of temporary measures.'

FINAL ADVICE

Arrive well rested, well fed and well hydrated

HUMAT is an intensive test, so make sure you're ready for it! Be well hydrated before you go in. Make sure you're well rested and fed in order to be at your best!

Move On

If you're struggling, move on. Every question has equal weighting. **In the time it takes to answer one hard question, you could gain three times the marks** by answering the easier ones. Be smart to score points.

Afterword

Remember that the route to a high score is your approach and practice. Don't fall into the trap that "*you can't prepare for the HUMAT*"– this COULD NOT be further from the truth. With knowledge of the test, some useful time-saving techniques and plenty of practice you can dramatically boost your score.

Work hard, be persistent and do yourself justice.

Good luck!

WHAT'S NEXT?

Preparing for the HUMAT is just **one step** on your path to medical school.

To make the most of your preparation, we would strongly recommend that you ensure you perform at your very best in your **interviews** as well.

Don't worry though, we have you covered. Medical interviews can be unpredictable, and are *always* tough, but UniAdmissions is the UK's best medical admissions company for a reason, and our expertise is key to mastering your interviews.

The Ultimate Medical School Interview Guide is your next step – take control of your application, and your future, here and save up to 50%: https://amzn.to/3NJoJWI

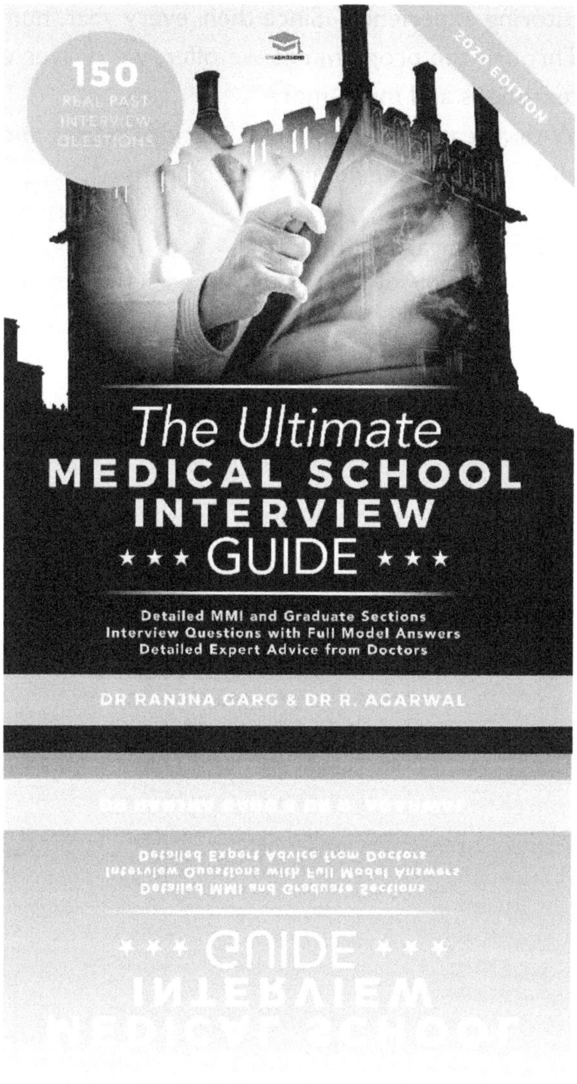

ABOUT US

We currently publish over 115 titles across a range of subject areas – covering specialised admissions tests, examination techniques, personal statement guides, plus everything else you need to improve your chances of getting on to competitive courses such as medicine and law, as well as into universities such as Oxford and Cambridge.

Outside of publishing we also operate a highly successful tuition division, called UniAdmissions. This company was founded in 2013 by Dr Rohan Agarwal and Dr David Salt, both Cambridge Medical graduates with several years of tutoring experience. Since then, every year, hundreds of applicants and schools work with us on our programmes. Through the programmes we offer, we deliver expert tuition, exclusive course places, online courses, best-selling textbooks and much more.

With a team of over 1,000 Oxbridge tutors and a proven track record, UniAdmissions have quickly become the UK's number one admissions company.

Visit and engage with us at:
Website (UniAdmissions): www.uniadmissions.co.uk
Facebook: www.facebook.com/uniadmissionsuk

YOUR FREE BOOK

Thanks for purchasing this Ultimate Book. Readers like you have the power to make or break a book –hopefully you found this one useful and informative. *UniAdmissions* would love to hear about your experiences with this book. As thanks for your time we'll send you another ebook from our Ultimate Guide series absolutely FREE!

How to Redeem Your Free Ebook

1) Find the book you have on your Amazon
purchase history or your email receipt to help find the book on Amazon.

2) On the product page at the Customer Reviews area, click 'Write a customer review'. Write your review and post it! Copy the review page or take a screen shot of the review you have left.

3) Head over to www.uniadmissions.co.uk/free-book and select your chosen free ebook!

Your ebook will then be emailed to you – it's as simple as that!
Alternatively, you can buy all the titles at

www.uniadmissions.co.uk

Printed and bound by CPI Group (UK) Ltd, Croydon, CR0 4YY
26/10/2026
02239367-0013